Abnormal Uterine Bleeding

Malcolm G. Munro
Professor
Department of Obstetrics and Gynecology
David Geffer School of Medicine
University of California, Los Angeles, and
Kaiser Permanente, Southern California

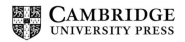
CAMBRIDGE
UNIVERSITY PRESS

CAMBRIDGE UNIVERSITY PRESS
Cambridge, New York, Melbourne, Madrid, Cape Town, Singapore,
São Paulo, Delhi, Dubai, Tokyo

Cambridge University Press
The Edinburgh Building, Cambridge CB2 8RU, UK

Published in the United States of America by
Cambridge University Press, New York

www.cambridge.org
Information on this title: www.cambridge.org/9780521721837

© M. Munro 2010

First published 2010

Printed in the United Kingdom at the University Press, Cambridge

A catalogue record for this publication is available from the British Library

Library of Congress Cataloguing in Publication data
Munro, Malcolm G.
  Abnormal uterine bleeding / Malcolm G. Munro
    p. ; cm.
  Includes bibliographical references and index.
  ISBN 978-0-521-72183-7 (pbk.)
  1. Menorrhagia.   2. Uterine hemorrhage.   I. Title.
  [DNLM: 1. Menorrhagia–therapy.   2. Menorrhagia–diagnosis.
  3. Metrorrhagia–diagnosis.   4. Metrorrhagia–therapy.
  WP 555 M968a 2010]
  RG176.M86 2010
  618.1′72–dc22   2009035699

ISBN 978-0-521-72183-7 Paperback

A book such as this reflects a lifetime of influence and guidance from colleagues and mentors alike, as well as tolerance and support from both family and friends. While there have been many important mentors, three stand out – Ralph Anderson, who sowed the seeds that led to my decision to enter the specialty; John Collins, who taught understanding of, and respect for evidence; and Victor Gomel, my friend and former chair, who encouraged and supported the early dreams and endeavors of a sometimes overzealous young faculty member. Many residents and colleagues have contributed to my involvement with abnormal uterine bleeding (AUB), but special mention should be made of Hilary Critchley, from Edinburgh, and Ian Fraser, from Sydney, who have partnered with me in the ongoing process of standardization of nomenclature and classification of causes of AUB that form much of the infrastructure of this book. Finally, I give thanks to my wife Sandra, and my children Justin, Megan and Tyler, from whom I borrowed the time to create this project.

Contents

Preface

It is a privilege to be able to share my knowledge, experience, and passion for the pathogenesis, clinical presentation, investigation, treatment, and support of women with abnormal uterine bleeding (AUB), a problem that impacts uncounted millions worldwide. While in most countries precise data are currently scarce, in the United Kingdom heavy menstrual bleeding (HMB) affects more than 20% of premenopausal women over the age of 35 [1], and 5% of those in their thirties and forties receive care for HMB each year [2]. It is safe to assume that AUB similarly impacts the women of other countries, adversely affecting their families, their employers, and the resources of their health care systems.

Bleeding that women consider excessive or unacceptable and for which they seek care covers a broad range of volume and predictability. The diagnosis of "clinically significant" bleeding has been an issue of controversy, with some suggesting that bleeding that does not result in anemia is clinically irrelevant. This approach ignores the inconvenience experienced with unpredictable or periodic heavy bleeding that may not result in depletion of iron stores or reduction in measured levels of hemoglobin and hematocrit. For example, a woman with heavy bleeding of unpredictable onset may be unwilling to participate in routine activities, may require continuous access to pads and/or tampons, and may fear social activity or sexual relationships because she always perceives that she is on the precipice of a heavy period.

It is important for the clinician to remember that chronic AUB rarely is a life-threatening circumstance, and that, for the vast majority of women, appropriate counseling will allow them to make their own informed decision. The decision is made in the context of a strategy that is appropriate to her condition, her desires regarding current and future fertility, and her sense of perceived side effects and risks.

Why this book?

I am hoping that the reader will be able to use the written and electronic resources of this volume to support a better understanding of both the physiology of normal menstrual bleeding and the known pathogenesis of abnormal bleeding, which will together facilitate effective management of women with AUB. Knowledge of these basic principles should allow the clinician to elicit and clarify symptoms of AUB as a prelude to the creation of a judiciously applied, structured investigation, the results of which allow the development of a complete menu of treatment options that empowers the woman presenting with AUB to make choices consistent with her perceptions, needs, and goals, particularly with respect to the integrity of her reproductive tract. While many of the approaches are those that have been honed with decades of clinical service, self education, and the insightful opinions and practices of mentors, peers, and, yes, students, they are steeped in a context of basic science and clinical evidence that is critical to the contemporary practice of medicine. After all, if one does not know the depth, breadth, and quality of the scientific underpinnings of a clinical decision, there is a corresponding lack of ability to determine when and if a better choice or set of choices may exist.

What about evidence?

Many of my students and residents perceive that evidence-based medicine (EBM) is clinical practice based entirely upon randomized controlled trials (RCTs), an approach that would place all medical practitioners in a near perpetual state of clinical paralysis since only 5–10% of clinical situations and conditions have been evaluated in this way. In fact, EBM is actually the clinical integration of clinician experience and expertise and the best available external evidence from systematic research. Fortunately Sackett et al. has provided us with, in my opinion, the best definition of EBM and one that applies to all clinical conditions [3]:

> The conscientious, explicit, and judicious use of current best evidence when making decisions about the care of individual patients.

Each of the words, "conscientious," "explicit," and "judicious," are important to the concept of EBM. The *conscientious* clinician should acquire knowledge of the case-related external evidence for each and every patient in a careful and meticulous fashion that is facilitated by the wealth of available electronic resources such as the Cochrane Library, MEDLINE, and other sources. This evidence generally comes from either the basic sciences or, more commonly, from clinical research involving the accuracy of diagnostic tests, and the efficacy and safety of medical interventions. The best available external evidence generally comes from the RCT, which has its imperfections but the conclusions are generally more reliable than those derived from "lower quality" nonrandomized studies and case series. In some instances, there is no published external evidence applicable to the clinical presentation or condition, a circumstance where the best available evidence will be "Class III," residing totally in the experience of the clinician. Whatever the source, the therapeutic options and decisions should be made in the context of the best available external evidence, *explicitly* stating why that evidence does or does not apply. It is this clinical decision, the *judicious* application of the best available evidence, which is totally reliant on the clinical expertise of the practitioner, a resource that can be aided but never replaced by external evidence.

In this book, I will continuously remind the reader of the quality of evidence supporting the described approaches and techniques by inserting the classification of evidence in the text. I will use a modified version of the system developed by the Canadian Task Force on Preventive Health Care [4] that was adopted by the US Preventive Services Task Force [5], and which is shown in Figure 0.1. The modification is the division of Class I evidence into Class I-1, which is a systemic review (metaanalysis) of RCTs, and Class I-2, which describe a single RCT.

The book is organized into a number of sections that include Background, Anatomy and physiology, Classification and pathogenesis, Clinical management, and Procedures, with a Glossary of terms at the end. The Procedures section includes chapters that provide detail regarding some relatively simple diagnostic and therapeutic procedures and others, such as endometrial ablation, hysterectomy, and uterine artery embolization, which are designed only to familiarize the reader with the procedural concepts. Details on the performance of these procedures are outside the scope of this book. Each chapter starts with a synopsis or chapter summary that is designed to review, or preview, the highlights of that chapter's contents.

Finally, remember that effective clinical medicine requires the creation of a relationship with your patient that is established by effective communication. The ability to obtain an

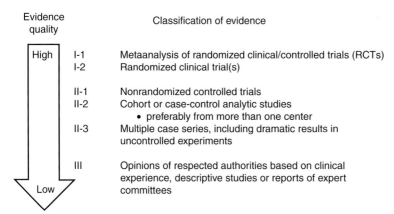

Figure 0.1 Evidence classification for clinical studies. Modification of the system designed by the Canadian Task Force on Preventive Health Care that has also been adopted by the US Preventive Services Task Force. The modification is the separation of Class I evidence into two components by adding metaanalysis of randomized controlled trials as the highest level achievable. While useful, this system is not applicable for basic science studies and is often not useful for studies that evaluate prognosis or diagnostic tests. (Based on the Canadian Task Force on Preventative Health Care 1979 [4].)

accurate history is a skill that cannot be replaced by evidence, tests, drugs, or devices, and without it, the clinician and patient will walk a precarious path. This approach can be summed up in a quote often attributed to Sir William Osler who said, "Listen to the patient – she is trying to tell you what is wrong."

References

1. Gath D, Osborn M, Bungay G, Iles S, Day A, Bond A, et al. Psychiatric disorders and gynaecological symptoms in middle aged women: a community survey. *Br Med J (Clin Res Ed)*. 1987;**294** (6566):213–18.
2. Peto V, Coulter A, Bond A. Factors affecting general practitioners' recruitment of patients into a prospective study. *Fam Pract*. 1993;**10** (2):207–11.
3. Sackett DL, Rosenberg WM, Gray JA, Haynes RB, Richardson WS. Evidence based medicine: what it is and what it isn't. *BMJ*. 1996;**312**(7023):71–2.
4. Canadian Task Force on the Periodic Health Examination. The periodic health examination. *Can Med Assoc J*. 1979;**121** (9):1193–254.
5. Grimes DA, Atkins D. The US Preventive Services Task Force: putting evidence-based medicine to work. *Clin Obstet Gynecol*. 1998;**41**(2):332–42.

Background
Historical context

Chapter summary

- Historically, our culture has traditionally viewed even normal menstruation as an aberration, ostracizing reproductive-aged women; this legacy impacts contemporary societal perceptions.
- Many contemporary religions specify behavior for individuals and couples during menstruation.
- A given woman's perception of her own symptoms may be impacted by her cultural and religious context; she may be embarrassed to present her symptoms, or may not know that they are indeed abnormal.
- Contemporary understanding of the pathogenesis of AUB is based on relatively new observations and evidence.
- Surgical and pharmacological therapy of AUB are currently in a state of relatively rapid evolution after changing little for a century.

Introduction

For the majority of those who have chosen to read this book, it is obvious that menstruation is a normal component of female reproductive physiology. However, perceptions of menstruation by our society at large may vary substantially by age, by culture, and by religious belief. Indeed, even in Western cultures, societal perceptions of normal menstruation may be impacted more than we'd like to think by our cultural legacies which, until relatively recently, were steeped in a context of medical naiveté. Indeed, as recently as the late nineteenth century, menstruation was described by the academic H. Beckwith Whitehouse as, "one of the sacrifices which women must offer at the altar of evolution and civilisation." [1]

Despite the acquisition of vast amounts of knowledge about the female reproductive system in general and an increasing capability to control menstruation and treat its disorders, many of these concepts continue to suffuse our culture, contributing to the plight of women affected by AUB. Understanding the historical and social underpinnings of menstrual mysticism is an important part of the education of any medical practitioner who deals with women in the reproductive years, or of any age, with both normal and abnormal uterine bleeding.

Similarly, it is useful for the practitioner to understand something of the historical evolution of the therapeutic agents and procedures in contemporary use. Such knowledge provides a context for understanding the continuous evolution of knowledge about the pathogenesis, investigation, and medical and surgical treatment of women with AUB.

Normal menstruation

The process of menstruation, itself unique to the female of the species, is associated with a range of symptoms and perceptions have been the subject of documents and publications that date to the beginning of recorded history [1–3]. Not surprisingly, this legacy has been influenced by a number of myths and societal taboos. In the first century AD, largely negative societal attitudes were depicted and perhaps influenced by a Roman historian named Pliny the Elder [4]. His *Historia Naturalis* includes a description of his perception of the menstruating woman, a vision that perhaps sets the stage for the perceptions of menstruation for the centuries that followed: "wine sours if they pass, vines wither, grass dies, and buds are blasted. Should a menstruating woman sit under a tree, the fruit will fall. A looking-glass will discolour at her glance, and a knife turn blunt. Bees will die, and dogs tasting her blood run mad."

Indeed, over 1500 years later, seventeenth-century descriptions of menstruation continued to reflect the perception of normal menstruation as a disorder and included terms such as "the monthly disease, the monthly infirmity, the sickness, monthly evacuations, natural purgations," or even, the "time of your unwonted grief," or, perhaps even worse, "the monthly flux of excrementitious and unprofitable blood." [2] One of the more poetic terms, "the flowers," was actually a pejorative term likening menstruation to the fermentation of malt liquors whereby the liquid flings up to the surface a sort of scum bounding with air, which is called "the flowers." [5] These seventeenth-century English perceptions of normal menstruation were captured by the Jacobean dramatist Barnabe Barnes who wrote, "thy soule foule beast is like a menstruous cloath, polluted with unpardonable sinnes."[6]

It is of interest that primitive societies quite independently usually have negative terms for menstruation, such as the "sik bilong mun" of the Pidgin language of Papua New Guinea. The phrase, "at those monthly periods", was used for the first time in the early seventeenth century [2]. Even in current times, certain religious and cultural beliefs surround the process of normal menstruation. For example, even for Modern-Orthodox Jews, the term *Niddah* refers to the ritually unclean period that comprises the days of menstruation and a week thereafter, when any physical contact between spouses is strictly forbidden [7]. Indeed, even mainstream women, and, in particular, adolescents, are often saddled with the notion that menstruation is an unhealthy time and one that shouldn't be the topic of open conversation [8]. Consequently, even contemporary practitioners must render care knowing that normal menstruation, for many, is rooted in a cultural context of shame.

Abnormal menstruation

It is likely that the first mention of heavy uterine bleeding (HUB) in the ancient literature was from Hippocrates, who was born in approximately 460 BC and wrote the first comprehensive medical textbooks. The English translations of Hippocrates' work date from the early nineteenth century and are, no doubt, influenced by the English language as it was used at the time. Consequently, interpretation of these translations should be undertaken in this context. Aristotle quoted Hippocrates in describing the process of HUB in the following fashion: "In quantity, bleeding is excessive, saith Hippocrates, when they flow about eighteen ounces." "In time when they flow about three days." "But it is inordinate flowing when the faculties of the body are thereby weakened." Aristotle also used a number of terms to describe abnormal menstruation and included variable, irregular, and often light bleeding in his descriptions, including the notation that such bleeding is often accompanied by pain [9]. It is worth noting that the 18 ounces is equivalent to about 540 mL of blood, a volume almost seven times what is considered the upper limit of normal today. Thomas Sydenham, writing in 1666 [10], describes "immoderate menstrual flow" and considered that "the natural flow of the menses would fill a vessel the size of a goose's egg," a volume more in keeping with contemporary understanding.

William Heberden, a very successful general physician and astute observer, practising in London in the mid 1700s, was also a capable gynecologist. He perhaps provided one of the earliest descriptions of acute anovulatory AUB:

> Sometimes, without any apparent cause the menses have exceeded the healthy limits … and have appeared in too great abundance. But these cases have been usually more alarming than dangerous, for among the many instances of excessive floodings which I have known, I have remarked only two, who, without being pregnant, have bled till they were exhausted and died. [11]

The word *menorrhagia*, which is derived from the Greek word "mene" meaning moon and the verb "regnumi" meaning to burst forth, appears to have come into use for the first time in the late 1700s in the lectures of Professor William Cullen, Professor of the Practice of Physic at the University of Edinburgh. Cullen wrote extensively about "menorrhagia," using the term "menorrhagia rubra" to describe immoderate bleeding in nongravid and nonpuerperal women, and "menorrhagia abortus" to describe heavy bleeding in pregnant or lying-in women [12].

The English physician Fleetwood Churchill, one of the first true specialists in obstetrics and gynecology, authored a textbook on the *Principal Diseases of Women* in which he devoted a full chapter to "menorrhagia," which he indicates "signifies an increase in the catamenia." He specifically states that the term "uterine haemorrhage should be applied exclusively to floodings connected with pregnancy and parturition." [13]

It seems probable that the term "metrorrhagia," used to describe irregular bleeding, came into usage at about the same time as "menorrhagia," since Cullen certainly used the term "maetrorrhagia" in his lectures [12]. However, "metrorrhagia" seems to have been less popular than "menorrhagia," and Churchill does not use this term at all – he uses "irregularity of bleeding" – although he does use other Latin-based terms like amenorrhea and dysmenorrhea [13].

The causes of abnormal uterine bleeding

Until the 1800s only Aristotle can be found to have opined on the causes of AUB, suggesting that one or a combination of "breaking of the veins, heating of the blood, and trauma" were at fault [9]. However, by the mid 1800s a number of authors began to suggest interesting hypotheses. Dewees penned the following perspective on the pathogenesis of heavy menstrual bleeding (HMB):

> Women are most obnoxious to menorrhagia: who live indolently and indulge in stimuli; who use little or no exercise; who keep late hours; who dance inordinately; who are intemperate; who have borne many children; who have been subject to febrile infections; who have much leucorrhoea; who are too prodigal in the joys of wedlock; who are advancing towards the nonmenstrual period; or, who yield too readily to passions or emotions of the mind. [14]

Similarities and differences can be found in the opinion of Mauriceau, in his *The Married Woman's Private Medical Companion*, where he suggested that AUB would manifest in women who have "great weakness, general debility of the uterus occasioned by tedious labour or frequent miscarriages, full habit (obesity), violent exercise, excess in venery or strong passions of the mind." [15] Not all of these opinions are as outrageous as they seem as obesity, stress, and proximity to menopause all may predispose to anovulation, a cause of AUB that will be discussed in Chapter 5.

Later in the nineteenth century a number of developments facilitated a better understanding of mechanisms involved in the pathogenesis of AUB. These included the introduction of anesthesia with its ability to allow more complete examinations, the development of safe surgery, and the advent of modern pathological examination of removed tissue specimens. Effective imaging had to await much more modern technologies with X-rays and ultrasound, although Pantaleone first described hysteroscopic evaluation of an endometrial polyp in 1869 [16]. The clinical and pathological appearances of uterine fibroids and adenomyosis were well described and defined by the early twentieth century [17, 18], but the symptomatic and clinical associations of endometriosis were not clearly described and defined until somewhat later, largely due to the efforts of Samson [19, 20]. The term adenomyosis was initially used by Frankl who was the first to describe the entity in detail [21].

The term "dysfunctional uterine bleeding" (DUB) appears to have been first used by Graves to describe regular or irregular cases of "menorrhagia or metrorrhagia" caused by "impairment of the endocrine factors" which normally control menstrual function [22]. These usages suggest that he was applying the term "dysfunctional uterine bleeding" to unexplained causes of a wide range of menstrual symptoms, whether or not they occurred in women with disturbances of ovulation or despite the presence of a normal ovulatory state.

Treatment of heavy menstrual bleeding

Medical therapy

The history of effective medical therapy for HMB is difficult to find, but seems to be a relatively recent development. The first available evidence of endocrine therapy for HMB seems to come from Germany, in 1953, where Leeb described the use of intravenous progesterone [23]. Shortly thereafter, in 1956, Rauscher and Rhomberg demonstrated that an intramuscular estrogen-progesterone combination could also be effective [24]. The first randomized controlled trial (RCT) of systemic hormonal therapy for acute uterine bleeding appears to be a comparison of intravenous conjugated equine estrogens to placebo, published by DeVore et al. from New Haven, Connecticut in 1983 [25].

With increased knowledge about the physiology and pathogenesis of HMB, other pharmaceutical interventions began to appear in the medical literature. In 1970, Callender et al. published a double-blind RCT on the use of tranexamic acid (TA), an agent that inhibits the activation of plasminogen to plasmin, and demonstrated that HMB could be successfully treated with an agent provided only during menses [26]. This was the first practical evidence that not only is there increased fibrinolytic activity in women with HMB, but also that targeting this mechanism can have positive therapeutic effects. The role of endometrial prostaglandins and their disorders in the genesis of HMB was exploited by Anderson et al. who reported on the treatment of seven patients with HMB (menorrhagia) using the cyclooxygenase inhibitor, mefenamic acid [27].

From Scotland, in 1970, Cameron et al. first published evidence that intrauterine progestins could reduce menstrual blood loss, a step that had significant and positive repercussions for women with HMB worldwide [28]. In Sweden, Andersson and Rybo demonstrated the value of the levonorgestrel-releasing intrauterine system (LNG-IUS) for the treatment of HMB [29]. For the first time, the systemic impact of hormonal agents was reduced while, at the same time, increasing the local impact in a very beneficial way.

Surgical therapy

Hysterectomy

The ability to perform surgery successfully was rather recent in medical history, but surgical intervention clearly preceded the advent of effective pharmaceutical agents for AUB. Hysterectomy was the first such surgery that could be applied to AUB, and, although the first mention of uterine extirpation in the literature appears to be by Soranus of Ephsus [30], the first successful, planned vaginal hysterectomy was by Langenbeck in 1813 [31]. This and most of the other vaginal hysterectomies performed prior to the midpoint of the nineteenth century were generally for cervical cancer, and the preoperative mortality was extremely high. In 1853, Walter Burnham, in Massachusetts, performed the first abdominal hysterectomy where the patient survived [32]. Despite these successes, deficiencies in technique, in anesthesia, and the absence of an understanding of the presence and role of bacteria in perioperative morbidity and mortality conspired to result in an operative mortality rate of about 70%. However, by around the turn of the twentieth century, a number of surgeons had abandoned these approaches and improved dissection, ligation, and aseptic techniques enough to reduce the mortality of both vaginal hysterectomy and abdominal supracervical hysterectomy to 5% or less [33–35]. By the end of the 1930s, renowned vaginal surgeons such as Green-Armytage in England and Heaney in the United States, achieved operative mortality rates of 1.2 and 0.5% respectively [35, 36].

To this point in history, and with the exception of surgery for cervical carcinoma, virtually all abdominal hysterectomies were supracervical. However, leaving the cervix in vivo allowed cervical carcinoma to occur in a small number of women, a factor that contributed to the rationale for Richardson's technique for total abdominal hysterectomy (TAH), which is still used by most contemporary gynecologists [37]. This approach, combined with improvements in anesthesia and, later, blood transfusion and antibiotics, minimized the morbidity and mortality associated with TAH, thereby reducing supracervical hysterectomy to a procedural curiosity.

There were no major changes in hysterectomy technique until later in the twentieth century with the introduction of laparoscopic hysterectomy, first conceived by Semm but first reported by Reich [38]. The concept was to reduce the morbidity associated with a laparotomy incision by converting a TAH to a hysterectomy performed under laparoscopic direction, either totally, or to the point where the procedure could be completed vaginally.

More recently, in an interesting "reverse" evolution of technique, laparoscopic supracervical hysterectomy has been introduced, essentially simultaneously by Lyons [39] and Semm [40].

Hysteroscopic procedures

As previously referred to, Pantaleone, in 1869, described the insertion of a hollow metal tube into the uterus through which, with the aid of an external candle for illumination, he successfully identified and treated an endometrial polyp with topical silver nitrate [16]. In France, David described the use of contact hysteroscopy in 1907 [41], and in 1925 Rubin improved visualization by using carbon dioxide gas to fill the uterus [42]. Surprisingly little progress was made with hysteroscopy throughout much of the twentieth century, perhaps in part because of technical limitations of imaging systems and partly because of a relative inability to treat pathology if it was encountered [43].

It wasn't until the last third of the twentieth century that changes in light sources, endoscope design, and creative use of fluid and gas distending media allowed predictable and effective imaging of the endometrial cavity [44, 45]. This establishment of an effective endoscopic viewing platform set the stage for the development of hysteroscopically-directed operative procedures for AUB such as radiofrequency submucosal myomectomy using a urological resectoscope [46]. Targeted destruction of the endometrium, now called endometrial ablation (EA), was first described by Milton Goldrath of Detroit, using neodymium: yttrium alumnum garnet (Nd:YAG) laser energy with a fiber passed through the instrument channel of an operating hysteroscope [47]. Subsequently, a number of investigators described series using the resectoscope to resect [48], electrodesiccate [49], or vaporize [50] the endometrium, which collectively replaced the more cumbersome and expensive laser-based approach to endometrial destruction.

Nonresectoscopic endometrial ablation

A published report describing EA without the use of an endoscope and using steam can be found in 1898 [51], and the first published series with clinical outcomes was introduced by Bardenheuer from Germany who, in 1937, described his experience with a monopolar radiofrequency intrauterine probe [52]. Hypothermic EA using a hypercooled intrauterine probe also preceded hysteroscopic and resectoscopic techniques as it was introduced by Cahan and Brockunier in 1967 [53]. These nonresectoscopic devices and the concept of EA were largely forgotten until it became apparent that both the clinical efficacy associated with resectoscopic EA and the minimization of complications was strongly related to the skill of the surgeon. As a result, the private sector industry developed a number of automated or semiautomated systems for EA based upon heated fluid, tissue freezing, and radiofrequency and microwave energy. These systems have undergone regulatory approval in many constituencies, and were released starting in 1995 in Europe and 1997 in the United States. Besides being mislabeled as "second generation," they have also been mislabeled as "global" for none of the systems even approximate predictable amenorrhea nor are any applicable to all women with HMB. Nevertheless, they seem to be effective, less risky than resectoscopic techniques, and associated with a high degree of patient satisfaction (Chapter 15).

Uterine-preserving procedures for leiomyomas

Interestingly enough, the first targeted therapy for uterine leiomyomas was selective removal following laparotomy, an operation first described by Atlee in 1845 [54]. The procedure was largely perfected by Victor Bonney in the 1930s, who introduced and described techniques still used today [55]. The advent of operative endoscopy added new surgical options for the woman with symptomatic leiomyomas. A number of previous candidates for abdominal myomectomy were afforded a less morbid approach with the introduction of hysteroscopically-directed resection of submucosal myomas by Neuwirth and Amin in 1976 [46]. By 1991 Dubuisson et al. published the first series of laparoscopically-directed myomectomies as a potentially less morbid alternative to a laparotomy-based approach [56].

In 1995, Ravina et al., from France, described the use of interventional radiology to perform bilateral uterine artery embolization with polyvinyl alcohol (PVA) microspheres positioned by a catheter passed through the right femoral artery [57]. This approach, has spawned controversy, in part for political reasons, and in part because of limited early critical assessment of the technique. However, Spies et al., from Washington DC have carefully evaluated a relatively large cohort of patients, reporting highly successful results in about three quarters of treated patients at five years after the index procedure [58].

Laparotomically-directed localized uterine artery resection was originally described in a small series of patients with HUB, most of whom had leiomyomas, by Bateman, from Toronto, in 1964 [59]. More than 35 years later, Liu et al., from Taiwan, reported a similar procedure using laparoscopically-directed technique to occlude the uterine vessels with electrodesiccation [60]. While still under evaluation, it is apparent that these techniques will likely have a permanent, if limited role to play in the future management of AUB associated with uterine leiomyomas.

The term "myolysis" was coined to describe the use of hypothermic (cryotherapy), laser, or radiofrequency electrical energy to ablate uterine leiomyomas by laparoscopic or hysteroscopically-directed approaches. The first such technique described was by Donnez et al. who used a Nd:YAG laser, first in 1990 via hysteroscopy [61], and then by laparoscopy [62]. Shortly thereafter other laparoscopically-directed myoma ablation techniques were described, including radiofrequency myolysis by Goldfarb [63] and cryomyolysis by Olive et al. [64]. More recently, Tempany et al., and then Stewart et al., reported initial results of the use of magnetic resonance imaging (MRI) to focus therapeutic ultrasound energy on leiomyomas [65, 66].

Summary

While we know that menstruation is a physiological event, elements of our society still frequently view the process in a way that is problematic for women young and old, for they frequently do not have a forum for discussing its impact on their lives. Contemporary clinicians should be alert to social and cultural issues that surround menstruation and its disorders so that they may facilitate the identification and treatment of problems that may not be appreciated even by the women themselves.

Over the past several decades, a number of advances in our understanding of normal and abnormal menstruation have occurred simultaneous with the development of improved diagnostic strategies and therapeutic techniques. Collectively, these resources provide the contemporary woman with AUB a set of options that even 50 years ago could not have been imagined.

References

1. Whitehouse HB. The physiology and pathology of uterine haemorrhage.
1. Physiogical uterine haemorrhage. *Lancet.* 1914;1:877–85.
2. Crawford P. Attitudes to menstruation in seventeenth century England. *Past and Present.* 1981;91;47–73.
3. Eccles A. *Obstetrics and Gynaecology in Tudor and Stuart England.* London: Croom Helm; 1982.
4. Bostock J, Riley HT. *Pliny the Elder.* London: Taylor and Francis; 1855.
5. Drake J. *Anthropologia Nova.* London: Sam. Smith and Benj. Walford; 1707.
6. Barnes B, De Somogyi N. *The Devil's Charter.* London: John Wright; 1607.
7. Guterman MA. Observance of the laws of family purity in Modern-Orthodox Judaism. *Arch Sex Behav.* 2008;37(2):340–5.
8. Stubbs ML. Cultural perceptions and practices around menarche and adolescent menstruation in the United States. *Ann N Y Acad Sci.* 2008;1135:58–66.
9. Aristotle. *Aristotle's Masterpieces.* London: G. Davis; 1845.
10. Sydenham T. *Medical Observations Concerning the History and the Cure of Acute Diseases.* London: The Sydenham Society; 1868.

11. Heberden. *Menstrua, Commentaries on the History and Cure of Diseases*. London: T. Payne; 1802.

12. Cullen W. *First Lines of the Practice of Physic*. Edinburgh: Balfour & Bradfute; 1816.

13. Churchill F. *Principal Diseases of Women*. Dublin: Martin Keene and Son; 1838.

14. Dewees WP. *Treatise on Diseases of Females*. Philadelphia: Blanchard & Lea; 1860.

15. Mauriceau AM. *The Married Woman's Private Medical Companion*. New York: 129 Liberty Street; 1852.

16. Pantaleone DC. On endoscopic examination of the cavity of the womb. *Medical Press and Circular*. 1869;8:26–7.

17. Kelly H, Cullen TS. *Myomata of the Uterus*. Philadelphia: W.B. Saunders; 1909.

18. Cullen TS. *Adenoma of the Uterus*. Philadelphia: W.B. Saunders; 1908.

19. Sampson JA. Perforating hemorrhagic (chocolate) cysts of the ovary. *Arch Surg*. 1921;3:245–323.

20. Sampson JA. Peritoneal endometriosis due to the menstrual dissemination of endometrial tissue into the peritoneal cavity. *Am J Obstet Gynecol*. 1927;14:411–69.

21. Frankl O. Adenomyosis uteri. *Am J Obstet Gynecol*. 1925;**10**:680–4.

22. Graves WP. Some observations on etiology of dysfunctional uterine bleeding. *Am J Obstet Gynecol*. 1930;**20**:500–18.

23. Leeb H. [Therapy of functional uterine hemorrhages with intravenous progesterone.] *Geburtshilfe Frauenheilkd*. 1953;13(4):322–6.

24. Rauscher H, Rhomberg G. [Successful treatment of functional uterine hemorrhage with a one-time administration of estrogen-progesterone solution in oil.] *Zentralbl Gynakol*. 1956;**78** (50):2002–10.

25. DeVore GR, Owens O, Kase N. Use of intravenous Premarin in the treatment of dysfunctional uterine bleeding – a double-blind randomized control study. *Obstet Gynecol*. 1982;**59**(3):285–91.

26. Callender ST, Warner GT, Cope E. Treatment of menorrhagia with tranexamic acid. A double-blind trial. *Br Med J*. 1970;4 (5729):214–16.

27. Anderson AB, Haynes PJ, Guillebaud J, Turnbull AC. Reduction of menstrual blood-loss by prostaglandin-synthetase inhibitors. *Lancet*. 1976;1(7963):774–6.

28. Cameron IT, Leask R, Kelly RW, Baird DT. The effects of danazol, mefenamic acid, norethisterone and a progesterone-impregnated coil on endometrial prostaglandin concentrations in women with menorrhagia. *Prostaglandins*. 1987; **34**(1):99–110.

29. Andersson JK, Rybo G. Levonorgestrel-releasing intrauterine device in the treatment of menorrhagia. *Br J Obstet Gynaecol*. 1990;**97**(8):690–4.

30. Temkin O, ed/trans. *Soranus'Gynecology*. Baltimore: Johns Hopkins University Press; 1956.

31. Langenbeck CJM. Geschichte einer von mir glucklich verichteten extirpation der ganger gebarmutter. *Biblioth Chir Opth Hanover*. 1817;**1**:557.

32. Burnham W. Extirpation of the uterus and ovaries for sarcomatous disease. *Nelson's Am Lancet*. 1854;**8**:147–51.

33. Garceau E. Vaginal hysterectomy as done in France. *Am J Obstet Dis Women Child*. 1895;**31**:305–46.

34. Ségond E. Considerations on the technique, the difficulties, and the dangers of vaginal hysterectomy. *Trans Am Gynecol Soc*. 1896;**21**:133–46.

35. Green-Armytage VB. Vaginal hysterectomy: a new technique and follow-up of 500 consecutive operations for haemorrhage. *J Obstet Gynaecol Br Emp*. 1939;**46**:848–56.

36. Heaney NS. A series of 627 vaginal hysterectomies performed for benign disease with three deaths. *Am J Obstet Gynecol*. 1935;**30**:269–72.

37. Richardson EH. A simplified technique for abdominal panhysterectomy. *Surg Gynecol Obstet*. 1929;**48**:248–51.

38. Reich H, de Caprio J, McGlynn F. Laparoscopic hysterectomy. *J Gynecol Surg*. 1989;**5**:213–15.

39. Lyons TL. Laparoscopic supracervical hysterectomy. A comparison of morbidity and mortality results with laparoscopically assisted vaginal hysterectomy. *J Reprod Med*. 1993;**38** (10):763–7.

40. Semm K. *Hysterectomy by Pelviscopy: an Alternative Approach without Colpotomy (CASH)*. Oxford: Blackwell Scientific Publications; 1993, pp. 118–32.

41. David C. Endoscopie de l'uterus apres l'avortement et dans les suites de couches normales et pathologiques. *Soc Obstet Paris*. 1907;**10**:288–97.

42. Rubin IC. Uterine endoscopy, endometroscopy with the aid of uterine insufflation. *Am J Obstet Gynecol*. 1925;**10**:313–27.

43. Valle RF. Development of hysteroscopy: from a dream to a reality, and its linkage to the present and future. *J Minim Invasive Gynecol*. 2007;**14**(4):407–18.

44. Lindemann HJ. Eine neue untersuchungsmethode fur die hysteroskopie. *Endoscopy*. 1971;**4**:194–7.

45. Edstrom K, Fernstrom I. The diagnostic possibilities of a modified hysteroscopic technique. *Acta Obstet Gynecol Scand*. 1970;**49**(4):327–30.

46. Neuwirth RS, Amin HK. Excision of submucus fibroids with hysteroscopic control. *Am J Obstet Gynecol*. 1976;**126**(1):95–9.

47. Goldrath MH, Fuller TA, Segal S. Laser photovaporization of endometrium for the treatment of menorrhagia. *Am J Obstet Gynecol*. 1981;**140**(1):14–19.

48. DeCherney AH, Diamond MP, Lavy G, Polan ML. Endometrial ablation for intractable uterine bleeding: hysteroscopic resection. *Obstet Gynecol*. 1987;**70**(4):668–70.

49. Vancaillie TG. Electrocoagulation of the endometrium with the ball-end resectoscope. *Obstet Gynecol*. 1989;**74**(3 Pt 1):425–7.

50. Vercellini P, Oldani S, DeGiorgi O, Cortesi II, Moschetta M, Crosignani PG. Endometrial ablation with a vaporizing electrode in women with regular uterine cavity or submucous leiomyomas. *J Am Assoc Gynecol Laparosc*. 1996;**3**(4 Suppl):S52.

51. Fritsch H.I. Uterusvapokauterisation, tod durch septische peritonitis nach spontaner sekundarer perforation. *Centralblatt fur Gynakologie*. 1898;**52**:1409–18.

52. Bardenheuer F. Elektrokoagulation der Uterusschleimhaut zur Behandlungklimakterischer Blutungen. *Zentralblatt fur Gynakologie*. 1937;**4**:209–11.

53. Cahan WG, Brockunier A, Jr. Cryosurgery of the uterine cavity. *Am J Obstet Gynecol*. 1967;**99**(1):138–53.

54. Atlee WL. Case of successful extirpation of a fibrous tumor of the peritoneal surface of the uterus by the large peritoneal section. *Am J Med Sci*. 1845;**9**:309–35.

55. Bonney V. *The Technical Minutia of Extended Myomectomy and Ovarian Cystectomy*. London: Cassel; 1946.

56. Dubuisson JB, Lecuru F, Foulot H, Mandelbrot L, Aubriot FX, Mouly M. Myomectomy by laparoscopy: a preliminary report of 43 cases. *Fertil Steril*. 1991;**56**(5):827–30.

57. Ravina JH, Merland JJ, Ciraru-Vigneron N, Bouret JM, Herbreteau D, Houdart E, et al. [Arterial embolization: a new treatment of menorrhagia in uterine fibroma.] *Presse Med*. 1995;**24**(37):1754.

58. Spies JB, Bruno J, Czeyda-Pommersheim F, Magee ST, Ascher SA, Jha RC. Long-term outcome of uterine artery embolization of leiomyomata. *Obstet Gynecol*. 2005;**106**(5 Pt 1):933–9.

59. Bateman W. Treatment of intractable menorrhagia by bilateral uterine vessel interruption. *Am J Obstet Gynecol*. 1964;**89**:825–7.

60. Liu WM, Ng HT, Wu YC, Yen YK, Yuan CC. Laparoscopic bipolar coagulation of uterine vessels: a new method for treating symptomatic fibroids. *Fertil Steril*. 2001;**75**(2):417–22.

61. Donnez J, Gillerot S, Bourgonjon D, Clerckx F, Nisolle M. Neodymium: YAG laser hysteroscopy in large submucous fibroids. *Fertil Steril*. 1990;**54**(6):999–1003.

62. Nisolle M, Smets M, Malvaux V, Anaf V, Donnez J. Laparoscopic myolysis with the Nd:YAG laser. *J Gynecol Surg*. 1993;**9**(2):95–9.

63. Goldfarb HA. Laparoscopic coagulation of myoma (myolysis). *Obstet Gynecol Clin North Am*. 1995;**22**(4):807–19.

64. Olive DL, Rutherford T, Zreik T, Palter S. Cryomyolysis in the conservative treatment of uterine fibroids. *J Am Assoc Gynecol Laparosc.* 1996;3(4 Suppl):S36.

65. Tempany CM, Stewart EA, McDannold N, Quade BJ, Jolesz FA, Hynynen K. MR imaging-guided focused ultrasound surgery of uterine leiomyomas: a feasibility study. *Radiology.* 2003;226(3):897–905.

66. Stewart EA, Rabinovici J, Tempany CM, Inbar Y, Regan L, Gostout B, et al. Clinical outcomes of focused ultrasound surgery for the treatment of uterine fibroids. *Fertil Steril.* 2006;85(1):22–9.

Anatomy and physiology
Uterine anatomy

Chapter summary

- A sound understanding of uterine anatomy is critical to understanding the pathogenesis of AUB as well as safe and effective evaluation of the presenting patient.
- The uterus results from the fusion and selective absorption of the embryologic Müllerian ducts; disorders of this process result in a spectrum of congenital abnormalities.
- The normal uterus may vary with respect to version, flexion, and other morphological features that are important considerations when instrumenting the cervical canal and endometrial cavity.
- The uterus has a rich and redundant blood supply from a number of arterial sources.
- The basal layer of the endometrium is responsible for generating the functionalis that sloughs with menstruation.
- The cervix and corpus are innervated separately, an issue that has clinical importance when administering local anesthetic agents for the performance of procedures.
- The uterus is abutted by the urinary bladder anteriorly. Nearby and laterally are the ureters; the sigmoid colon lies posteriorly; and small bowel typically surrounds the fundus. These relationships must be considered when instrumenting the uterus as they are vulnerable if mechanical or energy-based instruments perforate the uterine cervix or corpus.

Introduction

A sound knowledge of the embryology and anatomy of the uterus is critical to understanding the physiology of menstruation, the anatomic tenets of the various disorders that cause AUB, and for the effective and safe performance of necessary diagnostic and therapeutic procedures.

The purpose of the uterus is to contain and facilitate nourishment of the developing embryo and fetus until it has reached developmental maturity. At that point, the cervix, heretofore a relatively rigid barrier to delivery, becomes soft and pliable, while the uterine wall changes from the relatively passive function of a container, to that of a dynamic, coordinated, rhythmically contracting muscle designed to retract and dilate the cervix and expel the fetus through the open cervical canal and vagina.

For most women, the uterus supports pregnancy for only a small portion of their life, if at all. For the remainder it lies dormant, such as is the case prior to the menarche and following menopause, or it functions as an organ that uniquely, but in vain, prepares for the implantation of a pregnancy that does not occur. In such circumstances, it sheds the specially prepared endometrium in the process that we call menstruation.

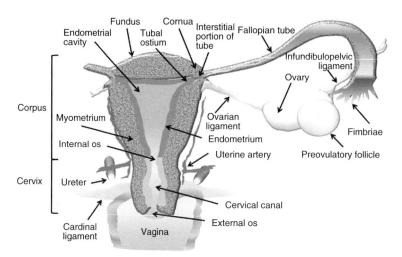

Figure 2.1 Uterus, fallopian tubes, and ovaries; coronal view.

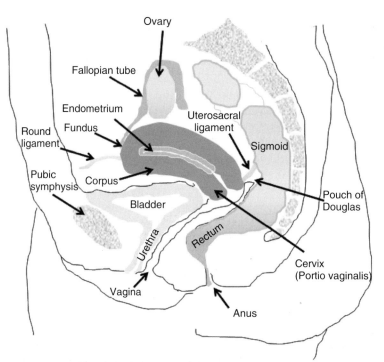

Figure 2.2 Uterus and adjacent pelvic organs; sagittal view.

Description of the normal uterus

The uterus is normally a hollow, pear-shaped organ, somewhat flattened anterioposteriorly. It is located entirely within the pelvis, comprising of a *cervix* and a body or *corpus*, which are joined at the *isthmus* (Figures 2.1and 2.2). The size, shape, and other features of both the corpus and cervix vary somewhat based upon one or a combination of factors which include individual variation, pregnancy history, and endocrine status.

For the newborn, the cervix and corpus are approximately equal in size, while for the adult woman in the reproductive years the corpus is typically two or three times the size of the cervix. For women in the reproductive years who have never been pregnant (at least much beyond the early second trimester), the normal uterine length is approximately 7.5–8.0 cm, 5–6 cm wide at the corpus, and 2–3 cm thick in an anteroposterior plane. The usual weight of the adult uterus in the reproductive years is 30–80 g, but this is typically much less prior to menarche and after menopause, and may be much more in the presence of pathological conditions such as adenomyosis or leiomyomas. In normal pregnancy, the uterus enlarges up to 20 times its nonpregnant size and weight.

In the pelvis, the uterus lies posterior and superior to the empty urinary bladder and anterior to the lower sigmoid colon. The uterine corpus is invested by the visceral peritoneum, also called the *serosa*, which is contiguous with the abdomen's peritoneal surface. Posteriorly, sometimes called the intestinal side, this peritoneal surface extends all the way to the vagina, covering the posterior vaginal fornix before it courses cephalad again over the sigmoid colon. The resulting space between the uterus and the colon and contiguous with peritoneal cavity is called the *pouch* or *cul-de-sac of Douglas*, which is frequently and loosely occupied by coils of small intestine. On the anterior side of the uterus, sometimes called the vesical side, and between the corpus and the dome of the bladder, the peritoneum forms a similar but less deep structure called the *vesicouterine pouch*. Directly inferior to the apex of this pouch, the anterior portion of the cervix is directly attached to the bladder with loose areolar tissue. At its most caudal point, the uterus is attached to the vagina at the level of the cervix.

The wall of the corpus is convex in all directions, and comprises a musculofibrous structure called the myometrium. The endometrial cavity is typically "T" or triangular shaped, flattened anteroposteriorly, and inferiorly continuous with the cervical canal, sometimes called the endocervical canal. The cavity extends laterally in the fundal region to the *cornua* where it becomes contiguous with the lumen of the interstitial segment of the fallopian tubes.

The endometrial cavity is lined by the endometrium that transitions inferiorly to the mucus producing endothelium of the cervical canal, and in the cornual regions, to the serous producing ciliated epithelium of the fallopian tube. The endometrium comprises two principal layers, the *basalis* and the *functionalis*, the latter being the component that dynamically responds to external stimulation by gonadal steroids and which is sloughed off in the absence of pregnancy following the withdrawal of progesterone and estradiol (Figure 2.3). This process, and the dynamic biochemical activity within, is described in more detail in Chapter 3.

The corpus is divided into several regions. The lower region, where the cervical canal opens to the endometrial cavity, is called the isthmus or *lower uterine segment*. The actual portal between the canal and the endometrial cavity is called the *internal cervical os*. In the normal uterus, there are two *cornual* regions located on each side of the upper part of the corpus. These roughly triangular shaped regions funnel at their apex to the attachment with the interstitial or intramural portion of the fallopian tube. The openings to the fallopian tube, visible from the endometrial cavity, are called the *tubal ostia*. The *fundus* refers to the region of the uterine corpus that is between and cephalad to the cornua. The walls of the corpus are collectively called the *myometrium*, comprising three muscular layers of alternating longitudinal and oblique smooth muscle groups.

The uterine cervix is approximately 3–5 cm long. The portion that protrudes into the vagina comprises half the normal length and is termed the *portio vaginalis* or the exocervix;

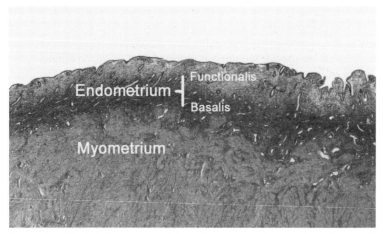

Figure 2.3 Histological appearance of the endometrium and superficial myometrium. The *functionalis* component proliferates in the follicular phase, under the influence of progesterone and estradiol from the corpus luteum, "matures" into an organ capable of accepting a pregnancy in the secretory phase, and then, absent pregnancy, sloughs in the menstrual phase of the cycle. The *basalis* component of the endometrium is permanent and serves as the source of cells, vessels, and other agents necessary for the reconstruction of the functionalis following menstruation.

it is surrounded by the vaginal fornices. Cephalically, the supravaginal portion, or portio supravaginalis, is attached to the pubis anteriorly with the pubocervical ligaments and to the bladder anteriorly, largely by loose areolar connective tissue. Laterally the cervix is supported by fibroconnective tissue including the cardinal ligaments and posteriorly with the uterosacral ligaments.

The opening between the vagina and the cervical canal, visible from the vagina, is called the *external cervical os*. The external os is generally closed in women who have not undergone vaginal delivery but, for those who have delivered vaginally, the opening gapes slightly. The cervical canal is flattened anterioposteriorly, and somewhat fusiform, being wider in the middle than at the ends that result in the internal and external os. Indeed there exists an anterior and posterior longitudinal ridge, a remnant of the fusion of the two Müllerian ducts (see below) that give rise to a number of oblique columns covered with columnar epithelium that bear resemblance to the branches of a tree.

The surface of the exocervix is usually covered with a nonkeratinized layer of squamous epithelium that is contiguous with that of the vagina and which changes to a mucus-producing, single layer of columnar epithelium, typically located at the level of the external os, a, transition referred to as the squamocolumnar junction.

Uterine position

The *position* of the uterus in the pelvis describes the orientation of the axis of the cervical canal and the corpus within the pelvis. It should be appreciated that both the cervix and corpus have intrinsic concavity or convexity and rarely are oriented in straight lines or planes. The terms *version* and *flexion* describe two distinct aspects of uterine positioning and orientation when viewed in the sagittal plane (Figure 2.4).

Version refers to the orientation of the long axis of the cervix to that of the vagina. Most commonly, this cervical axis is directed anterior to that of the vagina, an orientation that is

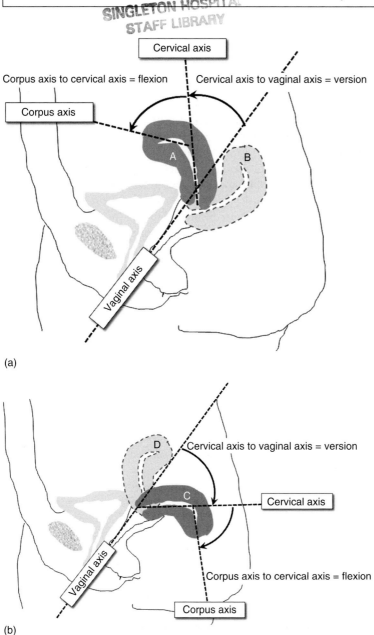

Figure 2.4 Uterine version and flexion. Uterine *version* is determined by the relationship of the long axis of the cervical canal to that of the vagina, while uterine *flexion* reflects the relationship of the long axis of the corpus to that of the cervix. Part (A) shows anteflexed uteri but one is anteverted while the other is retroverted. Anteflexed uteri are typically also anteverted, so a retroverted anteflexed uterus, particularly if it is fixed posteriorly, may indicate the presence of a posteriorly located adhesive process such as endometriosis. Part (B) demonstrates retroflexed uteri; one that is anteverted and the more commonly encountered retroverted/retroflexed configuration.

referred to as *anteversion*. Should this axis of the cervix be directed posterior to that of the vagina, the uterus is deemed to be *retroverted*. These angles may be particularly pronounced, approaching 90°; and, in such instances, the uterus may be deemed to be acutely anteverted or anteflexed. On the other hand, if the two axes are collinear in relationship to each other, the orientation is neutral or *axial*.

Flexion describes the relationship of the long axis of the corpus to that of the cervix. If this axial direction is anterior to that of the cervix, the corpus is referred to as *anteflexed*; if directed posterior to the axis of the cervix, it is *retroflexed*. Similar to version, the angle between the cervix and corpus may approach or even exceed 90°, a situation that may be deemed either acutely anteflexed or retroflexed. Position can also vary according to congenital individual variation, pregnancy history and attendant integrity of supporting structures, and the presence or absence of various disorders of the pelvis.

These two features of uterine anatomy and orientation are very clinically relevant, particularly when diagnostic or therapeutic procedures require instrumentation of the cervical canal and/or endometrial cavity. Consequently, clinicians performing such procedures must use one or a combination of careful manual examination and imaging to accurately define the version and flexion before instrumentation of the uterus. Failure to adapt the procedure to these anatomic characteristics may result in uterine perforation, incomplete or failed procedure, and, in some instances, related morbidity.

Supporting structures

The uterus is supported in the pelvis by a number of muscular, ligamentous, and fascial structures. The *uterosacral ligaments* are condensations of the endopelvic fascia that extend from the posterior inferior aspect of the cervix and upper vagina to the sacrum. The *cardinal ligaments* extend from the cervix to the pelvic fascia on the lateral walls of the pelvis. The *pubocervical ligaments* extend from the cervix anteriorly, around the bladder, to the posterior surface of the pubic symphysis. The *round ligaments* extend from the anterior cornual region of the uterus to the respective inguinal canals, which they traverse to attach to the labia majora. The broad ligaments are actually not ligaments at all – they are folds of peritoneum that extend from the uterus to each lateral sidewall and serve as conduits for the uterine nerves, lymphatics, and blood vessels.

Vascular anatomy of the uterus

The uterus receives its principal blood supply from the ovarian and uterine arteries (Figure 2.5). The paired uterine arteries are branches of the anterior division of the internal iliac arteries. The uterine artery crosses over the ureter as it courses medially and then bifurcates, usually just before its arrival at the uterus, into an ascending branch and a descending or cervical branch which anastamoses caudally with the vaginal artery. As the ascending branches course cephalad, they give rise to six to ten arcuate arteries, both posteriorly and anteriorly, each of which anastamose with corresponding vessels from the contralateral side, thereby forming a stacked series of vascular rings.

The myometrium receives its blood supply from centrifugal and centripetally oriented branches of the arcuate arteries that are oriented in a radial fashion, perpendicular to the serosal surface. When the centripetally oriented radial arteries cross the myoendometrial junction, they give rise to the smaller caliber basal arteries, but continue on toward the endometrial surface as the spiral arteries that provide blood supply to the functionalis layer of endometrium. The coiled spiral arteries have a cross sectional appearance that varies depending upon the time in the cycle, with increased coiling characteristic of progression through the progesterone dominated luteal phase. These arteries supply separate narrow, longitudinally oriented areas of the functional endometrium, each of which is 4–9 mm^2 in area [1].

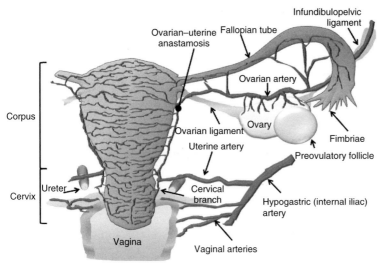

Figure 2.5 Principal arterial blood supply of the uterus. The uterus receives the majority of its blood supply from the uterine arteries, branches of the anterior division of the hypogastric (also called the internal iliac) artery. The ovarian arteries, branches of the abdominal aorta, supply most of the rest, and particularly the uterine fundus. Even if both the uterine and ovarian arteries were to be occluded, there is a rich anastamotic blood supply that is derived from some combination of the pudental, middle sacral, superior epigastric, middle hemorrhoidal, and other pelvic vessels.

The ascending branches also anastamose with their corresponding ovarian arteries that course through the broad ligament from the infundibulopelvic ligament after originating from the aorta. The contribution of the ovarian artery to the uterine blood supply is less well established, but seems to vary according to the time of the menstrual cycle and the location of the corpus luteum. Color Doppler sonography has been used to demonstrate that ovarian arterial blood flow increases during the luteal phase in the vessel ipsilateral to the ovary with the corpus luteum suggesting a gonadal steroid-related influence on arterial blood flow between the uterus and ovary [2].

Innervation

The innervation of the uterus is entirely autonomic with the sympathetic component arising from the inferior hypogastric plexus and the parasympathetic aspects deriving from the pelvic splanchnic nerves that have their roots in S 2, 3, and 4 (Figure 2.6). The afferent fibers travel with the sympathetic nerves to the T 10–12 and L 1 roots. Anatomically, the right and left hypogastric nerves link to the inferior hypogastric plexi over the posterolateral pelvis, passing behind the common iliac arteries before entering the uterosacral and cardinal ligaments where they then innervate the uterus and upper two thirds of the vagina [3]. The visceral plexi are derived from the inferior hypogastric plexi and provide innervations of the uterus and vagina in addition to the rectum and bladder. The primary innervation of the uterus comes from Frankenhauser's (uterovaginal) plexus that is located near the cardinal ligament. The myometrial innervation follows the branches of the uterine artery and may vary substantially with various disease processes such as adenomyosis and endometriosis [4]. Nerves extend through myometrium to the endometrial–myometrial interface where there exists a relatively well-defined plexus. Indeed the basal third of the

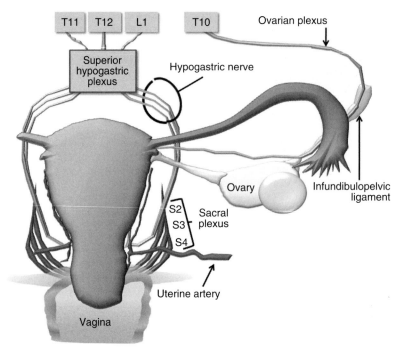

Figure 2.6 Innervation of the uterus. The cervix receives autonomic innervation from the S 2–4 components of the sacral plexus that appear to reach the uterus via Frankenhauser's plexus and the uterosacral ligaments. The corpus is innervated from the T 11, T 12, and L 1 components of the hypogastric plexus that also typically enter the uterus via Frankenhauser's plexus and the uterosacral and cardinal ligaments adjacent to the uterine arteries. The uterine corpus also receives innervation from T 10 via the infundibulopelvic ligament and the ovarian plexus. Not pictured is a rich plexus that exists at the endomyometrial interface.

endometrium is also innervated and neural fibers have been demonstrated in the superficial functionalis, particularly in women with symptomatic endometriosis [5]. There is also substantial innervation of the submucosal layer of the cervix, with an extensive plexus of nerves.

Lymphatics

There is some variation in lymphatic drainage, but, in general it follows a relatively predictable embryologically derived course that approximates the arterial blood supply. The cervix and most of the corpus drain to the internal iliac nodes while the fundus typically drains directly to the para-aortic chains.

Embryology

Like other anatomical structures, the uterus may be developmentally abnormal. Such abnormalities do not usually have anything to do with AUB, but they are important to both clinical evaluation and, in some instances, the viability of certain therapeutic options like intrauterine hormone releasing systems. The key to understanding the range of congenital uterine abnormalities that may be encountered is a basic knowledge of embryology.

The uterus, fallopian tubes, and upper vagina are derived from the *Müllerian* (or *paramesonephric*) ducts that are mesodermal in origin and are first seen by the seventh

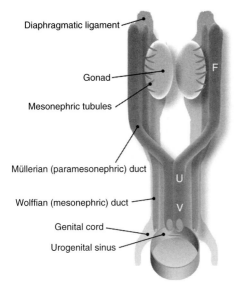

Diaphragmatic ligament

Gonad

Mesonephric tubules

Müllerian (paramesonephric) duct

Wolffian (mesonephric) duct

Genital cord

Urogenital sinus

Figure 2.7 Embryological origins of the uterus, fallopian tubes, and vagina. The Müllerian (paramesonephric) ducts propagate first caudally, then medially, and then, now adjacent to each other, caudally again until they reach the urogenital sinus. In the female, absent the H-Y antigen from the Y chromosome, Müllerian inhibiting factor is not manufactured, and the Müllerian ducts fuse in the regions destined to be the uterus and upper two thirds of the vagina. Subsequently, the fused walls absorb resulting in the formation of a single vagina, single cervix and cervical canal, and a single corpus and endometrial cavity. Partial or complete failure of fusion of the Müllerian ducts and/or absorption of the fused walls, can result in a spectrum of anatomical abnormalities ranging from a clinically insignificant "arcuate" uterus, to two parallel systems each comprising a single fallopian tube, endometrial cavity, cervix and cervical canal, and vagina.

embryological week (Figure 2.7). The ducts start as an invagination of the celomic epithelium (later to be the peritoneum), and positioned lateral to the most cranial aspect of the *Wolffian* (*mesonephric*) ducts and the metanephros (primordial kidney). Each duct propagates caudally and medially meeting the other in the midline and extending between the developing urinary bladder and rectum, to fuse with the urogenital sinus at a region called the Müllerian tubercle by eight embryological weeks. To this point, embryological development is identical in both genders, but in the male, the developing testes are responsible for the production of Müllerian inhibiting factor (MIF) that results in the cessation of Müllerian development. Indeed, the only remnants of the Müllerian duct in the normal male are the appendix testis and the prostatic utricle. In the female, absence of testosterone causes the Wolffian duct to cease development, but remnants generally remain including the epoophoron, the paraoophoron and the Gartner's ducts. In some instances, these structures become incorporated into the cervix or myometrium as these fibromuscular structures develop from surrounding mesoderm.

The fusion and continued development of the Müllerian ducts draw medially the two peritoneal folds that ultimately become the broad ligaments. The unfused cranial aspect of each duct develops into a fallopian tube, the middle fused portion becomes the uterus (corpus and cervix), and the lower fused ducts ultimately become the upper two thirds to four fifths of the vagina. Initially, these structures are solid, but they later become canalized.

Developmental abnormalities of this Müllerian system can be better understood. For example, persistence of a variable portion of the original double tube, beyond the fallopian tubes, may manifest in minor septae in the upper endometrial cavity, to entire failure of Müllerian fusion with a septum extending to the lower third or fifth of the vagina. Failure of canalization of the caudal end of the fused ducts results in a transverse septum or imperforate hymen. Alternatively, failure of development of one Müllerian duct can result in the unicornuate uterus and a single fallopian tube. Not surprisingly, such anomalies are frequently associated with coexistant absence or abnormalities in the development of the ipsilateral kidney and ureter.

References

1. Bartelmez GW. Histologic studies on the menstruating mucous membrane of the human uterus. *Contrib Embryol.* 1933;**142**:141–86.
2. Tan SL, Zaidi J, Campbell S, Doyle P, Collins W. Blood flow changes in the ovarian and uterine arteries during the normal menstrual cycle. *Am J Obstet Gynecol.* 1996;**175**(3 Pt 1):625–31.
3. Krantz KE. Innervation of the human uterus. *Ann N Y Acad Sci.* 1959;**75**:770–84.
4. Quinn MJ, Kirk N. Differences in uterine innervation at hysterectomy. *Am J Obstet Gynecol.* 2002;**187**(6):1515–9; discussion 9–20.
5. Tokushige N, Markham R, Russell P, Fraser IS. High density of small nerve fibres in the functional layer of the endometrium in women with endometriosis. *Hum Reprod.* 2006;**21**(3):782–7.

Physiology of menstruation

Chapter summary

- A sound understanding of female reproductive physiology including the mechanisms of normal menstruation is critical to understanding the pathogenesis of AUB.
- The endometrium responds predictably to ovarian production of estradiol and then, following ovulation, estradiol plus progesterone. Cessation of progesterone production results in endometrial ischemia and then menstrual bleeding.
- Endometrial ischemia is initiated by the local production release of a number of vasoactive substances that include prostaglandin (PG) $F_{2\alpha}$ and endothelin-1.
- The composition of menstrual discharge is only about 25% blood, with the remainder comprising fluid, endometrial cells, and tissue.
- Endometrial hemostasis following sloughing of the functionalis requires $PGF_{2\alpha}$ and endothelin-1 as well as an intact mechanism for the formation of an intraluminal vascular plug.

Introduction

Menstruation refers to the normal process of cyclical uterine bleeding that occurs in the reproductive years of the human female. It is always useful to remember that the sole purpose of the endometrium is to provide an environment for the delivery of nutrition and oxygen to the developing embryo and fetus. Consequently, and only from the perspective of propagation of the species, menstruation is a reflection of the "failure" of the woman to become pregnant.

The process is the result of a carefully orchestrated systemic endocrine relationship involving the hypothalamus, the pituitary, and the ovary that results first in follicular maturation, then ovulation, and, finally, in the absence of conception and implantation, sloughing of the superficial endometrium. Worldwide, the mean age at first menses (*menarche*) is 13.5 (SD ± 0.98) years, while menstruation ceases with menopause at a mean age of 49.24 (SD ± 1.73) years as the ovaries cease normal production of gonadal steroids [1, 2]. In developed countries, the mean age of menarche is lower – approximately 12.0–12.6 years in US Caucasians and Blacks respectively – and that of menopause higher than the international mean – as the average age at natural menopause in the United States is 51.4 years [3].

The process of menstruation requires the existence of a contiguous pathway that starts in the endometrial cavity and extends through to the cervical canal and vagina that allows the components of the menstrual discharge to be externalized. The onset of true menstruation is initiated by the withdrawal of ovarian estradiol and progesterone, while cessation of each episode of menstrual flow seems to be largely a local function, with the endometrium itself responsible for the production of many of the factors required for endometrial hemostasis.

In the reproductive years, following menarche, cyclic ovulation results in the onset of menstrual periods every 22–35 days [4–6]. While there is variation amongst women; the cycle length in a given individual should remain reasonably constant. Understanding this process requires a working knowledge of the mechanisms involved in the relationships among the hypothalamus, pituitary, ovary, and endometrium. Such knowledge is critical to understanding the pathogenesis of AUB, as well as many of the interventions designed to treat the disorder.

The hypothalamic-pituitary-ovarian axis

Systemic regulation of menstrual function is controlled by the hypothalamus, anterior pituitary gland, and ovary, which intercommunicate via a number of hormones including gonadotropin releasing hormone (GnRH), follicle stimulating hormone (FSH), luteinizing hormone (LH), 17-β estradiol, and progesterone. Gonadotropin releasing hormone is secreted by the hypothalamus, while FSH and LH are produced in and secreted from the anterior pituitary (Figure 3.1). Estradiol is made in the preovulatory follicle while, following ovulation, both estradiol and progesterone are secreted from the corpus luteum (Figure 3.2). The ultimate goal is to stimulate to ovulation a dormant *primordial follicle,* one of the thousands located in the ovary that are derived from the primordial germ cells, and arrested in prophase of the first meiotic division while the woman was still a developing fetus.

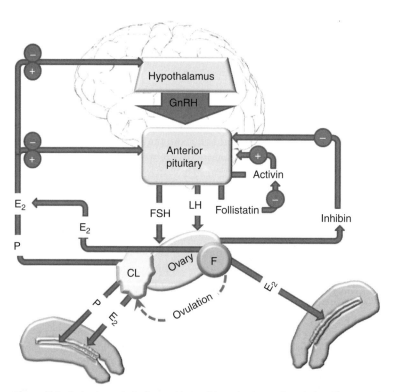

Figure 3.1 Systemic control of gonadal steroid production and ovulation. CL, corpus luteum; E_2, estradiol; F, follicle; FSH, follicle stimulating hormone; GnRH, gonadotropin releasing hormone; LH, luteinizing hormone; P, progesterone.

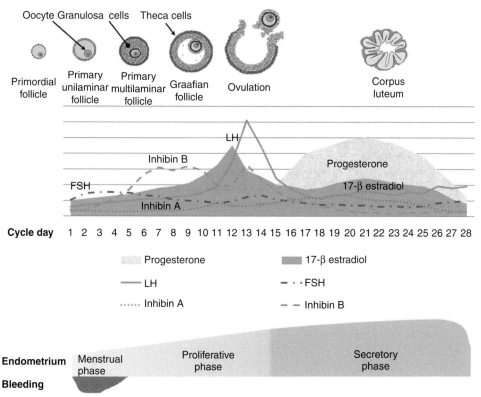

Figure 3.2 Stylized relationship of gonadal steroids, follicular development, and macroscopic appearance of the endometrium. The top layer demonstrates follicular development, ovulation, and then the corpus luteum. The second or middle layer shows the relative levels of estradiol, progesterone, follicle stimulating hormone (FSH), luteinizing hormone (LH), and inhibin A and B by cycle day. The bottom layer demonstrates a stylized endometrial profile with distinct menstrual, proliferative, and secretory phases.

A convenient place to start the description is early in the cycle where, following loss of the inhibitory effects of estradiol and progesterone, the pulsatile release of GnRH from the hypothalamus stimulates systemic release of FSH from the anterior pituitary, a process that is likely facilitated by the locally produced peptide *activin*. When FSH reaches the ovaries it begins to stimulate a selected number of primordial follicles, usually between 15 and 20, which subsequently mature into *primary follicles*. Ultimately one of these will become the dominant or Graafian follicle, the source of the mature ovum released at mid cycle. The mechanisms involved in the "selection" of primary follicles from the ovarian reserve of primordial follicles are unclear, but may involve members of the transforming growth factor-beta (TGF-β) superfamily such as endogenously secreted *activin*, which may increase FSH receptor expression in a given primordial follicle. The remaining primary follicles will ultimately be inactivated by the process of *atresia*.

The primary follicles initially comprise a primary oocyte surrounded by a single layer of granulosa cells (Figure 3.2). Between the granulosa cells and the oocyte exists a thick glycoprotein layer called the *zona pellucida* which, nevertheless, allows passage of nutrients and waste to and from the surrounding granulosa cells.

23

Following growth of the oocyte, the granulosa cells proliferate into multiple layers under the influence of FSH, which amplifies its own effect by stimulating the production of more FSH receptors in each granulosa cell, perhaps through the local production of activin. These granulosa cells respond by producing *inhibin (A and B)* and *17-β estradiol*, which we are calling estradiol, the latter from *testosterone*, locally produced largely by the adjacent *thecal cells*. The thecal cells are developed from peripheral granulosa cells under the influence of estradiol, and then ultimately differentiate under the influence of LH into two layers: the theca interna and theca externa. Although testosterone is usually considered to be a "male" hormone, in the presence of the *aromatase* enzyme, produced in abundance in granulosa cells, it is converted to 17-β estradiol. In addition, FSH, estradiol, and *inhibin* appear to induce the formation of receptors on the granulosa cells that allow LH to stimulate the production of androgens and to exert other effects later in the cycle. These LH receptors are also increased by LH itself, which is required for further growth of the follicle, for ovulation, and for luteinization of both granulosa and thecal cells following ovulation. Finally, it is important to understand that inhibin, FSH, and, at low serum levels, estradiol, each provide negative feedback to the hypothalamus, reducing the production of GnRH and, thereby, the production and release of FSH. These lower levels of FSH are offset by the much higher levels of FSH receptors in the primary follicles, thereby allowing continued growth and development.

The process of ovulation typically occurs after about 14 days of stimulation of the follicles with estradiol (day 14 of the cycle), but there is considerable variation in this *follicular phase*, which is the principal reason for cycle length variations among individuals. Indeed, one of the earlier changes in women in the late reproductive years is a shortening of the follicular phase [7]. As serum estradiol levels rise, the negative feedback changes to become positive feedback initiating a burst of LH (the LH "surge") from the pituitary that results in final maturation of the oocyte in the dominant follicle (formation of a secondary oocyte) and, ultimately, ejection of the oocyte into the peritoneal cavity. The mechanisms of LH-induced ovulation include prostaglandin secretion; the development of progesterone receptors; release of proteolytic enzymes that degrade the cells at the surface of the follicle; and the stimulation of follicular wall angiogenesis. In the pelvis, the oocyte is picked up by the distal (*fimbriated*) end of the fallopian tube where it begins a three-day trip down the oviduct to the endometrial cavity of the uterus.

In the follicle, the granulosa, surrounding theca cells, and other nearby tissue continue to undergo a transformation called *luteinization* that results in the formation of a temporary structure called the *corpus luteum*. The corpus luteum produces both estradiol and progesterone. The estradiol and progesterone production peak at about five to seven days postovulation, a time coincident with anticipated implantation of a fertilized ovum, which, by this time, would be considered a *blastocyst*. These high progesterone levels exert negative feedback on GnRH secretion and pulse frequency thereby reducing secretion of both FSH and LH.

The principle role of ovarian progesterone is to prepare the endometrium for implantation and initial hormonal support of an embryo should conception occur. If no such pregnancy ensues, the corpus luteum ceases to function about 12–14 days following ovulation, largely via the process of apoptosis that results in a dramatic reduction of both estradiol and progesterone levels in the systemic circulation. The resulting atretic corpus luteum evolves to a nonfunctional entity called the *corpus albicans*. With declining levels of both FSH and LH, their negative feedback on the production of GnRH reduces and the cycle starts once again.

Endometrial response

How does the cyclic production of estradiol and progesterone impact the endometrium? First, let's review the anatomy. As described in Chapter 2, the permanent *basalis*, that resides next to the myometrium, actually has two layers itself, zones 1 and 2. On the other hand the overlying and regenerative functionalis, that also has two layers (zones 3 and 4), normally and cyclically is separated from the basalis and sloughs if a pregnancy does not occur, and, consequently, progesterone levels fall.

Macroscopic response

In the reproductive years, it is useful to consider that the endometrium of an ovulatory woman undergoes three relatively distinct phases that reflect the changing estrogen-progesterone milieu: an estradiol-stimulated preovulatory follicular or *proliferative* phase; a progesterone-dominated, postovulatory luteal or *secretory* phase; and a *menstrual phase* (Figures 3.2 and 3.3). Grossly, these three phases of the cycle manifest in a spectrum of endometrial thickness that ranges from about 2 mm in the early proliferative phase, to about 5 mm in the late proliferative phase, and about 6 mm in the late luteal phase [8, 9]. These changes can be appreciated and even measured using diagnostic ultrasound (Chapter 23).

Molecular impact

So how do gonadal steroids impact the endometrium on a molecular level? On a simplified basis, the hormonal molecule travels to the endometrial cells, is allowed to cross the cell membrane, migrate into the nucleus, and then attach to specific nuclear receptors where gene transcription is initiated resulting in a number of profound molecular and cellular events (Figure 3.3).

Gonadal steroids and receptors

The principal nuclear gonadal steroid receptors include those for estrogens (ER), progesterone (PR), and androgens (AR). Indeed it is now recognized that there are two receptor isoforms for both progesterone (PRA and PRB) and for estrogens (ERα and ERβ). The differential roles for PRA and PRB are not yet clearly defined, but ERα is identified in glandular and stromal cells while ERβ is the only steroid receptor found in the endothelium and smooth muscle walls of endometrial vessels [10]. Androgen receptors can be found in endometrial tissue and, when activated by androgen molecules, seem to result in endometrial atrophy.

Following menstruation and the attainment of hemostasis, to be discussed presently, the only gonadal steroid of import that impacts the endometrium is estradiol, which is responsible for "priming" the endometrial cells in a number of ways, including the expression of increasing numbers of both estradiol and progesterone receptors. Following ovulation, the estradiol-primed endometrium is exposed to both the estradiol and progesterone produced from the corpus luteum that interact with the abundant estradiol and progesterone receptors created in the follicular phase. The physiological goals of this gonadal steroid pairing are to prepare the endometrium for implantation and initial development of the embryo via myriad local molecular and ultrastructural changes that are not within the scope of this book. Nevertheless, it is worth noting that continued exposure to progesterone results in down-regulation of both estrogen and progesterone receptors [11].

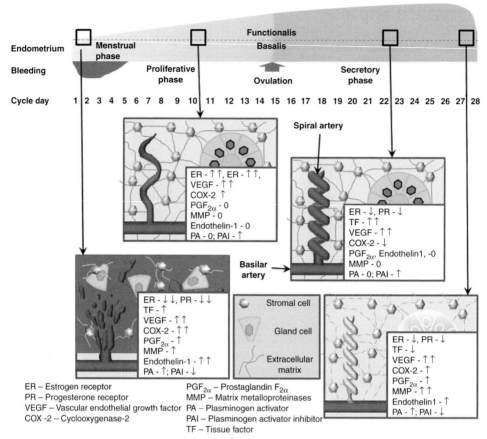

Figure 3.3 The induction and control of normal menstruation. A stylized endometrial profile is at the top of the figure demonstrating cycle days 1–28 with ovulation occurring late in the 14th day. The small boxes over the endometrium are blown up in the four panels which depict up- or downwards pointing arrows that depict the level and trend in concentration of the particular molecule. *Proliferative phase*: Vascular endothelial growth factor (VEGF) and both estrogen receptor (ER) and progesterone (PR) are increasing under the influence of estradiol. *Early secretory phase*: Both ER and PR have reached a maximum and even have started to decline under the influence of progesterone. *Late secretory phase*: There is a marked reduction in both ER and PR, and the endometrium is beginning to manifest the impact of progesterone withdrawal as the corpus luteum begins to involute. The levels of cyclooxygenase-2 (COX-2) are increased and contribute to the increased level of vasoconstricting $PGF_{2\alpha}$, which, in combination with endothelin-1, results in spiral artery vasoconstriction and endometrial ischemia. The proteolytic activity that results in separation of the ischemic functionalis from the basalis is related in large part to the expression of matrix metalloproteinases (MMPs) following progesterone withdrawal. In the early menstrual phase, blood, endometrial stromal and glandular cells, and transudate comprise the menstrual discharge, levels of prostaglandin (PG) $F_{2\alpha}$ and endothelin-1 are high and now contribute to hemostasis, and tissue factor (TF), generated in the decidualized endometrium under progesterone influence, contributes to the formation of the hemostatic plugs by acting as a receptor for factor VII to ultimately convert prothrombin to thrombin (Figure 3.4). Plasminogen activator levels are high in the early menstrual phase but should decline in the later phase so clot integrity is maintained.

Endometrial prostaglandins

Prostaglandins are produced in the endometrium throughout the menstrual cycle, but are seen in increased concentrations in the late luteal and menstrual phases, coincident with the declining levels of systemic and local progesterone. It is clear, without knowledge of the specific mechanism, that this process is intimately related to the local levels of estradiol and progesterone.

The endometrium is rich in the phospholipases necessary for the conversion of fatty acid precursors to arachadonic acid and, especially in the late luteal phase, the cyclooxygenase (COX) necessary for transforming arachadonic acid to prostaglandins [12]. A dominant player in the milieu of the immediate premenstrual luteal phase is $PGF_{2\alpha}$, a potent vasoconstrictor produced predominantly in the endometrium, particularly in the gland cells [13, 14]. It is likely that the mechanisms involved in creating $PGF_{2\alpha}$ require the presence of progesterone for it is found in low levels in anovulatory women [15]. We will see that the potent vasoconstricting actions of $PGF_{2\alpha}$ are one of the principle mechanisms responsible for the induction of menstruation and for endometrial hemostasis.

The endometrial stroma also produces prostaglandin E_2 (PGE_2) [16] and prostacyclin (PGI_2) [17] with platelet inhibiting and vasodilating activity. They may be found in greater abundance in ovulatory women with HMB as discussed in Chapter 5.

Endothelin-1

Another vasoconstrictive agent, endothelin-1 (ET-1) has been discovered in the late luteal and premenstrual decidualized endometrial stroma that clusters around the spiral arteries [18]. It is likely that ET-1, produced in quantity with the withdrawal of progesterone, is a potent contributor to spiral artery vasospasm.

Matrix metalloproteinases

Matrix metalloproteinases (MMPs) and other proteolytic enzymes can be found in the stroma of late secretory endometrium and also appear to be associated with the onset of menstruation [19]. There exist a number of MMPs, at least three of which seem to be involved with the induction of menstruation by a process of degradation of specific components of the endometrial stromal extracellular matrix (ECM). Matrix metalloproteinase-1 functions as an interstitial collagenase (types I, II, and III) by cleaving the helical structure of the molecule. Matrix metalloproteinase-2 is a gelatinase, attacking basement membrane collagens (types IV and V) as well as already denatured interstitial collagens, or gelatins. Matrix metalloproteinase-3 is a stromolysin that degrades ECM proteins like proteoglycans, glycoproteins, fibronectin, and laminin, as well as basement membrane collagens type IV and V [20–22]. Each of the MMPs are derived from precursor zymogens manufactured by endometrial stromal cell (proMMP-1, proMMP-2, and proMMP-3), the secretion of which is inhibited by progesterone (MMP-1, 3) and increased with the withdrawal of progesterone, at least in in-vitro models [23]. Consequently, the current hypothesis is that estradiol and progesterone stabilize the perivascular endometrial ECM by suppressing the expression of MMPs from endometrial stromal cells until late in the luteal phase. At that time, local mast cells may become involved by increasing production of cytokines, including interleukin-1 (IL-1) and tumor necrosis factor alpha (TNF-α), which individually and collectively increase the production of MMPs in vitro [24].

Vascular endothelial growth factor

It has been demonstrated that endometrial vascular endothelial growth factor (VEGF) expression is present throughout the cycle but increases with the onset of hypoxia. This occurs in association with an increased expression of VEGF receptors (KDR) in the superficial endometrium in the late luteal phase. The observation that VEGF may up-regulate MMP production lends credence to the notion that VEGF may be a contributor to the induction of menstruation.

Plasminogen activator

There exist other substances produced in abundance in the late luteal phase stroma that possess proteolytic activity. The family of plasminogen activators (PA) is a group of proteases that increase with MMP in the late luteal and early menstrual phases of the cycle, while their inhibitors (plasminogen activator inhibitors – PAI) decrease around menses. Indeed, PA may even contribute to the activation of at least some of the MMPs and potentially are involved in the induction of menstruation in a way that is synergistic with the action of MMPs [25, 26].

Tissue factor

Progesterone exposure results in decidualized cells surrounding the endometrial vessels that contain tissue factor (TF), a cell membrane-bound glycoprotein that acts as a receptor for factor VII and which supports hemostasis [27]. High levels of TF are present in the mid luteal phase, a function that inhibits bleeding during trophoblastic invasion should pregnancy occur. The levels reduce in the late luteal phase in keeping with the reduction in progesterone and PR levels and the upcoming induction of menstruation. However, during menstruation, TF is likely still important for hemostasis because of its influence on factor VII activation and subsequent thrombin formation.

Menstruation

If pregnancy does not occur, the programmed luteolysis that occurs 12–14 days following ovulation results in rapid reduction of local endometrial levels of estradiol and, most importantly, progesterone. As we have seen, progesterone is intimately related to the local production of molecules that are responsible for inducing menstruation and for the attainment of initial endometrial hemostasis. Progesterone is also responsible for delaying the local release of these substances until it is clear that pregnancy has not occurred.

Induction of bleeding

Progesterone withdrawal is thought to trigger menstrual bleeding in part by initiating the local production of large amounts of $PGF_{2\alpha}$ and ET-1 that, in turn, cause profound spiral artery vasoconstriction and resulting endometrial ischemia [28] (Figure 3.3). Immediately prior to the onset of menstruation there is loss of extracellular fluid from the endometrial stroma, with markedly increased coiling of the spiral arterioles, and slowing of local blood flow. These events have been very well described in the rhesus monkey by Markee [29], and seem to be very similar in the human.

Endometrial MMP expression also increases dramatically with the decline in progesterone activity. With the release of the local MMPs described previously, endometrial ECM degrades, facilitating sloughing of the now ischemic functionalis layer of the endometrium. With sloughing of the functionalis, bleeding occurs, likely in large part from venules in the endometrium [29]. However, there is undoubtedly some arterial bleeding that may be augmented by the presence of vasodilatory PGE_2 and PGI_2, particularly in the first two days of menses.

Composition of menstrual flow

It may come as a surprise to some that menstrual flow is actually a combination of blood, endometrium, and a serous endometrial "transudate." While menstrual content clearly contains some of the elements of whole blood, with red cells and leukocytes (particularly polymorphonuclear leukocytes), it has virtually no platelets. The proportion of menstrual fluid that is red cells is about 25% with the remaining fluid volume likely derived from the serous, endometrial "transudate" [30]. In women with HMB the mean whole blood component is increased to around 50% [31].

Whereas menstrual fluid is greatly deficient in platelets and clotting factors [11], fibrin monomer fibers can be recognized under the electron microscope even if a true blood clot with mature fibrin does not form, a finding that begs a question regarding the composition of the clots that some women experience with HMB. It is apparent that these clots are aggregations of red cells held together loosely by mucinous proteins that become more prominent when bleeding becomes heavy [14]. Grossly, one can sometimes see tissue fragments in the flow, but on histopathological evaluation these substances comprise a spectrum of material ranging from endometrial cells, to clumps of endometrial glandular and stromal tissue, to nonviable and unrecognizable tissue fragments and cellular material [11]. The larger tissue fragments are typically seen around 12 hours after the onset of bleeding. The cellular content of the flow has not been well studied, and there is limited information on the day-to-day changes in composition.

Hemostasis

With the onset of menstrual sloughing and bleeding comes the requisite need for local hemostasis, a process that depends upon a variety of factors. Whereas in other tissues, the initial process involves formation of the primary platelet plug (primary hemostasis), studies of endometrial clots in animal models suggest that platelet involvement is relatively low while features dependent upon the clotting cascade are of greater importance [32]. While these findings cannot necessarily be applied to the human, it is likely that local vasoconstriction plays the dominant role in securing early hemostasis. Thromboxane (from vascular endothelial and platelet origins), ET-1, and $PGF_{2\alpha}$ each contribute to the induction of vasospasm in the spiral arteries of the endometrium (Figure 3.3). As previously described, PGE_2 and PGI_2 can result in vasodilation of the same vessels and high ratios of PGI_2 and/or PGE_2 to $PGF_{2\alpha}$ are seen in women with HMB [33].

The coagulation cascade is likely important for secondary hemostasis following day one of the cycle. Historically, the coagulation cascade was depicted as comprising two distinct pathways, extrinsic and intrinsic, each of which was independently capable of activation of factor X (to Xa), which ultimately, under the influence of activated factor V, catalyzes the conversion of prothrombin to thrombin [34]. In this model the intrinsic pathway is initiated by factor XII and other contact agents, while the extrinsic pathway is activated by tissue factor, which, together with factor Xa, results in factor VII activation. Recently, the concepts of the coagulation cascade have been modified to be consistent with recently recognized regulatory steps and pathways [35] (Figure 3.4). Most important is the recognition of the important role of the factor VII/tissue factor complex of the extrinsic pathway which appears to activate factor IX of the intrinsic pathway, a feature that provides "crosstalk" between the two, formerly distinctly perceived systems.

Fibrinolysis

An important part of the natural history of an endometrial vascular clot is the process of fibrinolysis that is mediated by the generation of plasmin from plasminogen following

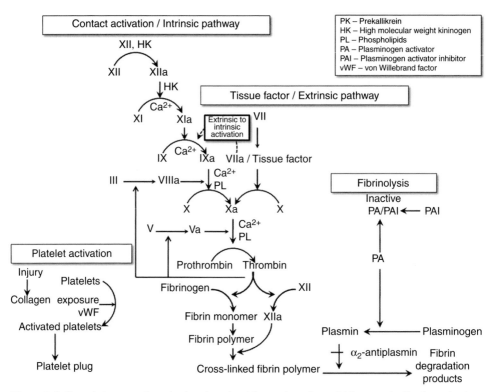

Figure 3.4 Coagulation cascade and other clot-related factors in endometrial hemostasis. Platelet activation that includes von Willebrand factor is shown in the lower left, while the contact activation (formerly intrinsic) and tissue factor mediated (formerly extrinsic) pathways are shown starting at the top. In the lower right, the fibrinolytic component is depicted where plasmin production varies according to the amount of local plasminogen activator.

its activation by plasminogen activator [36, 37]. While such fibrinolysis is physiological, and therefore necessary, enhanced fibrinolysis may impede the attainment of local hemostasis, a mechanism involved in HMB of endometrial origin, to be discussed in Chapter 5.

Endometrial regeneration

Surface repair and remodeling of the epithelium, stroma, and vasculature are complex processes about which remarkably little is known. These processes appear to be triggered to begin within hours of the start of endometrial breakdown. Regeneration of the functionalis probably begins from the mouths of opened glands as well as from pluripotential cells in the superficial stroma. It is likely that migratory leukocytes and a range of growth factors and cytokines play important roles in the repair process [28, 38]. Endothelial repair is complete within four to five days, and the menstrual discharge declines rapidly into the fourth and fifth days as the repair process ends. Estradiol is not essential for basic repair, but becomes important within the first few days to stimulate active endometrial proliferation.

References

1. Thomas F, Renaud F, Benefice E, de Meeus T, Guegan JF. International variability of ages at menarche and menopause: patterns and main determinants. *Hum Biol.* 2001; **73**(2):271–90.

2. Morabia A, Costanza MC. International variability in ages at menarche, first livebirth, and menopause. World Health Organization Collaborative Study of Neoplasia and Steroid Contraceptives. *Am J Epidemiol.* 1998;**148**(12):1195–205.

3. Gold EB, Bromberger J, Crawford S, Samuels S, Greendale GA, Harlow SD, et al. Factors associated with age at natural menopause in a multiethnic sample of midlife women. *Am J Epidemiol.* 2001;**153**(9):865–74.

4. Treloar SA, Martin NG, Heath AC. Longitudinal genetic analysis of menstrual flow, pain, and limitation in a sample of Australian twins. *Behav Genet.* 1998;**28**(2):107–16.

5. Chiazze L, Jr., Brayer FT, Macisco JJ, Jr., Parker MP, Duffy BJ. The length and variability of the human menstrual cycle. *JAMA.* 1968;**203**(6):377–80.

6. Belsey EM, Pinol AP. Menstrual bleeding patterns in untreated women. Task Force on Long-Acting Systemic Agents for Fertility Regulation. *Contraception.* 1997;**55**(2):57–65.

7. Van Zonneveld P, Scheffer GJ, Broekmans FJ, Blankenstein MA, de Jong FH, Looman CW, et al. Do cycle disturbances explain the age-related decline of female fertility? Cycle characteristics of women aged over 40 years compared with a reference population of young women. *Hum Reprod.* 2003;**18**(3):495–501.

8. Bakos O, Lundkvist O, Bergh T. Transvaginal sonographic evaluation of endometrial growth and texture in spontaneous ovulatory cycles – a descriptive study. *Hum Reprod.* 1993;**8**(6):799–806.

9. Grow DR, Iromloo K. Oral contraceptives maintain a very thin endometrium before operative hysteroscopy. *Fertil Steril.* 2006;**85**(1):204–7.

10. Critchley HO, Kelly RW, Baird DT, Brenner RM. Regulation of human endometrial function: mechanisms relevant to uterine bleeding. *Reprod Biol Endocrinol.* 2006;**4**(Suppl 1):S5.

11. Bouchard P. Progesterone and the progesterone receptor. *J Reprod Med.* 1999;**44**(2 Suppl):153–7.

12. Rees MC, Parry DM, Anderson AB, Turnbull AC. Immunohistochemical localisation of cyclooxygenase in the human uterus. *Prostaglandins.* 1982;**23**(2):207–14.

13. Abel MH, Baird DT. The effect of 17 beta-estradiol and progesterone on prostaglandin production by human endometrium maintained in organ culture. *Endocrinology.* 1980;**106**(5):1599–606.

14. Lumsden MA, Brown A, Baird DT. Prostaglandin production from homogenates of separated glandular epithelium and stroma from human endometrium. *Prostaglandins.* 1984;**28**(4):485–96.

15. Smith SK, Abel MH, Kelly RW, Baird DT. The synthesis of prostaglandins from persistent proliferative endometrium. *J Clin Endocrinol Metab.* 1982;**55**(2):284–9.

16. Hoffman MS, Lynch CM. Minilaparotomy hysterectomy. *Am J Obstet Gynecol.* 1998;**179**(2):316–20.

17. Smith SK, Abel MH, Kelly RW, Baird DT. A role for prostacyclin (PGI2) in excessive menstrual bleeding. *Lancet.* 1981;**1**(8219):522–4.

18. Word RA, Kamm KE, Casey ML. Contractile effects of prostaglandins, oxytocin, and endothelin-1 in human myometrium in vitro: refractoriness of myometrial tissue of pregnant women to prostaglandins E2 and F2 alpha. *J Clin Endocrinol Metab.* 1992;**75**(4):1027–32.

19. Marbaix E, Kokorine I, Moulin P, Donnez J, Eeckhout Y, Courtoy PJ. Menstrual breakdown of human endometrium can be mimicked in vitro and is selectively and reversibly blocked by inhibitors of matrix metalloproteinases. *Proc Natl Acad Sci U S A.* 1996;**93**(17):9120–5.

20. Woessner JF, Jr. The family of matrix metalloproteinases. *Ann N Y Acad Sci.* 1994;**732**:11–21.

21. Birkedal-Hansen H, Moore WG, Bodden MK, Windsor LJ, Birkedal-Hansen

B, DeCarlo A, et al. Matrix metalloproteinases: a review. *Crit Rev Oral Biol Med*. 1993;4(2):197–250.

22. McDonnell S, Wright JH, Gaire M, Matrisian LM. Expression and regulation of stromelysin and matrilysin by growth factors and oncogenes. *Biochem Soc Trans*. 1994;22(1):58–63.

23. Lockwood CJ, Krikun G, Hausknecht VA, Papp C, Schatz F. Matrix metalloproteinase and matrix metalloproteinase inhibitor expression in endometrial stromal cells during progestin-initiated decidualization and menstruation-related progestin withdrawal. *Endocrinology*. 1998;139(11):4607–13.

24. Zhang J, Nie G, Jian W, Woolley DE, Salamonsen LA. Mast cell regulation of human endometrial matrix metalloproteinases: A mechanism underlying menstruation. *Biol Reprod*. 1998;59(3):693–703.

25. Littlefield BA. Plasminogen activators in endometrial physiology and embryo implantation: a review. *Ann N Y Acad Sci*. 1991;622:167–75.

26. Gleeson NC. Cyclic changes in endometrial tissue plasminogen activator and plasminogen activator inhibitor type 1 in women with normal menstruation and essential menorrhagia. *Am J Obstet Gynecol*. 1994;171(1):178–83.

27. Schatz F, Krikun G, Caze R, Rahman M, Lockwood CJ. Progestin-regulated expression of tissue factor in decidual cells: implications in endometrial hemostasis, menstruation and angiogenesis. *Steroids*. 2003;68 (10–13):849–60.

28. Jabbour HN, Kelly RW, Fraser HM, Critchley HO. Endocrine regulation of menstruation. *Endocr* Rev. 2006;27 (1):17–46.

29. Markee JE. Menstruation in intraocular endometrial transplants in the rhesus monkey. *Contrib Embryol*. 1940;177: 220–30.

30. Fraser IS, McCarron G, Markham R, Resta T. Blood and total fluid content of menstrual discharge. *Obstet Gynecol*. 1985;65(2):194–8.

31. Fraser IS, Warner P, Marantos PA. Estimating menstrual blood loss in women with normal and excessive menstrual fluid volume. *Obstet Gynecol*. 2001;98 (5 Pt 1):806–14.

32. Gelety TJ, Chaudhuri G. Haemostatic mechanism in the endometrium: role of cyclo-oxygenase products and coagulation factors. *Br J Pharmacol*. 1995;114(5): 975–80.

33. Smith SK, Abel MH, Kelly RW, Baird DT. Prostaglandin synthesis in the endometrium of women with ovular dysfunctional uterine bleeding. *Br J Obstet Gynaecol*. 1981;88(4):434–42.

34. Roberts HR, Lozier JN. New perspectives on the coagulation cascade. *Hosp Pract (Off Ed)*. 1992;27(1):97–105, 9–12.

35. Broze GJ, Jr. The role of tissue factor pathway inhibitor in a revised coagulation cascade. *Semin Hematol*. 1992;29(3): 159–69.

36. Gleeson N, Devitt M, Sheppard BL, Bonnar J. Endometrial fibrinolytic enzymes in women with normal menstruation and dysfunctional uterine bleeding. *Br J Obstet Gynaecol*. 1993;100 (8):768–71.

37. Christiaens GC, Sixma JJ, Haspels AA. Hemostasis in menstrual endometrium: a review. *Obstet Gynecol Surv*. 1982; 37(5):281–303.

38. Salamonsen LA. Tissue injury and repair in the female human reproductive tract. *Reproduction*. 2003;125(3):301–11.

Classification and pathogenesis
Nomenclature and classification
of abnormal uterine bleeding

Chapter summary

- A number of historical terms of Latin origin that are used to describe abnormal menstruation have been used in an inconsistent and often confusing fashion, which limits their effective use in medical communication.
- It is recommended that many of these terms be replaced by simple terms describing four variables; regularity, frequency, duration, and volume, which can be translated easily and consistently into other languages.
- These terms require the establishment of normal parameters of menstruation, which are determined at the lower and upper limits by the 5th and 95th percentiles respectively.
- A classification system is proposed to categorize the different etiologies for AUB in a given patient to facilitate communication among health care professionals and to improve the design and interpretation of research.

Background

With any organ system and disease state, it is important to have a clearly defined nomenclature to describe anatomy, normal physiology, and the spectrum of symptoms, signs, and disorders that may be encountered. Unfortunately, in many aspects, the terminologies concerning both normal and abnormal menstrual bleeding vary substantially, by and even within different countries and medical cultures [1–3]. Consequently, the existence of different words and definitions describing symptoms and underlying causes undermines communication amongst both the lay and health care professional community, and has the potential to cause confusion concerning the interpretation of data from clinical trials regarding AUB.

The evolution of many of the Latin and traditional terms used to describe AUB were reviewed in Chapter 1. The most frequently used terms such as "menorrhagia," "metrorrhagia," and "dysfunctional uterine bleeding (DUB)" now have different meanings in different environments; textbooks and even published clinical studies often fail to unambiguously define such terms, or even provide conflicting descriptions and definitions [3]. For example, the term "DUB" may be used to indicate the presence of only ovulatory or only anovulatory cycles or both depending on where in the world, or the country, or the city, the patient is seen. For some, menorrhagia and DUB are used as symptoms, for others they are diagnoses, while some use them to describe both symptoms and diagnoses [2]. On the other hand, the term "abnormal uterine bleeding" (AUB) has received greater acceptance and encompasses a wide range of uterine bleeding symptoms [2].

A number of the causes of AUB have now been relatively well defined with the use of modern imaging, histopathological, and molecular biology techniques. Most would agree that many cases of AUB could fit within three discernible categories: (1) those with definable uterine pathology; (2) the existence of systemic medical disease; and (3) the use of medical therapy that impacts normal endometrial function. The fourth general category is reserved for those women with AUB unrelated to definable pelvic pathology, systemic medical disease, or exogenous medical therapy – in short, given current diagnostic tools, there is no identified cause. This category of women with AUB is currently defined as a "diagnosis of exclusion," which many have labeled as "dysfunctional uterine bleeding" or DUB. Unfortunately, applying the DUB label to those who, on clinical evaluation, do not have definable pelvic pathology, allows the inclusion of women with discrepant diagnoses ranging from disturbances in ovulation to local disorders of endometrial hemostasis. This is not a satisfactory environment for clinical, educational, or research activity.

This situation fostered the development of a process designed to address these issues. The entities and individuals involved included relevant international and national organizations, as well as journal editors and a number of scientists and clinician investigators with expertise in investigation and clinical management of women with AUB. The outcome, recently simultaneously published in both European- and North American-based peer review journals, reported almost universal agreement that the poorly defined terms of classical origin used in differing ways in the English medical language should be discarded. There was agreement that these should be replaced by simple, descriptive terms with clear definitions, translatable into most languages, and easily understood by health professionals and patients alike. The major recommendations were to abolish and replace terms such as menorrhagia, metrorrhagia, hypermenorrhoea, and dysfunctional uterine bleeding [2, 4]. Subsequent, but not-yet-completed and important components of this iterative process include the classification of etiology as well as cultural and quality of life measures.

The ultimate aim of this initiative was to ensure that we are all talking the same "language," which should not only allow for better communication between doctors and with patients, but will also facilitate the design of multi-institutional and multinational clinical trials allow more clear interpretation of the meaning of basic research studies on specific subgroups of patients.

Definitions of normal menstruation

Before defining AUB, the parameters of normal uterine bleeding must be determined, including cycle length, cycle predictability, and the duration and volume of blood flow. The group process determined that both menstrual cycle length and the duration of menstrual flow, below or above the 95th and 5th percentiles respectively, should be classified as abnormal.

Cycle length

The length of a menstrual cycle is determined by the number of days from day 1 of one menstrual period, to day 1 of the next menstrual period.[1] Using these parameters, the range of normal cycle length has been determined to be from 22–35 days in the mid-reproductive years [5]. The length of the cycle also changes with a number of other parameters of the population being evaluated, particularly age. Later in the reproductive years, cycle length tends to become shorter [6, 7].

---

[1] Many women mistakenly measure and report their cycle as the number of days from the end of one period to the beginning of the next, an important point to understand when taking a menstrual history.

Predictability and consistency in cycle length are also considered important normal parameters and, consequently, persistent variability in cycle length for a particular woman can be abnormal even if the interval remains within the 5th and 95th percentile. However, at this time there is no evidence to provide a threshold for determining an unacceptable level of variability.

Duration of menstrual flow

In the United Kingdom, a guideline for the management of heavy menstrual bleeding (HMB) was launched in 2007 by the National Institute for Health and Clinical Excellence (NICE) [8]. The guideline provides a definition of HMB that takes into account the evidence available on normal menstrual patterns including length of cycle and duration of bleeding. Using the typical duration in the reported four observational studies, [6, 9–11], it was determined that the range of normal duration should be from three to eight days. While duration can be considered a surrogate for menstrual volume, it is clear that periods of the same duration may be associated with substantial differences in menstrual volume. Some clinicians attempt to define menstrual volume by the patient's perception of volume, often including the number of tampons or pads used in a given period; unfortunately, there is a great degree of variation in what an individual considers to be a soaked menstrual item, making this a somewhat unreliable model [12, 13].

Describing normal and abnormal uterine bleeding

The recently published international meeting on terminologies for the symptoms and signs of spontaneous AUB has been described above. There was agreement that AUB is not a diagnosis but, instead, should be considered a symptom and in some instances a sign; and women with this sign should be regarded as a subset of the group of clinical problems encompassed by "abnormal reproductive tract bleeding," recognizing that such bleeding may sometimes come from other parts of the reproductive tract.

As a result of the definitions of "normal menstruation" described above, it is possible to describe a methodology for describing abnormal menstruation, at least based on history. The participants in the agreement process[2] strongly agreed that it was important to describe uterine bleeding in the reproductive years using a limited set of four dimensions, and only three choices of descriptive words for each dimension that depict "normal," "above normal," and "below normal" as previously defined (Table 4.1). Consequently, for a given individual, each of the four key menstrual dimensions should be described using one of the following terms: cycle regularity, frequency of menstruation, duration, and volume of menstrual flow:

1. *Regularity of menstruation:* irregular, regular, or absent.
2. *Frequency of menstruation:* frequent, normal, or infrequent.
3. *Duration of menstrual flow:* prolonged, normal, or shortened.
4. *Volume of menstrual flow:* heavy, normal, or light.

Any additional abnormality should be specified, such as intermenstrual bleeding and premenstrual spotting.

The term "heavy menstrual bleeding" appears to have been introduced to the medical literature by the New Zealand Guideline Group in 1999 [14] and, as described above, has

Table 4.1 Nomenclature for normal menstruation. Menstruation is described using the four categories of regularity, frequency, duration, and volume. The first three are quantified by days based on the 5th and 95th centiles. Volume is subjectively categorized by the patient as being normal, light, or heavy [2]. Those with one or a combination of prolonged and heavy bleeding may be said to have heavy menstrual bleeding.

		Abnormal uterine bleeding	
Feature	Normal	Abnormality 1	Abnormality 2
Regularity	Regular ± 2 20 days	Irregular Variation > 20 days	Absent
Frequency	Normal q 24–38 days	Frequent < 24	Infrequent > 38
Duration	Normal 4.5–8 days	Prolonged > 8	Shortened < 4.5
Volume	Normal	Heavy	Light

been adopted by the UK-based NICE guidelines [8]. Unfortunately a consensus definition of HMB has yet to be determined, in part related to the clinical impracticality of using direct measurements of menstrual loss. Consequently, and at present, the clinical definition must be achieved somewhat empirically by the health care provider, interpreting the patient's perspective of bleeding volume and its impact on her life. Nevertheless it is my opinion that it is useful to have a term that identifies women who are experiencing AUB of sufficient monthly volume to deplete iron stores without some medical or surgical intervention, even if it is only simple iron therapy and even if anemia has not yet occurred. As a result, in this book, I will use the term "HMB" to refer to the subset of women with chronic AUB (for three months or more) that in the opinion of the clinician are determined to have chronically prolonged duration and/or heavy volume or both, regardless of the frequency or regularity which will be separately classified as described below.

Intermenstrual bleeding

Uterine bleeding that occurs between cyclically normal menstrual periods will be called intermenstrual bleeding (IMB). Typically the term "metrorrhagia" has been used but the international process described above determined that metrorrhagia has an inconsistent definition and should be discarded. Intermenstrual bleeding may be related to contact, or if spontaneous, may be cyclical or occur at random times between periods.

Breakthrough bleeding

Breakthrough bleeding is unscheduled uterine bleeding that occurs in association with the use of gonadal steroids or other agents designed to suppress endocrine regulation of endometrial function. This is not to be confused with the withdrawal bleeding experienced, for example, with cyclically administered estrogen and progestin-containing oral contraceptives, or the use of cyclical progestins in the context of postmenopausal estrogen replacement. On the other hand, continuous exposure to progestins or to estrogen-progestin combinations tends to produce the least predictable patterns varying from complete amenorrhoea, through infrequent, light bleeding to frequent or prolonged episodes, although heavy bleeding tends to be unusual. Chapter 11 is dedicated to the pathogenesis, evaluation, and management of breakthrough bleeding.

Classification of causes of abnormal uterine bleeding

A universally accepted system of nomenclature and classification seems a necessary step for medical education, the evolution of collaborative research for the, and for optimal evidence-based application of results to clinical practice. The system presented here has not been previously published, but is based upon the preliminary discussions of the menstrual disorders group described above [2]. However, unlike the nomenclature criteria, the classification system has not been ratified by this group.

Acute and chronic abnormal uterine bleeding

It is recognized that the available literature has not formally distinguished between acute and chronic AUB in nonpregnant women. It is recommended that chronic AUB be defined as bleeding from the uterine corpus that is abnormal in volume, regularity, and/or timing, and which has been present for at least three months. Chronic AUB does not require urgent or emergent intervention. Acute AUB, on the other hand, is AUB that, in the opinion of the clinician, is an episode of sufficient volume to require urgent or emergent intervention. Acute AUB may present with or without a history of chronic AUB. Women in the reproductive years with acute AUB require unique interventions, but their followup care may largely be dependent upon whether or not they require investigation and ongoing care for underlying chronic AUB.

Classification of causes of abnormal uterine bleeding

Included in a classification system is the need for a standardized approach to nomenclature of causes of AUB in the reproductive years that includes room for both known and generally accepted entities, as well as those that are less well clarified.

The classification system is shown in Figure 4.1. It has been entitled the "PALM-COEIN" system, an acronym that can be pronounced "Palm-Coin" with each letter unique and representing one of the classification groups. Generally speaking, the PALM group represents entities that are currently clearly definable by gross and/or histopathological anatomic evaluation. On the other hand, the COEIN group includes those entities that are not definable as histopathological entities, so that they may occur in a structurally normal uterus. The one exception to this is the "Not classified" category that includes rare or ill-defined entities such as arteriovenous malformations or endometritis. The leiomyoma category is subdivided into "S" or "O" depending upon the presence of at least one submucosal leiomyoma, when the subclassification of "S" is applied, or "O" should all the myomas be either intramural or subserosal. A more detailed subclassification of leiomyomas is also included, but probably has its greatest value as a research tool.

The intention is that the identified cause(s) of the bleeding are identified by placing the appropriate letter following the designation "AUB," "IMB," or "HMB," with HMB taking precedence if the bleeding is consistently heavy or prolonged. For example, if a woman is determined to have an endometrial polyp that manifested with intermenstrual light bleeding, she would be designated as IMB-P. If, in addition, she was shown to have adenomyosis, the designation would be IMB-P,A, with additional causes added should they be identified. A woman with cyclical HMB thought to be of endometrial origin would be labeled HMB-E. For purposes of classification, the clinician is not asked to determine which, if any, of these definable entities is responsible for the bleeding, just to document their presence. Further discussion of these causes will be found in Chapter 5.

Polyp		Coagulopathy
Adenomyosis		Ovulatory dysfunction
Leiomyoma	Submucosal	Endometrial
	Other	Iatrogenic
Malignancy & hyperplasia		Not classified

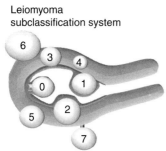

Leiomyoma subclassification system	S - Submucosal	0	Pedunculated intracavitary
		1	>50% intracavitary
		2	≤50% intracavitary
	O - Other	3	Contacts endometrium; 0% intracavitary
		4	Intramural
		5	Subserosal ≥50% intramural
		6	Subserosal <50% intramural
		7	Subserosal pedunculated
		8	Other

Figure 4.1 The PALM-COEIN classification system for causes of abnormal uterine bleeding (AUB). In the primary system, leiomyomas are classified as being either submucosal or "other," reflecting current perceptions of those that are likely (S) or unlikely (O) to contribute to AUB. The exact type of myoma can be categorized from the leiomyoma subclassification system. Understanding that more than one potential mechanism may be present following investigation of a given patient, each applicable letter is placed after the letters AUB, IMB, or HMB as appropriate.

References

1. Fraser IS, Inceboz US. *Defining disturbances of the menstrual cycle.* In O'Brien PMS, Cameron IT, MacLean AB, eds. *Disorders of the Menstrual Cycle.* London: RCOG Press; 2000.
2. Fraser IS, Critchley HO, Munro MG, Broder M. A process designed to lead to international agreement on terminologies and definitions used to describe abnormalities of menstrual bleeding. *Fertil Steril.* 2007;87(3):466–76.
3. Woolcock JG, Critchley HO, Munro MG, Broder MS, Fraser IS. Review of the confusion in current and historical terminology and definitions for disturbances of menstrual bleeding. *Fertil Steril.* 2008;90(6):2269–80.
4. Fraser IS, Critchley HO, Munro MG, Broder M. Can we achieve international agreement on terminologies and definitions used to describe abnormalities of menstrual bleeding? *Hum Reprod.* 2007; 22(3):635–43.
5. Snowden R, Christian B. *Patterns and Perceptions of Menstruation, a World Health Organization International Collaborative Study.* London: Croom Helm; 1983.
6. Treloar AE, Boynton RE, Behn BG, Brown BW. Variation of the human menstrual cycle through reproductive life. *Int J Fertil.* 1967;12(1 Pt 2):77–126.
7. Brodin T, Bergh T, Berglund L, Hadziosmanovic N, Holte J. Menstrual cycle length is an age-independent marker of female fertility: results from 6271 treatment cycles of in vitro fertilization. *Fertil Steril.* 2008;90(5):1656–61.
8. National Clinical Guidelines 44. *Heavy Menstrual Bleeding.* United Kingdom: National Institute for Health and Clinical Excellence; 2007.

9. Matsumoto S, Nogami Y, Onhkuri S. Statistical studies on menstruation; a criticism on the definition of normal menstruation. *Gunma J Med Sci.* 1962;**11**:294–318.

10. Campbell H, Edstrom K, Engstrom L. World Health Organization multicenter study on menstrual and ovulatory patterns in adolescent girls. II. Longitudinal study of menstrual patterns in the early postmenarcheal period, duration of bleeding episodes and menstrual cycles. *J Adolesc Health Care.* 1986;**11**(4):236–318.

11. Harlow SD, Campbell BC. Host factors that influence the duration of menstrual bleeding. *Epidemiology.* 1994;**5**(3):352–5.

12. Fraser IS, McCarron G, Markham R. A preliminary study of factors influencing perception of menstrual blood loss volume. *Am J Obstet Gynecol.* 1984;**149**(7):788–93.

13. Higham JM, Shaw RW. Clinical associations with objective menstrual blood volume. *Eur J Obstet Gynecol Reprod Biol.* 1999;**82**(1):73–6.

14. Working Party for Guidelines for the Management of Heavy Menstrual Bleeding. An evidence-based guideline for the management of heavy menstrual bleeding. *N Z Med J.* 1999;**112**(1088):174–7.

5 Pathogenesis of abnormal uterine bleeding

Chapter summary

- Nongestational acute or chronic AUB may be caused or contributed to by deficiencies in systemic hemostasis, by abnormalities in endometrial hemostasis, by disturbances of ovulation, by structural pathology, or by the use of drugs or devices that may impact the endometrium.
- Systemic disorders of hemostasis, most commonly von Willebrand disease, may be identified in about 13% of women with HMB.
- Structural pathology, including polyps, leiomyomas, and endometriosis may be the cause of AUB in a given patient, but they may, as well, be asymptomatic, with the actual cause of bleeding related to deficiencies in local hemostasis, ovulatory disturbances, or systemic disorders of hemostasis.

Introduction

In Chapter 3 the normal parameters of physiological uterine bleeding were described and in Chapter 4 both a nomenclature for describing AUB and a classification of causes was presented. This chapter is designed to familiarize the reader with the mechanisms that result in AUB – its pathogenesis – presented in the context of the classification system. This chapter will deal with AUB pathogenesis in the reproductive years. The pathogenesis (and management) of acute, premenarcheal, and postmenopausal bleeding are discussed in Chapters 10, 12, and 13 respectively.

In Chapter 4, the causes of chronic AUB were categorized according to the following "PALM-COEIN" system (Figure 4.1). An important consideration is that the individual may have more than one of the identified mechanisms contributing to the bleeding. For example, an individual with a submucosal myoma (L-s) may also be found to have ovulatory dysfunction (O). Alternatively an endometrial polyp (P) may coexist with asymptomatic adenomyosis (A). In Chapters 6 and 7, integration of these findings into a workable therapeutic strategy will be discussed.

Polyps (AUB-P)

Polyps are generally considered to be a localized tumor of the columnar epithelium of the endocervix or endometrial epithelium itself, each of which typically contain both glandular and stromal elements (Figure 5.1). Morphologically, they may be stratified into pedunculated lesions attached to the endothelium by a stalk and sessile lesions where a stalk is not present. The lesions may range from a few millimeters to several centimeters in maximal length and may vary from clearly three-dimensional lesions to those with a flattened morphology. These

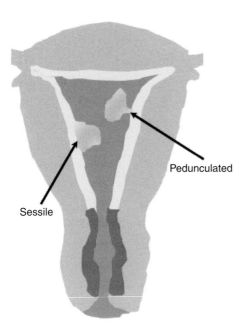

Figure 5.1 Endometrial polyps. Endometrial polyps may be tethered by a narrow stalk (pedunculated) or attached to the endometrium by a broad base (sessile). Their size varies from millimeters to several centimeters in diameter.

Pedunculated

Sessile

polyps are common and appear to be frequently asymptomatic, but have origins that are very poorly understood [1]. While the exact cause of endometrial polyps is unknown, one theory postulates that a limited portion of endometrium fails to be shed at menstruation and that this tissue continues to proliferate each month. Another, more tenable hypothesis, is localized abnormal proliferation of a group of cells in the basal layer of endometrium. Endometrial polyps usually have a single arterial blood supply that can often be clearly demonstrated on ultrasound scan using color Doppler flow techniques.

Symptomatic endometrial polyps may be associated with a history of increased volume of bleeding, but are more commonly thought to cause random, unpredictable intermenstrual spotting or bleeding (IMB-P). Observation of polyps suggests that some undergo patchy surface necrosis, while others can be seen to have prominent thin-walled surface vessels, which may be extremely fragile and therefore prone to result in spontaneous and erratic light bleeding. Women who experience random intermenstrual bleeding who are found to have endometrial polyps, improve following polypectomy. Images and videos of polyps and polypectomy can be found in Chapter 21.

Adenomyosis (AUB-A)

Adenomyosis has traditionally been defined as the existence of endometrial glands and stroma within the myometrium (Figure 5.2, [2]). The disorder may be diffuse, or, in some instances, may manifest with localized proliferations of adenomyotic tissue – so called *adenomyomas*. In most instances there is coexistent myometrial hypertrophy and hyperplasia. This condition has been associated with one or a combination of HMB (HMB-A), dysmenorrhea, and other pelvic pain; however, it is commonly found in women undergoing hysterectomy who have had no symptoms whatsoever [3].

Evaluation of the relationship between adenomyosis and AUB is confounded by its frequent coexistence with other causes of abnormal bleeding such as polyps and

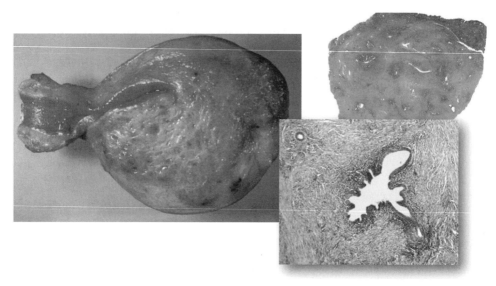

Figure 5.2 Adenomyosis. The typically thickened posterior myometrium is depicted in the sagittal section on the left. Low and high power micrographs demonstrate endometrial glands and stroma deeply in the myometrium. (From Bergeron et al. [2].)

leiomyomas that may or may not be symptomatic and which may or may not contribute to abnormal bleeding. Similar difficulty has been encountered when trying to link adenomyosis to pelvic pain.

Historically, critical evaluation of the relationship of adenomyosis to symptoms has been impeded by the absence of a method for diagnosis short of hysterectomy. However, even when the uterus is removed and examined, there is inconsistency regarding the histopathological definition of adenomyosis, particularly with respect to the threshold of "invasion" into the myometrium. Most suggest that adenomyosis exists when there is endometrium present half a low-power field (at least 2.5 mm) beneath the endomyometrial junction. However, others use one "low-power" field (at least 4 mm), some two such fields (at least 8 mm), and a few require that at least one third of the myometrial thickness to be involved [4]. These differences result not only in a substantial variation in the prevalence of the disorder, but also reflect the relative lack of knowledge regarding the relationship of these findings to symptoms.

Not surprisingly, the pathogenesis of adenomyosis is also unclear. Magnetic resonance imaging has demonstrated that disruption of the endometrial–myometrial interface and disorganization of the uterine junctional zone may play an integral role, but the mechanism is unknown. For reasons that are unclear, the posterior myometrial wall is more often involved than the anterior wall.

Biologically, adenomyosis appears to be an estrogen-dependent entity [5], as there is abundant expression of the α estrogen receptor. Additionally, adenomyotic tissue has been shown to contain progesterone receptors, as well as the capacity to synthesize its own aromatase and sulphatase enzymes. This combination of functions almost certainly contributes to the growth and function of the abnormal tissue.

There have been attempts to measure adenomyosis "disease burden" using grading systems based on depth of myometrial penetration and/or to the numbers of endometrial islets identified on histopathological examination. Using the ≥ 2.5 mm definition, 25% of over 1334 patients undergoing hysterectomy were found to have adenomyosis, and its presence in women with endometrial cancer, pelvic prolapse, and cervical cancer were similar to that for women with HMB [6]. Other investigators have also found that while the prevalence of adenomyosis is high, it seems equally high in the uteri of women with HMB and dysmenorrhea as it is when such symptoms are not present.

As a result of the above, it is unclear if the relationship between adenomyosis and HMB is one of cause and effect, or of coincidence. If the relationship is causal, there exists an hypothesis that disruption of the normal cycle-dependent contraction waves of the junctional zone has been linked to dysmenorrhea and HMB. Radiological images of adenomyosis can be found in Chapter 23 (Figures 23.10 and 23.16).

Leiomyomas (AUB-L)

Uterine leiomyomas are exceedingly common neoplasms that by the age of 50 can be found in almost 70% of Caucasian and more than 80% of women of African ancestry [7]. Clearly, not all – or even most – of these women suffer from AUB, leading to the conclusion that the vast majority of leiomyomas are asymptomatic, an observation that likely reflects features of the myomas, particularly their location with respect to the endometrium (Figure 5.3). Furthermore, it is also clear that when AUB exists in association with leiomyomas, the relationship may not be one of cause and effect. So which leiomyomas do cause AUB and what are the mechanisms involved?

Relationship to abnormal uterine bleeding

The mechanisms involved in leiomyoma-associated AUB are yet to be determined, so there is ample room for speculation based upon what is known. First, it should be understood

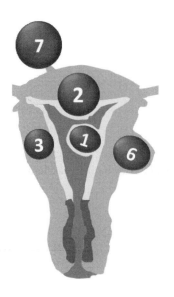

Figure 5.3 Leiomyomas by type. Those myomas that undermine the endometrium and distort the endometrial cavity are thought to contribute to heavy menstrual bleeding while those that do not contact the endometrium likely do not cause abnormal uterine bleeding.

that leiomyomas themselves are typically and strikingly solid and relatively avascular, so bleeding from the myoma itself is rare. On the other hand, the myoma may be surrounded by a relatively rich vasculature. When hysteroscopy demonstrates submucosal leiomyomas in women with HMB (HMB-Ls), in most instances the tumors are covered by endometrium, while in the others, endometrium seems thin or even absent, with a variable amount of perimyoma vasculature overlying the tumor [8].

The search for biochemical mechanisms of leiomyoma-associated uterine bleeding has demonstrated a number of differences between leiomyoma cells and normal myometrium. Myoma smooth muscle cells release angiogenic and growth factors, such as VEGF, basic fibroblast growth factor (BFGF) and TGF-β as well as plasminogen activators and inhibitors [9]. Leiomyoma MMP-2 and MMP-11 activity have been demonstrated to be increased, but MMP-1 and MMP-3 remain unchanged. Unfortunately, the relationship of these findings to myoma-related AUB remains unclear [10, 11].

The overwhelming clinical impression is that those myomas that cause bleeding are submucosal. The site of bleeding is usually the adjacent and/or overlying endometrium, or less commonly, the blood vessels that surround the myoma. This observation makes careful evaluation of the endometrial cavity important in determining the cause of AUB in a given woman. Clinically obvious myomas may have nothing to do with the bleeding; while submucosal tumors not detectable on manual examination may be the responsible pathologic entity (Figure 5.4).

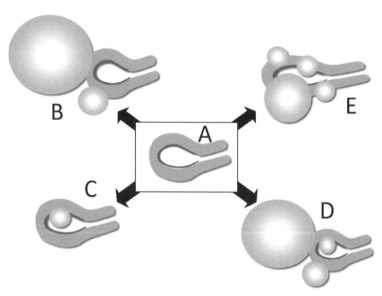

Figure 5.4 Leiomyomas and abnormal uterine bleeding. Given the prevalence of leiomyomas, it is important for the clinician to perform and interpret the investigation properly. The cause of heavy menstrual bleeding (HMB) in uterus "A" is clearly not related to leiomyomas, but the same could be said of uterus "B," which contains large fibroids but has a normal endometrial cavity. The type 1 myoma in uterus "C" is a likely cause of HMB and, despite the two large subserosal myomas, removing the type 1 myoma in uterus "D" would likely also treat the bleeding symptoms successfully. The patient with uterus "E" likely has bleeding symptoms related to the two myomas that distort the endometrium.

Leiomyoma growth and development

Understanding medical therapy of leiomyomas requires some understanding of the myriad genetic factors and growth and steroid hormones that potentially influence leiomyoma development and growth.

Unfortunately, estrogens have been perceived by many clinicians as the key stimulators to myoma growth, largely perhaps, because of the recognition that leiomyoma volume decreases following menopause, an event that is largely considered to be simply hypoestrogenic but which is also a time when other gonadal steroid hormones are relatively absent, most importantly progesterone.

Indeed, progesterone receptor concentrations in leiomyomas are much higher than in normal myometrium. Interestingly, progesterone has been demonstrated to upregulate factors associated with leiomyoma growth including Bcl-2 protein, proliferating cell nuclear antigen and epidermal growth factor [12, 13]. There is evidence that progestins may result in growth of leiomyoma and that antiprogestational agents have the opposite effect [14].

Patients treated with GnRH agonist enter a temporary "medical" menopause, frequently requiring that estrogen and/or progestin "add-back" therapy be provided to treat vasomotor symptoms, vaginal atrophy, and to protect against osteopenia. Women so treated have been subjected to randomized trials comparing progestin only add-back to estrogen-progestin regimens. In most instances, myoma growth has been demonstrated only in association with progestin use and not seen with estrogen-progestin therapy [15] (Class I-2). Another clue to the influence of progestins on myoma growth is that antiprogestational therapy has been demonstrated to reduce myoma volume in conjunction with reductions in progesterone receptor levels [14, 16, 17] (Class I-2). All of these findings suggest that progestins play a significant if not a dominant role in the growth of leiomyomas and that estrogens are important but are themselves unlikely to directly cause the growth of leiomyomas.

Malignancy and hyperplasia (AUB-M)

Whereas it is obvious that premalignant and malignant lesions in the uterus are important causes of AUB at any age (AUB-M), this text is not designed as a guide for the treatment of these conditions. However it is important to understand basic concepts about the spectrum of hyperplastic and malignant disease that can be encountered.

Clearly the most relevant premalignant condition that is associated with AUB in the developed world is endometrial hyperplasia, which actually comprises a spectrum of histopathologically-defined entities that range from the very benign simple hyperplasia, without cytological atypia, to atypical endometrial hyperplasia, a known precursor to endometrial adenocarcinoma that often coexists with endometrial malignancy [18, 19] (Table 5.1 [20]). The majority of women with endometrial hyperplasia have a coexisting state of unopposed estrogen, which, in the reproductive years, is the result of prolonged anovulation.

A result of the frequency of prolonged anovulation is the fact that endometrial adenocarcinoma is the most commonly-encountered uterine malignancy in the developed world [21]. A minority of women with endometrial carcinoma do not have pre- or coexisting endometrial hyperplasia and instead have one of a spectrum of entities ranging from adenocarcinoma within an endometrial polyp (Video 23.12), to papillary serous

Table 5.1 AUB-M. World Health Organization classification of endometrial hyperplasia and the risk of progression to adenocarcinoma.

Classification	Histopathology	Approximate risk of progression to endometrial carcinoma
Nonatypical hyperplasias	Simple hyperplasia without atypia	1%
	Complex atypical hyperplasia	2–3%
Atypical hyperplasias	Simple atypical hyperplasia	8–10%
	Complex atypical hyperplasia	29–52%

From Horn et al. [20]

Table 5.2 AUB-M. Endometrial carcinoma. The most common type is the "endometrioid carcinoma," which is largely related to unopposed estrogen, but type 2 carcinomas as well as the other rarely encountered carcinomas and sarcomas appear to be unrelated to hormonal etiology.

Type I	Endometrioid adenocarcinoma
Type II	Endometrial intraepithelial carcinoma (EIC)
	Endometrioid carcinoma (high grade)
	Papillary serous
	Clear cell
Rare	Squamous cell
	Transitional cell
	Sertoliform
	Neuroendocrine
Sarcomas	Endometrial stromal sarcoma (ESS)
Mixed tumors	Carcinosarcoma

endometrial carcinoma, a much more aggressive malignancy than "simple" adenocarcinoma [19] (Table 5.2). There seems to be clear evidence that women from families with hereditary nonpolyposis colorectal cancer syndrome (HNPCCS) have a lifetime risk of developing endometrial cancer that may be 60% with a mean age between 48 and 50 [22, 23].

Endometrial sarcomas are relatively rare malignancies that may exist either on their own, or in combination with endometrial adenocarcinoma, a group of entities that are termed malignant mixed Müllerian tumors reflecting the different cellular progenitors of each malignant cell line. In the endometrium, such malignancies are often called *adenosarcomas*.

Sarcomas of myometrial origin may also manifest and, not infrequently, present with AUB. Perhaps the most common of these sarcomas is the *leiomyosarcoma*, an entity which morphologically looks like a leiomyoma. There exists controversy regarding the genesis of these sarcomas, with some perceiving that they arise de novo while others supporting the notion that they develop from leiomyomas. Regardless, the fraction of lesions that on palpation or imaging appear to be leiomyomas but are actually malignant is exceptionally small – much less than 1/1000 based on evidence from a number of clinical studies [24, 25]. It should be remembered that these frequencies are from myomas removed, as the denominator does not include the vast number of myomas in the population that are not surgically extracted.

Coagulopathy (AUB-C)

Disorders of systemic hemostasis, often called coagulopathies, can interfere with control of menstrual bleeding typically manifesting in HMB (HMB-C). These disorders may be inherited, acquired, or iatrogenic, and manifest by their impact on the coagulation "cascade" (Figure 5.5). In particular, the inherited versions seem to be far more common than generally recognized as the most commonly encountered such disorder, von Willebrand disease (vWD), was found in 13% of women with "menorrhagia" in a metaanalysis of large studies of women from a number of countries and a spectrum of cultures [26].

There exist three recognized variants of vWD with the majority (60–80%) a form (type 1) that is mild and commonly overlooked because it can only be diagnosed with certainty using specific testing for von Willebrand factor (vWF) levels [27, 28]. The type 2 variant is actually a quantitative deficiency that may solely manifest with bruising or HMB without impaired

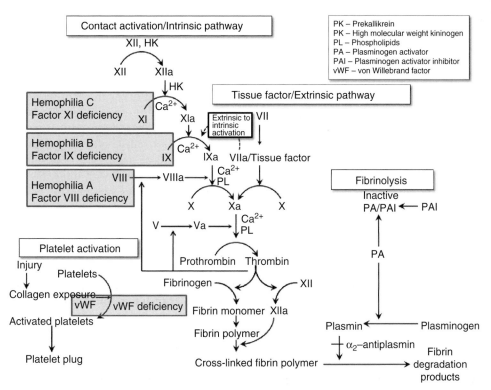

Figure 5.5 Systemic disorders of hemostasis. The location of the most common inherited defects in systemic hemostasis is shown in the shaded boxes. Abnormalities in von Willebrand factor can be found in 13% of women with heavy menstrual bleeding.

clotting. Affected individuals typically are identified to have vWF levels that are 10–45% of normal. The most severe form is type 3 where the paucity of available vWF generally manifests with serious bleeding from even mild injury. Individuals affected with type 3 vWD generally present in childhood or at the time of menarche when menstruation is found to be excessively heavy. These variants in vWD probably reflect abnormalities in related but different genes.

It is not absolutely clear to what degree these relatively commonly encountered (but less often diagnosed) disorders of hemostasis actually contribute to the genesis of AUB/HMB in a given woman, but it is likely that a substantial subset are actually subclinical. This underscores the need to perform a complete evaluation even if a previously unsuspected coagulopathy is detected on laboratory examination.

Although platelets play a lesser role in physiological endometrial hemostasis than in other body tissues, HMB may also be associated with severe thrombocytopenia and thrombocytopathies such as Glanzmann disease. Other factor deficiencies, while rare, include factors II, V, VII, VIII, IX, X, XI, and XII [29]. These disorders may be more commonly encountered in specific ethnic groups where intermarriage is associated with a higher risk of these abnormalities.

Finally, AUB/HMB or HMB-C can be caused by iatrogenic means secondary to the use of anticoagulants in women with recent thromboembolic disease or who are at enhanced risk for such a disorder based upon a spectrum of clinical conditions. In these circumstances, the mechanisms involved with AUB/HMB are obvious. Because this is clearly an iatrogenic cause of the bleeding, I have actually categorized this mechanism under AUB-I (below).

Ovulatory dysfunction (AUB-O)

Failure of consistent and predictable ovulation results in absent or inconsistent release of progesterone from the ovary (Figure 5.6). Such ovulatory disturbances are the result of systemic endocrinological disorders that range from complete absence of ovulation to frequent or isolated instances of anovulation (sometimes called "oligoanovulation") in the context of otherwise normal function. The absence of progesterone of corpus luteal origin may result in amenorrhea, but is frequently associated with unpredictable bleeding, a circumstance that can negatively affect the woman's lifestyle due to the constant concern about unexpected bleeding. Women with isolated or chronic anovulation may only experience abnormalities in the timing of uterine bleeding (AUB-O), but, in some instances, the volume of bleeding may be profuse (HMB-O), likely because of the dependence of local endometrial hemostatic mechanisms on progesterone (Chapter 3).

Knowing the deficiencies in endometrial hemostatic mechanisms associated with anovulation helps one understand why there is difficulty in controlling bleeding once it starts. But why then does the endometrium bleed at all when there is no progesterone withdrawal to trigger the process of menstruation? It is surmised that there are a number of endometrial events that occur secondary to relatively prolonged exposure to unopposed estrogen and that may be related to the onset of AUB. These include changes in uterine vascular tone [30], increased local levels of VEGF with resulting disturbance of angiogenesis [31], disordered prostaglandin synthesis [32], and increased nitric oxide production [33].

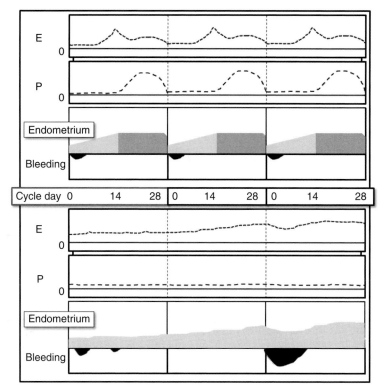

Figure 5.6 AUB/HMB-O. The endometrial profile in the top panel depicts the normal response of the endometrium to three months of cyclic ovulation with predictable production of estradiol (E) and progesterone (P). The profile in the bottom panel reflects the lack of influence of progesterone and the random episodes of bleeding, possibly related in part to transient reduction in the levels of circulating estrogens. Bleeding may be minimal but heavy bleeding may occur, in part because of the lack of progesterone-dependent production of endometrial prostaglandin (PG) $F_{2\alpha}$ and endothelin-1.

The etiology of ovulatory disturbances in any given woman varies extensively. Perhaps the majority are related to one or a combination of stress, rapid weight gain or loss, and obesity. Extreme weight loss or anorexia nervosa is also related to failure of ovulation but usually results in amenorrhea. Around menarche, the relative immaturity of the hypothalamic-pituitary-ovarian axis frequently results in a transient oligoanovulatory environment that typically lasts for six months [34].

Less frequently, the clinician will encounter one of a number of definable entities that are known or suspected to impact the normal function of the hypothalamic-pituitary-ovarian axis [35]. Polycystic ovarian syndrome is perhaps the most commonly encountered such entity that frequently results in AUB-O. Untreated hypothyroidism causes anovulation which typically manifests as amenorrhea, but may occasionally, and especially in older women, be associated with heavy, prolonged, and unpredictable bleeding [33]. Hyperprolactinemia also commonly causes anovulation, but this virtually always results in amenorrhea.

Finally, long-term chronic anovulation creates an endocrinologic endometrial milieu of chronic unopposed estrogen, known to facilitate the development of endometrial hyperplasia and endometrial carcinoma [36, 37].

Iatrogenic (AUB-I)

There are a number of mechanisms by which medical interventions or devices can cause or contribute to AUB (AUB-I). These include medicated or inert intrauterine systems and pharmacologic agents that directly impact the endometrium or interfere with blood coagulation mechanisms or the systemic control of ovulation. Detailed discussion of AUB associated with gonadal steroid use, also called "breakthrough bleeding" is the subject of Chapter 11.

Anticoagulants

Heavy menstrual bleeding is a relatively common consequence experienced by women on anticoagulant drugs such as heparin, low molecular weight heparin, and warfarin. The mechanism appears to be straightforward by prevention of the formation of an adequate "plug" or clot within the vascular lumen.

Drugs impacting ovulation

There are a number of pharmacological agents that are known to impact ovulatory function. Tricyclic antidepressants (e.g., amitriptyline, nortriptyline) and phenothiazines are two of a group of drug types that impact dopamine metabolism by reducing serotonin uptake. It is thought that the resulting reduced inhibition of prolactin release causes prolactin-related disruption in the hypothalamic-pituitary-ovarian axis and consequent disorders of ovulation, including anovulation. Consequently, any agent that impacts serotonin uptake is a candidate for causing ovulatory dysfunction and resulting amenorrhea or irregular uterine bleeding.

Systemically administered agents directly impacting the endometrium

Gonadal steroids, including estrogens, progestins, and androgens, either alone or in combination, have direct effects on the endometrium, in addition to their effect on ovulation. These agents frequently are associated with AUB, for a number of reasons including poor compliance, impaired absorption of the agent, ovarian estradiol production, and direct impacts on the endometrium. These mechanisms are described in more detail in Chapter 11.

Intrauterine systems

Medical devices which are placed in the uterus for a therapeutic purpose are often called intrauterine systems (IUS) or, in the United States and Canada, intrauterine devices (IUDs). There are two basic designs – "inert" devices that have no pharmacologically active substance, and "medicated" systems that are designed to continuously release a therapeutic agent. Currently available devices were designed for female contraception, which they achieve largely by impairing sperm transport. However, the local endometrial effects of these agents can contribute to the genesis of AUB.

Copper-wrapped devices are by far the most commonly used inert IUDs, and have been associated with one or a combination of HMB and intermenstrual bleeding, the latter more often in the first few weeks to months following insertion [38]. A local endometrial inflammatory (not infectious) process has been well described and there is evidence that this bleeding is associated with changes in the levels of local endometrial inflammatory cells and levels of prostaglandins [39, 40].

The *levonorgestrel-releasing intrauterine system* (LNG-IUS) secretes relatively high levels of the progestin levonorgestrel into the endometrial environment and relatively little into the systemic circulation. It is evident that there results a complex set of changes in local endometrial morphology, histopathology, and pharmacology that collectively can have a profound impact on uterine bleeding [41] (Figure 11.1). Typically, in women who are apparently ovulatory, there is a dramatic reduction in the volume of menstrual flow and, almost as often, the onset of intermenstrual spotting, a process that, in the majority of instances, resolves spontaneously after about six months [42].

Endometrial causes (AUB-E)

In a nonpregnant woman during her reproductive years, spontaneous AUB may occur within an ovulatory cycle (consistent cycle of 22–35 days) in the context of normal systemic hemostasis and a normal endometrial cavity (no structural abnormalities). In such circumstances, the cause of the abnormal bleeding is likely a disorder localized to the endometrium itself (Figure 5.7). There exists extensive evidence demonstrating a range of local disturbances of endometrial molecular mechanisms in women with HMB-E [43, 44].

In most instances, the manifestation is localized to the menses and the duration and/or volume of bleeding is increased, but in other instances, intermenstrual bleeding may be noted. HMB-E, previously termed "ovulatory dysfunctional uterine bleeding," appears to occur when there is loss of local control of the mechanisms which normally limit the volume of blood lost during menses and described in Chapter 3.

Impaired vasoconstriction

In Chapter 3 we learned that while endothelin-1 and $PGF_{2\alpha}$ stimulate local vasoconstriction, both PGE_2 and PGI_2 (prostacyclin) cause vasodilation of endometrial vessels with PGI_2 (prostacyclin) also a potent natural inhibitor of platelet aggregation. When the endometrium of women with HMB-E is studied, it is apparent that there tend to be reduced levels of endometrial endothelins and a number of alterations in prostaglandin metabolism and binding [43–45]. One important observation is an increase in local levels of cyclooxygenase, the enzyme that catalyzes the conversion of arachadonic acid to prostaglandin precursors, increased synthesis of PGE_2 compared with $PGF_{2\alpha}$ [46, 47], and increased expression of PGE_2 receptors [48]. There is also a local increase in the synthetic capacity for PGI_2 and the number of PGI_2 receptors [49]. Both individually and collectively, these features contribute to a reduction in the ability of the endometrium to attain effective hemostasis.

Enhanced fibrinolysis

Another component of local hemostasis is the process of clot breakdown – if lysis of the clot occurs too quickly, hemostasis may be impaired, resulting in HMB. Enhanced fibrinolysis, through increased endometrial levels of tissue plasminogen activator, have been demonstrated in women with HMB-E [50–52], who typically revert to reduced or even normal menstrual volumes when antifibrinolytic agents such as tranexamic acid are employed [53].

Impact on other local factors

There are a number of other alterations in endometrial function that may contribute to the genesis of HMB-E. The demonstrated increased synthesis of heparin-like activity may contribute to reduction in local hemostasis [54]. Other abnormalities have been

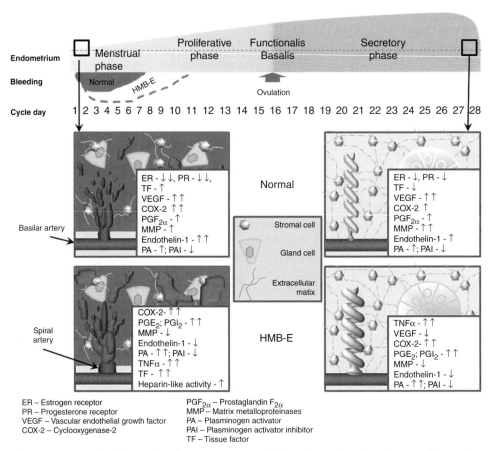

Figure 5.7 HMB-E. This figure is based upon Figure 3.3, with the endometrial profile at the top reflecting the response to the cyclically produced progesterone in the context of estradiol. HMB-E manifests with one or a combination of increased daily volume and prolonged duration of menses. On a molecular level, a number of changes may be seen in the late cycle endometrium of women with HMB-E (right panels). Frequently, levels of prostacyclin (PGI$_2$) and prostaglandin E$_2$ (PGE$_2$) are increased, and there is often an increase in plasminogen activator (PA) and/or a decrease in plasminogen activator inhibitor (PAI). These features favor vasodilation and increase the breakdown of clot. In the panels on the left, these and other changes can be shown to be associated with less efficient hemostasis and therefore increased bleeding duration and volume.

reported in the endometrium or menses of women with HMB-E including increased levels of TNF-α and reductions in the measured levels of VEGF-A and MMP-2 and MMP-9. The clinical significance of these observations is at present unclear, but it is evident that there is a wide and expanding range of endometrial regulatory molecules may be involved in AUB-E [55].

Genetic factors

Recent research has begun to focus on the activation of specific genes which may be associated with AUB/HMB-E. A novel gene called "endometrial bleeding-associated factor" (EBAF, also known as LEFTY-A) is transiently expressed in normal endometrium at menstruation and much more strongly expressed in HMB-E [56]. This gene is located on chromosome 1 and codes for a member of the TGF-β super-family. The concept of multi-gene activation patterns is now being explored as a possible explanation for complex functional disturbances of the type exemplified by HMB-E.

Not classified (AUB-N)

There exist other entities which are either extremely uncommon or less than adequately defined that may contribute to the genesis of AUB.

Arteriovenous malformations

An arteriovenous malformation (AVM) is a localized collection of abnormally connected arteries and veins. These lesions may be either congenital or acquired and, when they occur in the uterus, have been associated with episodes of acute and excessively heavy bleeding. Arteriovenous malformation-related bleeding is sometimes but not always associated with menstruation, and presumably relates to the superficial, thin-walled, and possibly fragile vessels.

In the past, hysterectomy was both the treatment and the mechanism by which a diagnosis was made – demonstrating coils of distended and thin-walled vessels in the myometrium and endometrium. With the advent of uterine imaging techniques, AVMs can be diagnosed in women through use of color Doppler transvaginal ultrasound.

Congenital AVMs are rare. They likely arise from abnormal embryological development of primitive vascular structures resulting in the localized existence of multiple abnormal connections between arteries and veins. Such lesions tend to possess multiple feeding arteries, numerous large draining veins, and a centralized tangle of vessels with characteristics of arteries and veins called a "nidus."

The more commonly encountered traumatic AVM may occur following uterine surgery, including curettage for retained placental tissue. These lesions comprise multiple small arteriovenous fistulae between intramural arteries and myometrial venous plexus and have a simpler construct with one or two feeding arteries and no nidus [57]. Arteriovenous malformations may be visualized using color Doppler scanning (Figure 5.8).

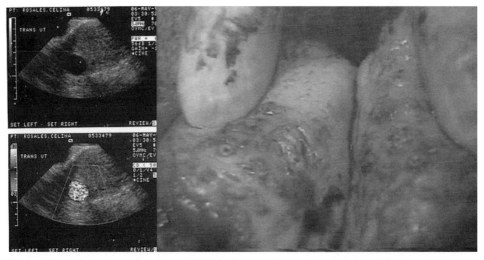

Figure 5.8 Arteriovenous malformation (AUB-N). In the two ultrasound images on the left the arteriovenous malformation is shown without (top) and with (bottom) Doppler color flow. At surgery the uterus is shown opened to the site with the transected localized collection of vessels visible.

Infection

Chronic endometrial infection and/or inflammation has been associated with both inter-menstrual bleeding and prolonged or heavy menses, and there exist some data supporting this relationship [58]. It is generally perceived that when inflammation of the columnar endothelial surfaces of the uterus exists, there is an associated disorder of angiogenesis that can result in abnormal bleeding from the distended thin walled, fragile vessels. Such inflammation tends to occur in the absence of a detectable organism, either in an idiopathic fashion or following instrumentation or pregnancy. Consequently, AUB may represent a manifestation of chronic, subacute, or acute pelvic inflammatory disease, in some instances a medically treatable condition.

References

1. Van Bogaert LJ. Clinicopathologic findings in endometrial polyps. *Obstet Gynecol.* 1988;**71**(5):771–3.
2. Bergeron C, Amant F, Ferenczy A. Best pathology and physiopathology of adenomyosis. *Best Pract Res Clin Obstet Gynaecol.* 2006;**20**:511–21.
3. Peric H, Fraser IS. The symptomatology of adenomyosis. *Best Pract Res Clin Obstet Gynaecol.* 2006;**20**(4):547–55.
4. Gordts S, Brosens JJ, Fusi L, Benagiano G, Brosens I. Uterine adenomyosis: a need for uniform terminology and consensus classification. *Reprod Biomed Online.* 2008;**17**(2):244–8.
5. Kitawaki J. Adenomyosis: the pathophysiology of an oestrogen-dependent disease. *Best Pract Res Clin Obstet Gynaecol.* 2006;**20**(4):493–502.
6. Vercellini P, Parazzini F, Oldani S, Panazza S, Bramante T, Crosignani PG. Adenomyosis at hysterectomy: a study on frequency distribution and patient characteristics. *Hum Reprod.* 1995;**10**(5):1160–2.
7. Day Baird D, Dunson DB, Hill MC, Cousins D, Schectman JM. High cumulative incidence of uterine leiomyoma in black and white women: ultrasound evidence. *Am J Obstet Gynecol.* 2003;**188**(1):100–7.
8. Patterson-Keels LM, Selvaggi SM, Haefner HK, Randolph JF, Jr. Morphologic assessment of endometrium overlying submucosal leiomyomas. *J Reprod Med.* 1994;**39**(8):579–84.
9. Stewart EA, Nowak RA. Leiomyoma-related bleeding: a classic hypothesis updated for the molecular era. *Hum Reprod Update.* 1996;**2**(4):295–306.
10. Palmer SS, Haynes-Johnson D, Diehl T, Nowak RA. Increased expression of stromelysin 3 mRNA in leiomyomas (uterine fibroids) compared with myometrium. *J Soc Gynecol Investig.* 1998;**5**(4):203–9.
11. Bogusiewicz M, Stryjecka-Zimmer M, Postawski K, Jakimiuk AJ, Rechberger T. Activity of matrix metalloproteinase-2 and -9 and contents of their tissue inhibitors in uterine leiomyoma and corresponding myometrium. *Gynecol Endocrinol.* 2007;**23**(9):541–6.
12. Shimomura Y, Matsuo H, Samoto T, Maruo T. Up-regulation by progesterone of proliferating cell nuclear antigen and epidermal growth factor expression in human uterine leiomyoma. *J Clin Endocrinol Metab.* 1998;**83**(6):2192–8.
13. Yin P, Lin Z, Cheng YH, Marsh EE, Utsunomiya H, Ishikawa H, et al. Progesterone receptor regulates Bcl-2 gene expression through direct binding to its promoter region in uterine leiomyoma cells. *J Clin Endocrinol Metab.* 2007;**92**(11):4459–66.
14. Murphy AA, Kettel LM, Morales AJ, Roberts VJ, Yen SS. Regression of uterine leiomyomata in response to the antiprogesterone RU 486. *J Clin Endocrinol Metab.* 1993;**76**(2):513–17.
15. Friedman AJ, Daly M, Juneau-Norcross M, Gleason R, Rein MS, LeBoff M. Long-term medical therapy for leiomyomata uteri: a prospective, randomized study of leuprolide acetate depot plus either oestrogen-progestin or progestin "add-back" for two years. *Hum Reprod.* 1994;**9**(9):1618–25.

16. Steinauer J, Pritts EA, Jackson R, Jacoby AF. Systematic review of mifepristone for the treatment of uterine leiomyomata. *Obstet Gynecol.* 2004;**103**(6):1331–6.

17. Fiscella K, Eisinger SH, Meldrum S, Feng C, Fisher SG, Guzick DS. Effect of mifepristone for symptomatic leiomyomata on quality of life and uterine size: a randomized controlled trial. *Obstet Gynecol.* 2006;**108**(6):1381–7.

18. Silverberg SG, Kurman RJ, Nogales GL, Mutter GL, Kubik-Huch RA, Tavassoli RA. *Tumors of the Uterine Corpus.* Tavassoli FA, Devilee P, editors. Lyon, France: IARC Press; 2003.

19. Trimble CL, Kauderer J, Zaino R, Silverberg S, Lim PC, Burke JJ, 2nd, et al. Concurrent endometrial carcinoma in women with a biopsy diagnosis of atypical endometrial hyperplasia: a Gynecologic Oncology Group study. *Cancer.* 2006; **106**(4):812–19.

20. Horn LC, Meinel A, Handzel R. Histopathology of endometrial hyperplasia and endometrial carcinoma: an update. *Ann Diagn Pathol.* 2007;**11**(4):297–311.

21. Jemal A, Siegel R, Ward E, Hao Y, Xu J, Murray T, et al. Cancer statistics, 2008. *CA Cancer J Clin.* 2008;**58**(2):71–96.

22. Lu KH, Broaddus RR. Gynecological tumors in hereditary nonpolyposis colorectal cancer: we know they are common – now what? *Gynecol Oncol.* 2001;**82**(2):221–2.

23. Lu KH, Dinh M, Kohlmann W, Watson P, Green J, Syngal S, et al. Gynecologic cancer as a "sentinel cancer" for women with hereditary nonpolyposis colorectal cancer syndrome. *Obstet Gynecol.* 2005;**105** (3):569–74.

24. Parker WH, Fu YS, Berek JS. Uterine sarcoma in patients operated on for presumed leiomyoma and rapidly growing leiomyoma. *Obstet Gynecol.* 1994; **83**(3):414–18.

25. Leibsohn S, d'Ablaing G, Mishell DR, Jr., Schlaerth JB. Leiomyosarcoma in a series of hysterectomies performed for presumed uterine leiomyomas. *Am J Obstet Gynecol.* 1990;**162**(4):968–74; discussion 74–6.

26. Shankar M, Lee CA, Sabin CA, Economides DL, Kadir RA. Von Willebrand disease in women with menorrhagia: a systematic review. *BJOG.* 2004;**111**(7):734–40.

27. Kouides PA, Conard J, Peyvandi F, Lukes A, Kadir R. Hemostasis and menstruation: appropriate investigation for underlying disorders of hemostasis in women with excessive menstrual bleeding. *Fertil Steril.* 2005;**84**(5):1345–51.

28. Lukes AS, Kadir RA, Peyvandi F, Kouides PA. Disorders of hemostasis and excessive menstrual bleeding: prevalence and clinical impact. *Fertil Steril.* 2005; **84**(5):1338–44.

29. Peyvandi F, Duga S, Akhavan S, Mannucci PM. Rare coagulation deficiencies. *Haemophilia.* 2002;**8**(3):308–21.

30. Fraser IS, McCarron G, Hutton B, Macey D. Endometrial blood flow measured by xenon 133 clearance in women with normal menstrual cycles and dysfunctional uterine bleeding. *Am J Obstet Gynecol.* 1987; **156**(1):158–66.

31. Smith SK. Angiogenesis, vascular endothelial growth factor and the endometrium. *Hum Reprod Update.* 1998; **4**(5):509–19.

32. Smith SK, Abel MH, Kelly RW, Baird DT. The synthesis of prostaglandins from persistent proliferative endometrium. *J Clin Endocrinol Metab.* 1982;**55**(2):284–9.

33. Krassas GE, Pontikides N, Kaltsas T, Papadopoulou P, Paunkovic J, Paunkovic N, et al. Disturbances of menstruation in hypothyroidism. *Clin Endocrinol (Oxf).* 1999;**50**(5):655–9.

34. Zhang K, Pollack S, Ghods A, Dicken C, Isaac B, Adel G, et al. Onset of ovulation after menarche in girls: a longitudinal study. *J Clin Endocrinol Metab.* 2008;**93** (4):1186–94.

35. Fraser IS, Michie EA, Wide L, Baird DT. Pituitary gonadotropins and ovarian function in adolescent dysfunctional uterine bleeding. *J Clin Endocrinol Metab.* 1973;**37**(3):407–14.

36. Schroder R. Endometrial hyperplasia in relation to genital function. *Am J Obstet Gynecol.* 1954;**68**(1):294–309.

37. Brown JB, Kellar R, Matthew GD. Preliminary observations on urinary oestrogen excretion in certain gynaecological disorders. *J Obstet Gynaecol Br Emp.* 1959;**66**(2):177–211.

38. Mishell DR, Jr. Intrauterine devices: mechanisms of action, safety, and efficacy.

Contraception. 1998;**58**(3 Suppl):45S–53S; quiz 70S.

39. Sheppard BL, Bonnar J. The effects of intrauterine contraceptive devices on the ultrastructure of the endometrium in relation to bleeding complications. *Am J Obstet Gynecol*. 1983;**146**(7):829–39.

40. Sheppard BL. Endometrial morphological changes in IUD users: a review. *Contraception*. 1987;**36**(1):1–10.

41. Guttinger A, Critchley HO. Endometrial effects of intrauterine levonorgestrel. *Contraception*. 2007;**75**(6 Suppl):S93–8.

42. Jensen JT, Nelson AL, Costales AC. Subject and clinician experience with the levonorgestrel-releasing intrauterine system. *Contraception*. 2008;**77**(1):22–9.

43. Livingstone M, Fraser IS. Mechanisms of abnormal uterine bleeding. *Hum Reprod Update*. 2002;**8**(1):60–7.

44. Jabbour HN, Kelly RW, Fraser HM, Critchley HO. Endocrine regulation of menstruation. *Endocr Rev*. 2006; **27**(1):17–46.

45. Salamonsen LA, Marsh MM, Findlay JK. Endometrial endothelin: regulator of uterine bleeding and endometrial repair. *Clin Exp Pharmacol Physiol*. 1999;**26**(2):154–7.

46. Smith SK, Abel MH, Kelly RW, Baird DT. Prostaglandin synthesis in the endometrium of women with ovular dysfunctional uterine bleeding. *Br J Obstet Gynaecol*. 1981;**88**(4):434–42.

47. Makarainen L, Ylikorkala O. Primary and myoma-associated menorrhagia: role of prostaglandins and effects of ibuprofen. *Br J Obstet Gynaecol*. 1986;**93**(9):974–8.

48. Adelantado JM, Rees MC, Lopez Bernal A, Turnbull AC. Increased uterine prostaglandin E receptors in menorrhagic women. *Br J Obstet Gynaecol*. 1988; **95**(2):162–5.

49. Smith SK, Abel MH, Kelly RW, Baird DT. A role for prostacyclin (PGI2) in excessive menstrual bleeding. *Lancet*. 1981;**1**(8219):522–4.

50. Rybo G. Plasminogen activators in the endometrium. II. Clinical aspects. Variation in the concentration of plasminogen activators during the menstrual cycle and its relation to menstrual blood loss. *Acta Obstet Gynecol Scand*. 1966; **45**(4):429–50.

51. Gleeson N, Devitt M, Sheppard BL, Bonnar J. Endometrial fibrinolytic enzymes in women with normal menstruation and dysfunctional uterine bleeding. *Br J Obstet Gynaecol*. 1993;**100**(8):768–71.

52. Gleeson NC. Cyclic changes in endometrial tissue plasminogen activator and plasminogen activator inhibitor type 1 in women with normal menstruation and essential menorrhagia. *Am J Obstet Gynecol*. 1994;**171**(1):178–83.

53. Gleeson NC, Buggy F, Sheppard BL, Bonnar J. The effect of tranexamic acid on measured menstrual loss and endometrial fibrinolytic enzymes in dysfunctional uterine bleeding. *Acta Obstet Gynecol Scand*. 1994;**73**(3):274–7.

54. Foley ME, Griffin BD, Zuzel M, Aparicio SR, Bradbury K, Bird CC, et al. Heparin-like activity in uterine fluid. *Br Med J*. 1978;**2**(6133):322–4.

55. Malik S, Day K, Perrault I, Charnock-Jones DS, Smith SK. Reduced levels of VEGF-A and MMP-2 and MMP-9 activity and increased TNF-alpha in menstrual endometrium and effluent in women with menorrhagia. *Hum Reprod*. 2006; **21**(8):2158–66.

56. Kothapalli R, Buyuksal I, Wu SQ, Chegini N, Tabibzadeh S. Detection of ebaf, a novel human gene of the transforming growth factor beta superfamily association of gene expression with endometrial bleeding. *J Clin Invest*. 1997; **99**(10): 2342–50.

57. O'Brien P, Neyastani A, Buckley AR, Chang SD, Legiehn GM. Uterine arteriovenous malformations: from diagnosis to treatment. *J Ultrasound Med*. 2006;**25**(11):1387–92; quiz 94–5.

58. Toth M, Patton DL, Esquenazi B, Shevchuk M, Thaler H, Divon M. Association between Chlamydia trachomatis and abnormal uterine bleeding. *Am J Reprod Immunol*. 2007;**57**(5):361–6.

Clinical management
Investigation of abnormal uterine bleeding

Chapter summary

- The first key to a successful investigation of women with chronic AUB is to obtain an appropriately accurate history that includes the establishment of the patient's normal menstrual pattern, the features of the abnormal bleeding including timing, volume, and associated symptoms, and the impact it has on her life.
- Physical examination is important to determine that the bleeding is not originating from visible lesions of the perineum, perianal area, or the lower genital tract, and is likely emanating from the uterus.
- All women with HMB should be screened for the presence of a systemic disorder of hemostasis using a structured history that will aid in the identification of a subset that should have laboratory testing.
- The presence or absence of intracavitary lesions potentially contributing to the bleeding can only be determined with uterine imaging including one or a combination of transvaginal ultrasound (TVS), saline infusion sonography (SIS), hysteroscopy, and magnetic resonance imaging (MRI).
- Endometrial sampling should be used liberally to evaluate high-risk patients for endometrial neoplasia, remembering that the technique frequently does not evaluate focal lesions.

Introduction

For a given woman with AUB, the identification of the appropriate therapeutic options requires a structured investigational strategy. For the patient, the problem usually comprises of one or a combination of disorders in frequency, predictability, duration, and/or volume of flow, and may be accompanied by other related symptoms such as dysmenorrhea. Some women do not appreciate that the collective volume of their uterovaginal bleeding is large enough to supercede dietary iron intake, and may present to their practitioner, not with the complaint of excessive bleeding, but one of fatigue, syncope, or other secondary effects of anemia.

While many women who do complain of heavy bleeding actually do not have excessive volume, others with normal blood loss (< 80 mL per month) experience anemia, likely because of inadequate nutritional intake [1–3] (Class II-1). In addition, there exist a number of other causes of iron deficiency anemia including malabsorptive syndromes, celiac disease, peptic ulcer disease, pulmonary hemosiderosis, and occult neoplasms, typically in the gastrointestinal tract. Other types of anemia may, superficially at least, be similar to iron deficiency anemia including thalassemia, sideroblastic anemia, and anemia related to chronic inflammatory disease. As a result, the clinician should ensure that the anemia is likely related to menstrual blood loss with a combination of history, a CBC including red cell indices (microcytic, hypochromic), and the peripheral blood smear that, collectively, will allow a presumptive diagnosis of iron deficiency anemia. Response of the patient to iron-based therapy helps to confirm the diagnosis.

Investigative strategy

The evaluation of a woman with chronic bleeding perceived to be from the vagina must first focus on confirming the origin of that bleeding. Bleeding perceived by the patient to be genital tract in origin instead may arise from extragenital sites, including urinary and gastrointestinal sources. In addition to the uterine corpus, genital tract bleeding may originate in the vulva, vagina, cervix, and even the fallopian tube which can be a rare source of abnormal vaginal bleeding. As a result, the history, the physical examination, and indicated ancillary tests should be conducted in a way that allows comprehensive evaluation of all possible sources of bleeding.

The presence or absence of ovulation is a key to the identification of the etiology of the bleeding, the appropriate investigations, and, in many instances, the choices for therapy. A picture consistent with a disorder of ovulation (AUB-O) should stimulate the clinician to expose causes of systemic malfunction. On the other hand, AUB associated with ovulation is an indication of disordered systemic (AUB-C) or local hemostasis (AUB-E), or to definable structural entities such as submucous myomas (AUB-Ls) or adenomyosis (AUB-A).

There exist a number of common, clinically identifiable entities such as adenomyosis and intramural or subserosal myomas that likely do *not* cause AUB. Consequently, when bleeding symptoms arise in the presence of such lesions, it is entirely possible, if not likely, that the etiology of the bleeding lies in the endometrium, a disorder of ovulation, or a disorder of systemic hemostasis. Assuming that such clinical "red herrings" are the cause of the bleeding may lead to the inclusion of ineffective treatment options in the therapeutic menu offered to the patient. As a result, there must always be an attempt to relate the findings to the pattern of bleeding and to consider all possible causes when constructing the menu of therapeutic options.

The evaluation of women with AUB may be divided into three components: the history and physical examination, the laboratory investigation, and evaluation of the uterus. In turn, uterine examination can be broken down into its three subcomponents: evaluation of the endometrium, the endometrial cavity, and the myometrium. While the history and physical examination are necessary for all women with AUB, the extent to which laboratory investigation and uterine evaluation are performed depend upon the specific clinical circumstances, the judgment of the clinician, and the desires of the patient.

History

A detailed menstrual history is important, not only to evaluate for pregnancy, ovulatory status, and frequency and duration of bleeding, but to determine the impact of the clinical problem on the woman's life and lifestyle. The timing, predictability, and volume of normal and abnormal uterine bleeding offer important clues to the potential cause of the AUB (Figure 6.1). Women with cyclical, predictable menses, starting every 22–35 days, will be demonstrated to be ovulatory in at least 95% of instances [4, 5]. Cycle-related molimina may provide clues additionally suggestive of ovulation, and include dysmenorrhea, mid-cycle unilateral pelvic pain suggestive of ovulation, and premenstrual symptoms, such as breast tenderness or bloating, that are relieved by menses. Anovulatory bleeding patterns are typically irregular in timing and flow, and are often, but not always, interspersed with episodes of amenorrhea of varying duration. Indeed, the first anovulatory bleed may be extremely heavy and can follow an extremely short or even nonexistent period of amenorrhea.

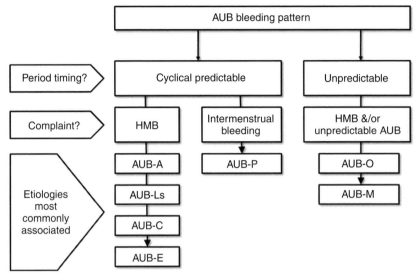

Figure 6.1 Historical features of abnormal uterine bleeding (AUB). The menstrual history is critically important to the evaluation of the woman with AUB in the reproductive years. Totally unpredictable bleeding, outside the context of regular and predictable menses is usually associated with ovulatory disturbances (AUB-O) but may be an indication of endometrial hyperplasia or malignancy (AUB-M). Women with cyclic and predictable menses with intermenstrual bleeding frequently have a polyp of the cervical canal or endometrium (IMB-P), while those with heavy menstrual bleeding may have one or a combination of AUB-E (endometrial), -C (coagulopathy), -Ls (submucosal leiomyoma), and -A (adenomyosis).

Table 6.1 Screening for coagulopathy (AUB-C). A positive screen comprises any of the following: (1) heavy bleeding since menarche, one from list; (2) two or more from list; (3) patients with a positive screen should be considered for further evaluation including consultation with a hematologist and/or testing of von Willebrand factor and ristocetin cofactor.

Initial screening for an underlying disorder of hemostasis in patients with excessive menstrual bleeding should be by a structured history:
1. Heavy menstrual bleeding since menarche
2. One of the following:
a. Postpartum hemorrhage
b. Surgical related bleeding
c. Bleeding associated with dental work
3. Two or more of the following symptoms:
a. Bruising one to two times a month
b. Epistaxis one to two times a month
c. Frequent gum bleeding
d. Family history of bleeding symptoms

From Kadir et al. [6]

Table 6.2 Hereditary nonpolyposis colorectal cancer syndrome (HNPCCS) (Lynch syndrome) is an autosomal dominant inherited cancer susceptibility syndrome that accounts for approximately 3% of colorectal and endometrial cancers. Despite the syndrome's name, the lifetime risk of endometrial cancer may exceed that of colon cancer, with a mean age of 48–50. The lifetime risk of ovarian cancer has been determined to be 12%. Because the Amsterdam criteria are so strict and because molecular biologic testing for microsatellite instability can identify tumors that are associated with the syndrome, there are new Bethesda criteria developed to identify patients who should be so tested.

Amsterdam criteria for diagnosis of HNPCCS

Patient must meet *all* of the following criteria:

- Three or more relatives with a histologically verified hereditary nonpolyposis colorectal-asociated cancer (colorectal cancer, cancer of the endometrium, ovary, small bowel, ureter, or renal pelvis), one of whom is a first-degree relative of the other two (familial adenomatous polyposis should be excluded); *and*

- Cancers involving at least two generations; *and*

- One or more cancer cases diagnosed before age 50

The revised Bethesda criteria for testing colorectal tumors for microsatellite instability

Tumors from individuals should be tested for microsatellite instability in the following situations:

- Colorectal cancer diagnosed in a patient who is less than 50

- Presence of synchronous, metachronous colorectal or other hereditary nonpolyposis colorectal cancer-associated tumors, regardless of age. (Hereditary nonpolyposis colorectal cancer-related tumors include colorectal, endometrial, stomach, ovarian, pancreas, ureter and renal pelvis, biliary tract, brain, usually glioblastoma as seen in Turcot syndrome tumors, sebaceous gland adenomas and keratoacanthomas in Muir–Torre syndrome, and carcinoma of the small bowel.)

- Colorectal cancer with the microsatellite instability high histology diagnosed in a patient who is less than 60. (Microsatellite instability – high in tumors refers to changes in two or more of the five National Cancer Institute-recommended panels of microsatellite markers. Histology indicated by presence of tumor-infiltrating lymphocytes, Crohn's-like lymphocytic reaction, mucinous/signet-ring differentiation, or medullary growth pattern.)

- Colorectal cancer diagnosed in one or more first-degree relatives with a hereditary nonpolyposis colorectal cancer-related tumor, with one of the cancers being diagnosed under age 50

- Colorectal cancer diagnosed in two or more first- or second-degree relatives with hereditary nonpolyposis colorectal cancer-related tumors, regardless of age

Women may also experience periodic episodes of unpredictable bleeding that vary in severity, but are superimposed upon a background pattern of predictable cyclical menses. While this story may suggest the presence of a lesion, it is more consistent with intermittent ovulation, often termed oligoanovulation. The history may provide clues to the cause of anovulation or oligoanovulation by searching for subjective features of the circumstances and clinical entities described in Chapter 5 in the discussion of anovulation.

Given the evidence regarding the relatively high prevalence of at least a chemical disorder of systemic hemostasis, not limited to adolescents, the clinician should review the personal, medical, and family history. It is evident that a structured history can be used as a screening tool with 90% sensitivity for the detection of these relatively common disorders (Table 6.1) [6].

The clinician should also determine if the patient has a genetically higher risk for endometrial carcinoma. There seems to be clear evidence that women from families with hereditary nonpolyposis colorectal cancer syndrome (HNPCCS) have a lifetime risk of developing endometrial cancer that may be 60%, with a mean age between 48 and 50 [7, 8]. The criteria for diagnosing HNPCCS are found in Table 6.2.

Physical examination

The physical examination is initiated with a general evaluation of the patient and should be directed in a way that allows comprehensive but efficient identification of potential causes of reproductive tract and other causes of bleeding that might be in the differential diagnosis. For women who appear to be ovulatory based upon the history, the exam should focus on acquiring evidence of systemic coagulopathy by looking for bruising and petechiae as well as for features such as hepatopathy and splenomegaly. For women who appear to have disorders of ovulation, the general bodily habitus may provide some clues as to the etiology of the disorder. Obesity is commonly associated with anovulation, and formerly obese women with relatively sudden weight loss may experience resultant amenorrhea and/or unpredictable bleeding. Extremely thin women and those who have rapidly lost weight will also be susceptible to anovulation. Recognition of these traits should cause the clinician to redouble efforts to identify sources of stress, psychiatric disorders, and systemic organic disease. The clinician should attempt to identify the discrete disease entities known to cause anovulation by seeking signs of hirsutism, thyroid enlargement, and galactorrhea. Acanthosis nigricans is frequently associated with insulin resistance and in combination with irregular bleeding is suggestive of polycystic ovarian syndrome.

Careful inspection of the perineum and perianal area should identify nongenital tract causes of bleeding such as lacerations, tumors, anal fissures, and urethral caruncles. A careful speculum examination will generally reveal vaginal sources that include lacerations and tumors. It is important to recognize that the blades of the speculum may obscure such lesions, particularly on the anterior and posterior vaginal walls. Consequently, the clinician should carefully visualize those areas as the speculum is slowly withdrawn.

Visual examination of the portio vaginalis ("vaginal part") of the cervix may demonstrate ectropion, a polyp, or a lesion suspicious of a malignant tumor. While a friable ectropion is most often related to chronic cervicitis, it may be a sign of trichomonas vaginalis, or *Chlamydia trachomatis*, the latter particularly if there is coexistent purulent cervical mucous. In such instances, an antigen test for *Chlamydia trachomatis* should be obtained.

If the clinician is a competent colposcopist, examination of the cervix under magnification with appropriate staining (acetic acid, Lugol's iodine) may be useful to reassure, or to allow the performance of a directed biopsy. Regardless, macroscopically visible cervical polyps or lesions suspicious for malignancy should be biopsied (Chapter 21).

Although the manual examination may be misleading and is therefore of limited value in determining the cause of uterine bleeding, a careful bimanual examination is conducted in a logical progression focusing it on the clinical problem at hand. The cul-de-sac and lateral fornices are examined for fullness that might suggest a pelvic mass and the corpus is assessed seeking evidence of symmetrical enlargement that might be found with pregnancy, adenomyosis, or a centrally located intramural myoma. Asymmetrical enlargement suggests leiomyoma(s) but can be a finding encountered in nodular adenomyosis.

Laboratory investigation

If heavy bleeding is known or suspected, measurement of hemoglobin and hematocrit should be considered the only routine laboratory assessments, with other ancillary investigations guided by the history and physical examination.

For those with a positive historical screen for coagulopathy (Table 6.1), factor VIII, vWF, and ristocetin cofactor assays should be considered [9]. If the diagnosis of ovulatory cycles is uncertain, it is appropriate to obtain a serum assay for progesterone taken in the presumed luteal phase. It should be remembered that, in women with disorders of ovulation, the assay will reflect only ovulatory status in that cycle. For women with ovulatory disturbances, a TSH will serve to screen for abnormal thyroid function and serum prolactin and/or serum free testosterone may be ordered as indicated by the clinical picture [10].

Evaluation of the uterus

Conceptually, it is useful to consider three components when evaluating the uterus: (1) the histolpathology of the endometrium; (2) the configuration of the endometrial cavity and cervical canal; and (3) the structure of the uterine wall including both the cervical stroma and the myometrium. Because not all components have to be evaluated in any, save every, patient, it is important for the clinician to learn when and how to perform uterine evaluation.

The endometrium

Histological assessment

Histological assessement of the endometrium requires that a sample of tissue be obtained (Chapter 16) (Video 16.1, 16.2, 16.3), and is frequently recommended as an initial part of the investigation of selected women with AUB [11, 12]. Unfortunately, there is inconsistency in the medical literature regarding the appropriate selection criteria for endometrial sampling in premenopausal women. A New Zealand group identified the following factors: (1) age over 45 years; (2) obesity (> 90 kg); (3) a history of chronic anovulation, infertility, or diabetes; (4) a family history of endometrial cancer; and (5) prolonged exposure to unopposed estrogens or tamoxifen [12]. In a smaller scale study, another group found that only irregular periods and age over 40 were associated with an increased risk of endometrial neoplasia [11]. As previously noted, women from families with HNPCCS have a lifetime risk of developing endometrial cancer that may be 60%, with a mean age between 48 and 50 [7, 8]. Consequently, women with AUB of any type who are known or suspected to be from affected families should be liberally investigated with endometrial sampling, regardless of age.

While blind sampling methodologies (endometrial biopsy; dilation and curettage) are reasonable screening techniques, they are very ineffective at diagnosing focal lesions. In one series evaluating institution-based dilation and currettage, 55% of polyps were missed by blind techniques, including a number of cases of focal atypical hyperplasia and carcinoma [13]. In another series where Pipelle-based endometrial sampling preceeded hysterectomy for known endometrial carcinoma, 11 of 65 cases were missed, including 5 that were confined to a polyp and 3 that occupied less than 5% of the endometrial surface [14]. Consequently, should symptoms persist; additional measures are recommended, generally involving imaging of the endometrial cavity as will be discussed below.

Imaging of the endometrium

As discussed in Chapter 3, the endometrium of the ovulating, reproductive-aged woman vascillates in thickness from about 2 mm in the early follicular phase to about 6 mm in the late luteal phase. At least in uteri of normal size, the endometrial thickness is easily discernible by TVS (Video 23.1). Typically, endometrial thickness is actually measured and reported as the sum of the two adjacent layers of endometrium – in essence, a double thickness; a measurement that is called the *endometrial echo complex* or EEC. Consequently, the EEC in the menstrual phase is typically about 4 mm and up to 12 mm in the late luteal phase (Chapter 23) (Figure 23.5).

The thickness of the EEC may vary in the presence of ovulatory disorders, typically being much greater than normal with prolonged exposure to estrogens in the absence of progesterone, an appearance that is also shared by the vast majority of instances of endometrial hyperplasia and endometrial carcinoma. As a result, TVS may be considered a component of initial triage of at-risk premenopausal women with AUB.

Unfortunately, there is some question as to the upper threshold for premenopausal women. One study has suggested that as long as the EEC thickness is 12 mm or less, there is a very low incidence of endometrial hyperplasia or neoplasia [15]. For postmenopausal women not on estrogen-containing hormone replacement therapy (HRT), the EEC should be much thinner (Chapters 13 and 23).

The endometrial cavity

Blind instrumentation has been demonstrated to be inadequate for precise depiction of the structure of the endometrial cavity [16–18]. Consequently, accurate structural evaluation of the endometrial cavity requires imaging, usually by ultrasonographic techniques and/or direct inspection with hysteroscopy. In instances when vaginal access is limited (virginal women for example) evaluation with MRI may be the best option.

Transvaginal sonography

In the nonpregnant woman with abnormal bleeding, a homogenously thin EEC (< 5 mm) in combination with an absence of adjacent or deflecting leiomyomas is usually associated associated with a negative hysteroscopic examination. However, while focal lesions such as polyps may be seen (Figure 23.7), they may have a compressed architecture and, consequently, may be present even with an EEC thickness of 5 mm [19, 20]. In the presence of an abnormally thick endometrium, when myomas exist suspiciously close to the EEC, or when abnormal bleeding occurs or persists despite a normal TVS, additional evaluation with SIS or hysteroscopy should be considered (Figures 23.2 and 23.8). Hysteroscopic evaluation is likely superior to SIS for evaluation of the cervical canal. Transvaginal sonography is discussed in detail in Chapter 23.

Saline infusion sonography

Saline infusion sonography (SIS; also known as sonohysterography) is the sonographic (usually transvaginal) evaluation of the endometrial cavity following the transcervical instillation of saline, an approach that is comparable to hysteroscopy in its sensitivity for the diagnosis of intracavitary polyps and submucosal myomas [21, 22] (Figure 23.2) (Video 23.2, 23.3). The major deficiency, compared to hysteroscopy, is limited evaluation of the endocervical canal and the inability to concurrently remove selected lesions unless additional instrumentation is performed.

Hysterography

Most studies, each based on infertility patients, suggest that contrast-based radiographic hysterography (the uterine imaging aspect of the hysterosalpingogram or HSG) is less

63

accurate than hysteroscopy for cavity evaluation with suboptimal sensitivity and specificity [23, 24].

Hysteroscopy

Hysteroscopy can usually be performed in an office environment (Figures 23.11–23.14) to identify and direct the biopsy of focal lesions which may represent hyperplasia or cancer (Videos 16.2 and 23.4). Endometrial carcinoma and especially endometrial hyperplasia (AUB-M) arising as a field defect may not be recognizable hysteroscopically, and endometrial biopsy is a more sensitive test for such field lesions [25] (Class II-2) [26] (Class I-1). Office hysteroscopy may be more cumbersome, involves a steeper learning curve than either TVS or SIS, and it may also be more uncomfortable for the patient. Patients with tortuous or stenotic cervices may be difficult to examine with office hysteroscopy, but, in our experience, even difficult cases can be performed successfully and comfortably provided the existence of adequate and sufficient local anesthesia (Video 21.2).

Magnetic resonance imaging

Magnetic resonance imaging is another modality that has been shown to be accurate in the evaluation of the endometrial cavity in women with AUB, although it can miss polyps otherwise detected by SIS [19] (Class I-2). Nevertheless, it may have value in selected patients in whom SIS or hysteroscopy are not feasible.

The myometrium

The myometrium may be assessed to determine the extent of submucous myoma involvement, to identify adenomyosis and arteriovenous malformations, and to distinguish between leiomyomas and adenomyomas.

Ultrasound

Two-dimensional (2-D) TVS is generally useful for the evaluation of myomas in the myometrium, although variations in echogenicity can, in some instances, reduce the sensitivity of the examination (Figure 23.17). Such 2-D imaging can provide challenges when the aggregate uterine and myoma mass is quite large, as it is difficult to adequately image and track the various lesions identified. In such instances, 3-D ultrasound may be of additional value.

In appropriately trained hands and with contemporary equipment TVS is quite sensitive for the diagnosis of diffuse adenomyosis [27] (Chapter 23). Available evidence suggests that TVS is nearly as sensitive as MRI for this purpose. There is less evidence evaluating the ability of TVS to distinguish focal adenomyosis (an adenomyoma) from a leiomyoma where MRI may be superior [27].

Color flow Doppler ultrasound

Color flow Doppler ultrasound is useful in detecting blood flow and, consequently, is useful for the detection of arteriovenous malformations (Figure 5.8). In addition, color Doppler has a place in distinguishing focal adenomyosis from leiomyomas, as myometrial vessels course around the lesion, while in adenomyosis the vessel retains its vertical orientation to the endometrial cavity [28].

Magnetic resonance imaging

Magnetic resonance imaging is relatively sensitive in the evaluation of the myometrium for leiomyomas and adenomyosis [29]. This modality is generally effective at distinguishing adenomyomas from leiomyomas (Class II-1) (Figure 23.16). It is important for the clinician to remember that these entities can coexist making it important to scrutinize carefully any imaging studies, particularly if surgery is to be undertaken.

Magnetic resonance imaging also appears superior to TVS, SIS, and hysteroscopy for measuring the myometrial extent of submucus leiomyomas [19].

Myometrial biopsy

Transcervical needle biopsy seems to have high specificity but poor sensitivity for the diagnosis of adenomyosis when compared to histopathological examination of hysterectomy specimens [30, 31] (Class II1).

Summary

The approach described in this chapter is summarized in the algorithms shown in Figures 6.2 and 6.3. It should be remembered that these are guidelines and that the exact order of investigation may appropriately vary depending upon the clinical situation. Finally, the clinician should remember that there may exist more than one contributor to the genesis of the AUB, and that, frequently, identified structural lesions such as adenomyosis, some polyps, and leiomyomas (≥ type 3) are asymptomatic. In these circumstances, clinical judgment and, in many instances, trials of therapy will be necessary to determine the clinically important findings.

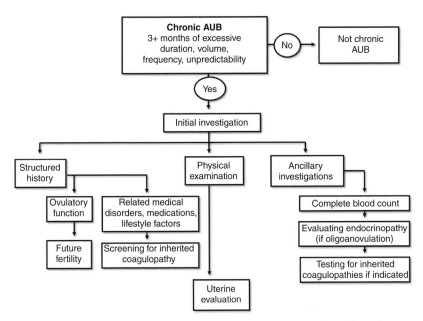

Figure 6.2 Investigation of chronic abnormal uterine bleeding. Women should have three or more months of symptoms. The three components include careful menstrual history, physical examination followed by detailed examination of the uterus, and appropriate ancillary investigation.

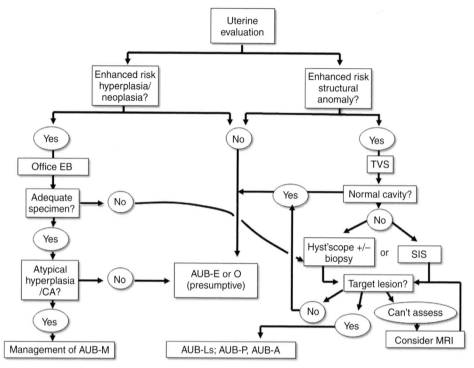

Figure 6.3 Initial uterine evaluation. The clinician uses the history, physical examination, and appropriate testing to determine if the patient is at increased risk for hyperplasia/neoplasia and/or a structural anomaly. For those at increased risk for neoplasia, office endometrial biopsy is performed, while those who are thought to have a greater risk for structural anomalies undergo sonographic evaluation followed by detailed evaluation of the endometrial cavity for selected patients. Initially, if the clinician determines that the patient is at low risk for either type of anomaly, a presumptive diagnosis of either AUB-E or -O can be made. Women who continue with abnormal uterine bleeding, despite therapy directed at the presumed diagnosis, must have a complete evaluation of the endometrium and endometrial cavity.

References

1. Janssen CA, Scholten PC, Heintz AP. Reconsidering menorrhagia in gynecological practice. Is a 30-year-old definition still valid? *Eur J Obstet Gynecol Reprod Biol.* 1998;**78**(1): 69–72.

2. Warner PE, Critchley HO, Lumsden MA, Campbell-Brown M, Douglas A, Murray GD. Menorrhagia I: measured blood loss, clinical features, and outcome in women with heavy periods: a survey with follow-up data. *Am J Obstet Gynecol.* 2004;**190** (5):1216–23.

3. Warner PE, Critchley HO, Lumsden MA, Campbell-Brown M, Douglas A, Murray GD. Menorrhagia II: is the 80-mL blood loss criterion useful in management of complaint of menorrhagia? *Am J Obstet Gynecol.* 2004;**190**(5):1224–9.

4. Malcolm CE, Cumming DC. Does anovulation exist in eumenorrheic women? *Obstet Gynecol.* 2003;**102**(2): 317–18.

5. Fraser IS, Critchley HO, Munro MG. Abnormal uterine bleeding: getting our terminology straight. *Curr Opin Obstet Gynecol.* 2007;**19**(6):591–5.

6. Kadir RA, Economides DL, Sabin CA, Owens D, Lee CA. Frequency of inherited bleeding disorders in women with menorrhagia. *Lancet.* 1998;**351** (9101):485–9.

7. Lu KH, Broaddus RR. Gynecological tumors in hereditary nonpolyposis colorectal cancer: we know they are

common – now what? *Gynecol Oncol.* 2001;**82**(2):221–2.

8. Lu KH, Dinh M, Kohlmann W, Watson P, Green J, Syngal S, et al. Gynecologic cancer as a "sentinel cancer" for women with hereditary nonpolyposis colorectal cancer syndrome. *Obstet Gynecol.* 2005; **105**(3):569–74.

9. Lusher JM. Screening and diagnosis of coagulation disorders. *Am J Obstet Gynecol.* 1996;**175**(3 Pt 2):778–83.

10. Krassas GE, Pontikides N, Kaltsas T, Papadopoulou P, Paunkovic J, Paunkovic N, et al. Disturbances of menstruation in hypothyroidism. *Clin Endocrinol (Oxf).* 1999;**50**(5):655–9.

11. Ash SJ, Farrell SA, Flowerdew G. Endometrial biopsy in DUB. *J Reprod Med.* 1996;**41**(12):892–6.

12. Farquhar CM, Lethaby A, Sowter M, Verry J, Baranyai J. An evaluation of risk factors for endometrial hyperplasia in premenopausal women with abnormal menstrual bleeding. *Am J Obstet Gynecol.* 1999;**181**(3):525–9.

13. Epstein E, Ramirez A, Skoog L, Valentin L. Dilatation and curettage fails to detect most focal lesions in the uterine cavity in women with postmenopausal bleeding. *Acta Obstet Gynecol Scand.* 2001; **80**(12):1131–6.

14. Guido RS, Kanbour-Shakir A, Rulin MC, Christopherson WA. Pipelle endometrial sampling. Sensitivity in the detection of endometrial cancer. *J Reprod Med.* 1995; **40**(8):553–5.

15. Farquhar C, Ekeroma A, Furness S, Arroll B. A systematic review of transvaginal ultrasonography, sonohysterography and hysteroscopy for the investigation of abnormal uterine bleeding in premenopausal women. *Acta Obstet Gynecol Scand.* 2003;**82**(6):493–504.

16. Valle RF. Hysteroscopic evaluation of patients with abnormal uterine bleeding. *Surg Gynecol Obstet.* 1981;**153**(4):521–6.

17. Gimpelson RJ, Rappold HO. A comparative study between panoramic hysteroscopy with directed biopsies and dilatation and curettage. A review of 276 cases. *Am J Obstet Gynecol.* 1988; **158**(3 Pt 1):489–92.

18. Loffer FD. Hysteroscopy with selective endometrial sampling compared with D&C for abnormal uterine bleeding: the value of

a negative hysteroscopic view. *Obstet Gynecol.* 1989;**73**(1):16–20.

19. Dueholm M, Lundorf E, Hansen ES, Ledertoug S, Olesen F. Evaluation of the uterine cavity with magnetic resonance imaging, transvaginal sonography, hysterosonographic examination, and diagnostic hysteroscopy. *Fertil Steril.* 2001; **76**(2):350–7.

20. Breitkopf DM, Frederickson RA, Snyder RR. Detection of benign endometrial masses by endometrial stripe measurement in premenopausal women. *Obstet Gynecol.* 2004;**104**(1):120–5.

21. Widrich T, Bradley LD, Mitchinson AR, Collins RL. Comparison of saline infusion sonography with office hysteroscopy for the evaluation of the endometrium. *Am J Obstet Gynecol.* 1996;**174**(4):1327–34.

22. Saidi MH, Sadler RK, Theis VD, Akright BD, Farhart SA, Villanueva GR. Comparison of sonography, sonohysterography, and hysteroscopy for evaluation of abnormal uterine bleeding. *J Ultrasound Med.* 1997;**16** (9):587–91.

23. Prevedourakis C, Loutradis D, Kalianidis C, Makris N, Aravantinos D. Hysterosalpingography and hysteroscopy in female infertility. *Hum Reprod.* 1994; **9**(12):2353–5.

24. Goldberg JM, Falcone T, Attaran M. Sonohysterographic evaluation of uterine abnormalities noted on hysterosalpingography. *Hum Reprod.* 1997;**12**(10):2151–3.

25. Lasmar RB, Barrozo PR, de Oliveira MA, Coutinho ES, Dias R. Validation of hysteroscopic view in cases of endometrial hyperplasia and cancer in patients with abnormal uterine bleeding. *J Minim Invasive Gynecol.* 2006;**13**(5):409–12.

26. Clark TJ, Voit D, Gupta JK, Hyde C, Song F, Khan KS. Accuracy of hysteroscopy in the diagnosis of endometrial cancer and hyperplasia: a systematic quantitative review. *JAMA.* 2002;**288**(13):1610–21.

27. Dueholm M. Transvaginal ultrasound for diagnosis of adenomyosis: a review. *Best Pract Res Clin Obstet Gynaecol.* 2006; **20**(4):569–82.

28. Chiang CH, Chang MY, Hsu JJ, Chiu TH, Lee KF, Hsieh TT, et al. Tumor vascular pattern and blood flow impedance in the differential diagnosis of leiomyoma and adenomyosis by color Doppler sonography. *J Assist Reprod Genet.* 1999;**16**(5):268–75.

29. Mark AS, Hricak H, Heinrichs LW, Hendrickson MR, Winkler ML, Bachica JA, et al. Adenomyosis and leiomyoma: differential diagnosis with MR imaging. *Radiology.* 1987; **163**(2):527–9.

30. Popp LW, Schwiedessen JP, Gaetje R. Myometrial biopsy in the diagnosis of adenomyosis uteri. *Am J Obstet Gynecol.* 1993;**169**(3):546–9.

31. Vercellini P, Cortesi I, De Giorgi O, Merlo D, Carinelli SG, Crosignani PG. Transvaginal ultrasonography versus uterine needle biopsy in the diagnosis of diffuse adenomyosis. *Hum Reprod.* 1998;**13**(10):2884–7.

Therapy: disorders of hemostasis (AUB-C)

Chapter summary

- Women with systemic disorders of hemostasis may best be managed in the context of a multidisciplinary clinic or program that includes the process of counseling of other family members.
- Many variants of vWD only mildly impact hemostasis, if at all, so that other causes of AUB must be considered.
- The management of AUB-I is frequently successful using agents and techniques that apply to AUB-E.

Introduction

Disorders of hemostasis may be inherited, can be acquired, or may be a consequence of medical therapy. Inherited systemic disorders of hemostasis ("coagulopathies") are more common than is generally appreciated, as they are detected in approximately 13% of women with HMB [1]. The clinical significance of many of the biochemically-identified inherited disorders is not clear but some obviously represent the principal cause of that patient's HMB (Chapters 5 and 6). Furthermore, knowledge of the existence of an inherited coagulopathy helps to guide the counseling and care of potentially affected family members. In many instances the internist or hematologist guides primary therapy but one or a combination of the medical and surgical approaches otherwise used for HMB-E or -O may be necessary and effective [2–4] (Class III).

Therapeutic environment

Ideally, inherited coagulopathies are managed in the context of a multidisciplinary clinic specifically designed to function within the network of hemophilia treatment centers (HTCs). This ensures capable on-site performance of the hemostasis testing important for confirmation of the diagnosis, and for the provision of well conceived and coordinated ongoing care. Hemophilia treatment centers are typically staffed by hemophilia specialists, obstetricians, gynecologists, hemophilia nurse specialists, family counselors and/or therapists, and other professionals who are involved when necessary. Such an environment also facilitates communication among professionals and allows an opportunity to address the psychosocial complications of HMB-C.

There exist preliminary data from the US Centers for Disease Control and Prevention (CDC), that supports the beneficial role of HTCs: 71 of 75 (95%) of affected women reported a high degree of satisfaction with their care at a HTC [5]. Other centers have reported similar positive findings including the multidisciplinary Katharine Dormandy Haemophilia Centre of the Royal Free Hospital in London, the Mary M. Gooley

Hemophilia Treatment Center (Rochester, NY), and the Women's Hemostasis and Thrombosis Clinic at the Duke University Medical Center (Durham, NC) [6].

Antifibrinolytic therapy

Tranexamic acid (TA) is an antifibrinolytic agent that is described in Chapter 8. Tranexamic acid has been widely used for women with bleeding disorders, and has been employed orally, intravenously, or topically, alone or as an adjuvant therapy, both for prevention and management of oral cavity bleeding, epistaxis, gastrointestinal bleeding, and HMB. However, there is a relative paucity of evidence regarding the efficacy of this treatment for reduction of menstrual blood loss in women with HMB-C. Kadir et al. from the Royal Free College, London, used 1 g four times per day during menses and observed a significant reduction of bleeding in 40% of 37 women with HMB-C [6]. There is also a report on successful use of a single TA dose of 4 g in a small series of women with vWD, but this regimen was frequently associated with severe nausea and vomiting [2] (Class III).

When TA is not available (not currently available in the United States), epsilon aminocaproic acid can be used, but optimal doses have not been established. Kabi 2161, a precursor of TA, is another antifibrinolytic that has been used for HMB [7]. It has the advantage of better gastrointestinal absorption and increased bioavailability, but there are no data on this agent in women with HMB-C.

Systemic gonadal steroid agents

Estrogen and progestin combinations

There is a paucity of evidence evaluating the impact of combined estrogen and progestin agents in the treatment of women with HMB-C. Theoretically, combined estrogen and progestin oral contraceptive compounds (COCs) containing at least 50 μg of ethinyl estradiol increase both factor VIII and vWF factor functional activity, and there is some evidence that there is clinical efficacy that may depend, in part, on the type of vWD [8]. The COCs were effective in 88% of women with HMB-C associated with type 2 and 3 vWD, but for type 1 patients only 24% reported improvement, 37% if high dose oral contraceptives were used [8] (Class II-3).

At least theoretically, the use of continuous COCs would be associated with the induction of amenorrhea and a beneficial therapeutic impact; however, there are no published data using this approach. It should be noted that while continuous COCs frequently cause amenorrhea, there is also a relatively high incidence of spotting and breakthrough bleeding early in the course of therapy, a side effect that could be a source of anxiety for the patient, but this bleeding is uncommonly heavy.

Progestin-only therapy

The use of systemic progestins for HMB-E and AUB-O is described in Chapter 8. There are no studies specifically evaluating progestins for the treatment of HMB-C, but there are some seemingly logical conclusions that might be made. First of all, while the short cycle use of progestins will likely be ineffective, there could be value in women with disorders of ovulation associated with coagulopathy (HMB-C, -O). This is a relatively common circumstance when faced with adolescents, or women in the late reproductive years with vWD who frequently have ovulatory disturbances. The use of depot medroxyprogesterone acetate (DMPA) frequently causes amenorrhea in contraceptive doses, but patients should be counseled that irregular bleeding is frequent, particularly in the first year of therapy. While this bleeding is typically not severe, the problem with DMPA is that the patient is committed to the approach for months after the injection.

Danazol

Danazol (Chapter 8) has a relatively unique application for the treatment or prevention of HMB-C for patients with idiopathic thrombocytopenia purpura (ITP). In one study, 84% attained amenorrhea or occasional light bleeding within 2 months of initiation of therapy, while the majority experienced an elevation in their platelet levels [9]. Typical dosing is between 400 and 600 mg/day, levels that are generally and unfortunately frequently associated with the side effects of acne, oily skin, and hirsutism.

Intrauterine progestins

Whereas there has been extensive high quality investigation on the use of the LNG-IUS in women with apparently normal coagulation status (Chapter 8), there is a paucity of studies on those with HMB-C. In a series evaluating 16 women with HMB-C (13 with vWD), all were shown to have objective improvement of blood loss compared with baseline, 9 (56%) became amenorrheic, and mean hemoglobin concentrations rose [10]. Intermenstrual spotting was noted by most but it did not become a clinical problem. Another study looked at seven women and demonstrated that the majority (five) experienced a reduction in bleeding while two did not [11].

The LNG-IUS has also been evaluated in 23 women with HMB-C secondary to warfarin and most, but not all, had substantial improvement [12].

One important issue with the LNG-IUS is the relatively high incidence of intermenstrual spotting and bleeding in the first six months of therapy, at least in normal women (Chapter 11). The concern about IUS-associated infection risk is not thought to be clinically important in the vast majority of women [13].

Gonadotropin releasing hormone agonists

One concern with the induction of gonadotropin releasing hormone agonist (GnRHa) therapy in women who are anemic or who are at increased risk of bleeding is the so called "flare" reflecting the initial prolonged release of FSH that results in a transient elevation of ovarian estradiol, and which may be mitigated with short-term use of a progestin such as medroxyprogesterone (MPA) or megestrol acetate for the first three weeks [14] (Class III). While there are no available data on dosing, I use MPA 10–20 mg twice daily, depending, in part, on patient weight.

Generally, GnRHa therapy is seen as a short-term approach (3–6 months), largely because of cost and the risk of osteopenia and osteoporosis with long-term therapy. Consequently, it is generally considered an interim measure allowing women to build iron stores and formulate a long-term therapeutic plan. In some instances, however, GnRHa may be a viable long-term alternative using "add-back" gonadal steroid therapy, both to treat vasomotor symptoms and to prevent bone loss. Continuous use of norethindrone acetate, 5 mg/day, has been demonstrated efficacious in this regard without the breakthrough bleeding often associated with regimens employing both estrogens and progestins [15]. In addition, GnRH agonists have also been described for women about to undergo stem cell transplantation and myelosuppressive chemotherapy [14, 16].

Desmopressin acetate (DDAVP)

An analog of the vasoactive agent *vasopressin* is 1-deamino-8-D-arginine vasopressin, also known as desmopressin or "DDAVP." Desmopressin has been demonstrated effective in type 1 and sometimes type 2 vWD, and in mild to moderate hemophilia A, because it increases plasma levels of factor VIII and vWF. Desmopressin has been evaluated for the treatment of HMB-C, both in a subcutaneous and a nasal spray formulation, but efficacy for reduction in menstrual volume is not clear, as the only RCT showed equivocal results [17] (Class I-2). As a result, use of desmopressin in this clinical situation must be individualized, usually treating the patient for the first three days of the menses, when volume is usually the greatest. The typical dose is 300 μg/day.

Endometrial ablation

Endometrial ablation offers a therapeutic option for women with HMB-C provided they have no desire for future fertility. The evidence of the efficacy of this approach is conflicting as, in one small study, three of seven treated patients still required hysterectomy within one year [4]. In another, more recent case control study from the Mayo Clinic, only 2 of 41 women with HMB-C underwent hysterectomy or reablation up to 60 months following EA [18] (Class II-2). Consequently, EA may have a role in patients with HMB-C.

References

1. Shankar M, Lee CA, Sabin CA, Economides DL, Kadir RA. Von Willebrand disease in women with menorrhagia: a systematic review. *BJOG*. 2004;**111**(7):734–40.

2. Ong YL, Hull DR, Mayne EE. Menorrhagia in von Willebrand disease successfully treated with single daily dose tranexamic acid. *Haemophilia*. 1998;**4**(1):63–5.

3. Mohri H. High dose of tranexamic acid for treatment of severe menorrhagia in patients with von Willebrand disease. *J Thromb Thrombolysis*. 2002;**14**(3):255–7.

4. Rubin G, Wortman M, Kouides PA. Endometrial ablation for von Willebrand disease-related menorrhagia – experience with seven cases. *Haemophilia*. 2004;**10**(5):477–82.

5. Kirtava A, Crudder S, Dilley A, Lally C, Evatt B. Trends in clinical management of women with von Willebrand disease: a survey of 75 women enrolled in haemophilia treatment centres in the United States. *Haemophilia*. 2004;**10**(2):158–61.

6. Kadir RA, Lukes AS, Kouides PA, Fernandez H, Goudemand J. Management of excessive menstrual bleeding in women with hemostatic disorders. *Fertil Steril*. 2005; **84**(5):1352–9.

7. Edlund, M., Andersson K, Rybo G, Lindoff C, Astedt B, von Schoultz B. Reduction of menstrual blood loss in women suffering from idiopathic menorrhagia with a novel antifibrinolytic drug (Kabi 2161). *Br J Obstet Gynaecol*. 1995; **102**(11):913–17.

8. Beller FK, Ebert C. Effects of oral contraceptives on blood coagulation. A review. *Obstet Gynecol Surv*. 1985; **40**(7):425–36.

9. Ambriz, R., Pizzuto J, Morales M, Chávez G, Guillén C, Avilés A. Therapeutic effect of danazol on metrorrhagia in patients with idiopathic thrombocytopenic purpura (ITP). *Nouv Rev Fr Hematol*. 1986; **28**(5):275–9.

10. Kingman CE, Kadir RA, Lee CA, Economides DL. The use of levonorgestrel-releasing intrauterine system for treatment of menorrhagia in women with inherited bleeding disorders. *BJOG*. 2004; **111**(12):1425–8.

11. Lukes AS, Reardon B, Arepally G. Use of the levonorgestrel-releasing intrauterine system in women with hemostatic disorders. *Fertil Steril*. 2008;**90**(3):673–7.

12. Pisoni CN, Cuadrado MJ, Khamashta MA, Hunt BJ. Treatment of menorrhagia associated with oral anticoagulation:

efficacy and safety of the levonorgestrel releasing intrauterine device (Mirena coil). *Lupus.* 2006;**15**(12):877–80.

13. Farley TM, Rosenberg MJ, Rowe PJ, Chen JH, Meirik O. Intrauterine devices and pelvic inflammatory disease: an international perspective. *Lancet.* 1992; **339**(8796):785–8.

14. Lhomme C, Brault P, Bourhis JH, Pautier P, Dohollou N, Dietrich PY, et al. Prevention of menstruation with leuprorelin (GnRH agonist) in women undergoing myelosuppressive chemotherapy or radiochemotherapy for hematological malignancies: a pilot study. *Leuk Lymphoma.* 2001;**42**(5):1033–41.

15. Surrey ES, Hornstein MD. Prolonged GnRH agonist and add-back therapy for symptomatic endometriosis: long-term follow-up. *Obstet Gynecol.* 2002; **99**(5 Pt 1):709–19.

16. Chiusolo P, Salutari P, Sica S, Scirpa P, Laurenti L, Piccirillo N, et al. Luteinizing hormone-releasing hormone analogue: leuprorelin acetate for the prevention of menstrual bleeding in premenopausal women undergoing stem cell transplantation. *Bone Marrow Transplant.* 1998;**21**(8):821–3.

17. Kadir RA, Lee CA, Sabin CA, Pollard D, Economides DL. DDAVP nasal spray for treatment of menorrhagia in women with inherited bleeding disorders: a randomized placebo-controlled crossover study. *Haemophilia.* 2002; **8**(6):787–93.

18. El-Nashar SA, Hopkins MR, Feitoza SS, Pruthi RK, Barnes SA, Gebhart JB, et al. Global endometrial ablation for menorrhagia in women with bleeding disorders. *Obstet Gynecol.* 2007; **109**(6):1381–7.

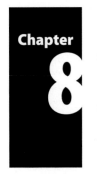

Chapter

8 Therapy: endometrial causes (AUB-E) or disorders of ovulation (AUB-O)

Chapter summary

- Therapies effective for AUB-E may be less effective or ineffective for AUB-O and vice versa.
- For anemic women, iron therapy is critically important and, for some, this may be the only necessary intervention.
- For HMB-E, the LNG-IUS is the reversible intervention associated with the greatest degree of therapeutic success and patient satisfaction.
- There exist many other medical interventions that are highly effective, but, for some women, the side effects have a substantial impact on their quality of life.
- Endometrial ablation is a surgical procedure associated with reduced morbidity and short-term costs when compared to hysterectomy, but a substantial number of women ultimately have their uterus removed.

Introduction

This chapter deals with the treatment of women found to have AUB unrelated to structural causes, systemic coagulopathies, or to iatrogenic causes. Often called "dysfunctional uterine bleeding," such patients actually have AUB related to endometrial causes (AUB-E) or to disorders of ovulation (AUB-O). The clinician should be aware that asymptomatic lesions such as polyps, leiomyomas, or adenomyosis may be present in such women. The algorithm in Figure 8.1 summarizes the contents of this chapter.

Medical options

Iron

For many women with AUB there is associated depletion of iron stores or frank anemia, a circumstance that makes iron an essential component of any therapeutic strategy. For some, it may be the only treatment required, while for others iron replacement is combined with temporary or long-term medical therapy, or is part of a strategy that includes surgery.

Iron intake can be optimized with dietary counseling in an attempt to increase the ingestion of iron-rich foods, which include legumes, whole grain bread, raisins, and meats including fish, poultry, beef, and, especially, liver. To supplement dietary intake, oral iron can be administered, in optimal doses that range from 150 to 200 mg of elemental iron per day. Optimal gastrointestinal absorption is achieved with the ferrous (Fe^{2+}) form and the concomitant use of 250 mg/day of ascorbic acid.

Oral iron therapy is associated with gastrointestinal symptoms in approximately 10–20% of women. Symptoms may include one or a combination of nausea, constipation, epigastric

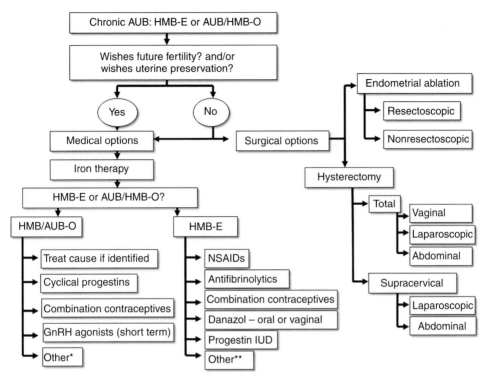

Figure 8.1 Treatment algorithm for HMB-E or AUB-O. A critical determination is the desire of the patient for future pregnancies, as surgical options for this category permanently impact future fertility. Medical options include simple iron therapy, which should be a component of any regimen if the patient is anemic. The menu of medical options depends in large part on whether the patient has AUB-O or HMB-E. *,** It is possible that other medical interventions may be effective in a given patient.

distress, and vomiting. Reduction in the amount of elemental iron ingested or the use of a liquid preparation generally is effective, and the patient can try to slowly escalate the dose as tolerated and needed. Ingestion with meals may help as well, but is often associated with decreased absorption. Despite these measures, some women remain intolerant to therapy, or have a malabsorption syndrome that precludes the use of oral iron. In such instances, parenteral iron may be administered either intramuscularly or intravenously, with the latter approach preferred. There are a number of available preparations including iron dextran, ferric fluconate complex, and iron sucrose, the latter two approved only for intravenous use. Iron dextran has been associated with both local and systemic side effects in about 5% of cases and occasionally can be severe, including pain, muscle necrosis, phlebitis, and anaphylaxis. Ferric gluconate and iron sucrose may be associated with fewer side effects. Further discussion of parenteral iron therapy is outside the scope of this book [1].

Following restoration of the hemoglobin and hematocrit levels, it is generally considered preferable to continue iron therapy for 6–12 months in order to replenish depleted iron stores.

Antifibrinolytics

The role that fibrinolysis plays in the process of endometrial hemostasis was described in detail in Chapter 3 and the impact of excess fibrinolytic activity on the pathogenesis of HMB-E was described in Chapter 5.

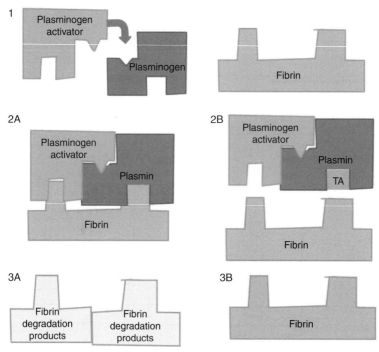

Figure 8.2 Tranexamic acid. Normally, plasminogen activator binds to plasminogen (1) converting it to plasmin which then couples to fibrin monomers (2A) causing them to break down into fibrin degradation products (3A). Tranexamic acid binds to plasmin (2B) in a way that prevents attachment to the fibrin thereby leaving the fibrin monomer, and, as a result, the clot, intact (3B).

Tranexamic acid (TA) is an antifibrinolytic agent that functions by inhibiting plasminogen activator from converting plasminogen to plasmin (Figure 8.2). When administered orally, 1 g every 6 hours, for the first 4 days of the cycle, TA is associated with a 40–60% reduction in bleeding volume [2] (Class I-1). It is important to note that no study has evaluated the use of TA in the treatment of HMB-O.

Placebo-controlled RCTs show no increase in gastrointestinal side effects when TA is compared to other medical therapies [2] (Class I-2). Available evidence suggests that TA does not increase the incidence of thromboembolic disease, even when used in women at high risk [3] (Class II-2). Consequently, TA therapy not only should be considered safe, but should be one of the first line treatments for HMB-E. While in some countries, TA is available as an "over-the-counter" preparation, in most it remains a prescription item, and in the United States it is still unavailable at the time of writing.

Cyclooxygenase inhibitors

Local prostaglandin activity has a major role in the initiation of menses and a profound impact on local endometrial hemostasis (Chapter 3). Ovulatory women with HMB-E typically have excess levels of PGE_2 and PGI_2 along with reduced relative and absolute levels of $PGF_{2\alpha}$, features that could reflect disorders in local cyclooxygenase (COX) activity (Chapter 5).

Cyclooxygenase inhibitors, often referred to as nonsteroidal anti-inflammatory drugs (NSAIDs), generally reduce endomyometrial prostaglandin levels via the inhibition of the

COX-mediated conversion of arachadonic acid to prostaglandins [4]. Theoretically, COX inhibitors from the fenamate family of drugs, such as mefenamic acid, should have the greatest impact because of their dual action – inhibition of prostaglandin synthesis and impairment of PGE_2-receptor binding [5].[1]

In a Cochrane Review of women treated for "menorrhagia" with COX inhibitors, the mean reduction of blood flow was 20%, with 5 of 7 RCTs demonstrating benefit and 2 no significant difference [6] (Class I-1). Although most of the published reports evaluated mefenamic acid, and despite its theoretical advantages, there is no currently available evidence that one formulation is superior to the other. Optimal dose and dose scheduling is more difficult to discern, although most studies have analyzed regimens that start with the first day of menses and continue for five days or until the cessation of menstruation. Mefenamic acid and naproxen are typically prescribed in a dose of 250–500 mg 2–4 times daily while ibuprofen has been studied in dose regimens ranging from 600 to 1200 mg/day. It is to be emphasized that there are no available data for women with HMB-O.

Randomized trials comparing COX inhibitors with other regimens for HMB-E suggest that both danazol [7] and TA [8] are superior at reducing menstrual volume (Class I-2). However, for some, the reduction is quite profound, and, for those with accompanying primary dysmenorrhea, itself mediated by $PGF_{2\alpha}$, COX inhibitors may provide an effective, low cost, and safe approach for the management of both problems.

Gonadal steroids

Gonadal steroids, including estrogens, progestins, and androgens, alone or in combination, exert a profound impact on the endometrium and, depending on how they are administered, can regulate the timing and volume of bleeding. Some approaches to dosing and administration can eliminate bleeding altogether.

Progestins

Most therapeutic progestational agents are either the 19-nortestosterone derivatives such as norethindrone (NET) or 21-carbon molecules such as medroxyprogesterone acetate (MPA). There exists a variety of routes of administration and dose schedules, ranging from intermittent (cyclical) oral administration designed to simulate the luteal phase, to continuous administration either orally, through intramuscular injection, or using a LNG-IUS (Mirena®, Bayer Schering Pharma AG, Berlin, Germany).

Cyclical administration

As discussed in Chapter 5, anovulatory women do not make physiologically significant, cyclical, circulating levels of progesterone. Consequently, at least 50% of women with AUB-O experience successful regulation of their menses and reduction in menstrual volume with oral NET or MPA administered approximately 10 days per month [9] (Class I-2). On the other hand, women with HMB-E ovulate, do make cyclical progesterone, and do not benefit from the administration of progestins in the luteal phase of the cycle [10, 11] (Class I-2) [12] (Class I-1).

Progestins can also be administered in a "long" cyclical fashion, 3 weeks or more of each month, and may be effective for women with HMB-E, reducing menstrual volume by 87%

---

[1]   It can also be hypothesized that COX inhibitors would further reduce levels of the vasoconstricting $PGF_{2\alpha}$ as well, thereby counteracting the otherwise beneficial impact on PGE_2 production and activity. This may explain the modest and somewhat inconsistent results of COX inhibitors in the context of RCTs.

in one clinical trial [13] (Class I-2). This regimen of 5 mg of NET 3 times daily from day 5 to day 26 of the cycle has more in common with continuous regimens that usually suppress ovulation. It should be noted that in this study, which compared oral NET to a LNG-IUS, women generally preferred the intrauterine to the oral therapy, as only 22% of those assigned to the NET were willing to continue with their treatment after 3 months.

Continuous systemic administration

Continuous administration of progestins may be effective for HMB-E or AUB-O but there are no clinical trials to provide guidance regarding dosage or efficacy. Potential options include continuous oral NET or NET acetate 5–15 mg/day; oral MPA 30–40 mg/day; and depot MPA 150–200 mg q 2–3 months (Class III). Caution should be exerted in the use of injectable or implantable systemic progestins for chronic AUB therapy as the most evaluated agent, depot MPA, is associated with irregular bleeding in about 50% of women so treated (Chapter 11). Other options, such as implantable progestins, have not been evaluated in the treatment of AUB but may provide successful therapy for some women. With these agents, similar caution has to be conveyed to the patient, for irregular bleeding is a frequent symptom associated with such therapy. I often use NET-acetate, 5 mg once or twice per day and, in many instances, find it to be an acceptable approach.

Local administration

Intrauterine progestins have proven to be a very effective option for HMB-E as was first reported in 1990 [14]. Changing the route of progestin administration from a systemic source to one directly applied to the target tissue, in this case the endometrium, provides an opportunity to increase the local impact of the agent while simultaneously reducing important impediments to success such as inadequate absorption, suboptimal tissue delivery due to body mass and other variables, and systemic side effects such as bloating and breast tenderness. The LNG-IUS seems to produce a profound impact on bleeding volume with a 81.6% reduction in blood loss at 3 months and 95.8% at 12 months as reported in one RCT [15] (Class I-2).

Intrauterine progestins compare favorably with resectoscopic endometrial ablation (REA) [16, 17] (Class I-2), and the LNG-IUS has also been compared with nonresectoscopic endometrial ablation (NREA). One clinical trial used balloon ablation as the NREA technique and showed similar impact of the two interventions on hemoglobin levels, but, at one year, the LNG-IUS was associated with a greater frequency of systemic symptoms and a less profound reduction of bleeding volume [18] (Class I-2). Another study from Australia found no differences in clinical and quality of life outcomes at 15 months in women treated with NREA and the LNG-IUS [19] (Class II-2).

The LNG-IUS has also been compared to hysterectomy. In one RCT of women waiting for hysterectomy for HMB, 64.3% of those randomized to the LNG-IUS chose to cancel surgery compared to only 14.3% of those who continued with systemic medical management [20] (Class I-2). In another RCT, 42% of those allocated to the LNG-IUS had a hysterectomy with 5 years of follow up, a number that may seem high on first assessment, but, given that all women in this study were willing to be randomized to hysterectomy, it suggests a significant therapeutic result [21] (Class I-2). Furthermore, despite the hysterectomy rate, the direct costs associated with the LNG-IUS were less than that of routine hysterectomy, even when the "failures" were considered.

There are side effects associated with the use of the LNG-IUS; the most common of which is intermenstrual spotting that typically lasts for months following insertion of the device (Figure 11.1). Despite the local administration, there is still some systemic absorption that causes progestin-related symptoms that some women find unacceptable. In addition, by one year, approximately one third of women will be amenorrheic; an impact which some find a "side effect" while others find a welcome therapeutic outcome.

At the time of this publication, there were no trials evaluating the use of the LNG-IUS in the treatment of women with HMB-O, but there is little reason to think that the device will not be associated with reduced menstrual volume in this population. Finally, accumulating evidence of efficacy in the context of dysmenorrhea related to adenomyosis or endometriosis makes the LNG-IUS a very useful option, if not the treatment of choice, for women with such a symptom complex [22] (Class I-2).

Estrogens plus progestins

Combined (estrogen and progestin) oral contraceptive (COC) products are generally considered effective for the treatment of both AUB-E and AUB-O; however, there are few available data supporting this approach, and there are none evaluating the use of other combination contraceptive products such as the patch (Ortho Evra®, Ortho-McNeil-Janssen Pharmaceuticals Inc, Raritan, NJ, USA) and the transvaginal ring (NuvaRing®, Organon BioSciences NV, Oss, the Netherlands).

There exists a single RCT that included a group of women assigned to a monophasic COC that demonstrated menstrual flow to be reduced by about 50% in women with either HMB-E or AUB-O [23] (Class I-2). However, the sample size of this study is small and precludes any further conclusions. A larger RCT from the United States did not identify ovulatory status (therefore the group comprises mixed HMB-E and HMB-O, and possibly some with HMB-C) but, overall, almost 80% were substantially improved with COCs compared to about 26% of those receiving placebo [24] (Class I-2).

For women who desire contraception, and for whom there is no contraindication to the use of estrogen-containing compounds, a trial of oral, transdermal, or transvaginal combination estrogen and progestin contraceptive agents seems to be a reasonable approach. It is not clear whether or not there are advantages of continuous over cyclical therapy; the former may be associated with fewer bleeding days but more unpredictable bleeding. Cyclical administration is associated with more bleeding days in total, but fewer episodes of "intermenstrual" bleeding [25].

Androgens

Danazol is the most investigated such androgenic agent, a synthetic isoxazol derivative of 17-α ethinyl testosterone. Depending upon the dose, danazol can manifest with a combination of actions that include suppression of ovulation, reduced ovarian production of 17-β estradiol, and/or direct effects on estrogen receptors in the endometrium and elsewhere, and has been demonstrated to reduce menstrual blood loss more effectively than mefenamic acid [26] (Class I-2).

Higher doses of danazol (200+ mg/day) seem to be more successful, possibly because of their inhibitory affect on ovulation [27]. In RCTs, about 50% of subjects experience a successful decrease in menstrual volume with either a 200-mg daily dose or a declining daily dose regimen (200-mg, month 1; 100-mg, month 2; 50-mg, month 3) [28] (Class I-2). However, adverse side effects such as weight gain, oily skin, acne, and deepening of the voice make the medication unacceptable for many. On the other hand, small doses of daily danazol are less effective at treating HMB-E, but have shown utility for chronic mastalgia

[29] (Class I-1). Consequently, women who have HMB-E or AUB-O in conjunction with mastalgia may be good candidates for the use of danazol.

Vaginal danazol in a dose of 200 mg/day has been evaluated in a small case series with reduced blood loss by 3 months of therapy [30]. Nonetheless, half asked to discontinue therapy by six months because of symptoms that include spotting, bloating, and weight gain, but not androgenic side effects. Vaginal danazol should be considered an option, particularly in individuals for whom oral administration of gonadal steroids is not tolerated or unsuccessful and for whom intrauterine progestins are not a viable option [29].

Gonodotropin releasing hormone agonists

As discussed in Chapter 3, GnRH is a decapeptide neurohormone produced in the hypothalamus that is essential for the release of anterior pituitary's trophic hormones, follicle stimulating hormone (FSH), and luteinizing hormone (LH). Physiologically, GnRH is secreted in a pulsatile fashion, but, when GnRHs are administered continuously, the pharmacologic effect is a reversible hypogonadotropic state. This circumstance is created by down-regulation of GnRH receptors that, in turn, results in dramatically decreased gonadotropin production from the anterior pituitary. The use of GnRH agonist (GnRHa) has been described for women with HMB-E, in conjunction with "add back" treatment of vasomotor symptoms and prevention of osteopenia using a cyclical estrogen-progestin regimen [31]. Not surprisingly, the women experienced a significant reduction in bleeding volume, and tolerated the regimen well, with 90% willing to continue for longer than 12 months. For women with AUB-O, 3 months of GnRHa resulted in improved bleeding in 21 of 38 women evaluated in the 4th *post-treatment* cycle (Class I-2). The reasons for this apparent prolonged impact are unclear.

Women's satisfaction with medical therapy for HMB

A fundamental question regarding medical treatment of HMB-E/O is just "How successful is it?" In the case of AUB, investigators have traditionally relied upon measures of success that include bleeding duration, frequency, and volume. However, even if such measures are improved with a certain therapy, the degree of patient satisfaction may be influenced by factors such as cost, inconvenience, and treatment side effects.

Measures of patient satisfaction and health-related quality of life, including the Medical Outcomes Study Short Form-36 (SF-36) [32], have been integrated into some RCTs comparing medical therapy for HMB with surgery. An RCT from Aberdeen's Royal Infirmary in Scotland randomized women with HMB-E to either medical therapy or REA and found that bleeding and pain were significantly reduced by both surgical and medical therapy, but those treated with surgery were more likely to be totally satisfied (76% vs 27%), and to find the intervention acceptable (93% vs 36%) [33] (Class I-2). It is worth noting that the highly effective LNG-IUS was not one of the medical interventions, but these studies serve to underscore the fact that "success" with respect to bleeding may not translate into success for the patient.

Surgery for HMB-E and HMB/AUB-O

Surgery for chronic AUB-E and AUB-O is generally utilized when medical therapy fails, is not tolerated by the woman, or because of patient or surgeon choice.

Endometrial ablation

Surgery that attempts selective destruction of the endometrium is commonly known as endometrial ablation (EA). Endometrial ablation performed under direct vision with a resectoscope, termed *resectoscopic endometrial ablation* (REA), was introduced in the late 1980s as a surgical alternative to hysterectomy for women with chronic HMB with the potential advantages of shortened hospital stay, absence of surgical incisions, and subsequent rapid return to normal activity (Video 15.1, 15.2, 15.3). Early EA studies demonstrated that optimal outcomes with REA required a level of skill and experience that may not be achieved by the average surgeon. Consequently *nonresectoscopic endometrial ablation* (NREA) techniques were reintroduced in the later 1990s; these procedures were conceived much earlier with the first reports noted in the late 1800s [34] and the first series published in the 1930s [35]. Currently available NREA devices include those using hypothermic techniques (cryotherapy, Video 15.6) and those that destroy tissue by elevating temperature using radiofrequency (RF) electricity (Video 15.4), microwaves (Video 15.8), or heated fluid, either freely flowing (Video 15.5) or contained in a balloon (Video 15.7). Detailed discussion of EA techniques and devices is found in Chapter 15. In this section I will deal with the clinical effectiveness of the techniques.

Effectiveness of endometrial ablation

For the clinician, it is important to understand the clinical utility of EA compared to alternative approaches to HMB including both medical therapy and surgical techniques, especially hysterectomy. In addition, given the relative plethora of available techniques, there should be an understanding of the relative performance of one EA technique to another.

Resectoscopic endometrial ablation compared to hysterectomy

Comparisons of REA to hysterectomy are probably best accomplished in the context of RCTs, although it should be understood that women who choose to participate in such studies likely have important differences from those who would rather select their surgical intervention. At this time, there exist six RCTs comparing EA to hysterectomy; four from the United Kingdom [36–39], one from Italy [40], and one from North America [41] that collectively comprise the core of the Cochrane Systematic Review [42] (Class I-1).

Although satisfaction with REA is high, it is, on average, slightly lower than that associated with hysterectomy, which is the only approach guaranteed to produce amenorrhea. It should be noted that women vary somewhat with respect to their desire for amenorrhea – some see it as a primary goal while others would prefer to continue to menstruate, albeit with normal flow [43]. Women treated by REA have shorter hospital stays, fewer postoperative complications, and resume normal activities much earlier than those who undergo hysterectomy. In the 2 RCTs with 4 years of follow up, assignment to EA was associated with accumulating re-operation rates, either with repeat ablation or hysterectomy, reaching 30–40% at 4 years [41, 44] (Class I-2). Both hysterectomy and EA were associated with positive outcomes with respect to mental health and depressive symptoms, and, importantly, there were no apparent differences in postprocedural sexual function.

Some of these trials have been designed to compare the direct and indirect resources consumed in delivering the two procedures. *Direct costs* are those immediately associated with the procedure such as institutional fees, professional services, and equipment and supplies, *indirect costs* are those associated with items such as lost income, job replacement, and child care, for example. In the Aberdeen RCT the direct costs of EA were about half that of hysterectomy within months of the procedure [44] (Class I-2). However as the frequency of visits and reoperation increased, the two became virtually equivalent at four years. Nevertheless, although indirect costs vary widely with the patient's economic situation, the Aberdeen trial suggests that it is likely that those associated with EA likely remain substantially lower than for hysterectomy.

Comparisons of NREA devices to REA

Hyperthermic balloons (Video 15.7): There are four such devices available worldwide, although by far the Thermachoice® (Ethicon Inc, Somerville, NJ, USA) device, currently in its third embodiment, is the most commonly used. Balloon ablation was compared to REA in a RCT involving 275 subjects using the original ("Thermachoice I") device [45]. At 1 year, patient satisfaction and success rates were equally good, but amenorrhea rates were higher for REA (27.2%) than for Thermachoice (15.2%). At 5 years, with only half of the original group available for evaluation, 21 of the evaluable women in each group had undergone hysterectomy; 3 and 2 respectively underwent repeat ablation [46]. For any study with the high attrition (loss to follow up) that is reported based on the evaluable patients, there exists the possibility that there is selection bias and that repeat surgery rates could be higher in the subset of women not available for evaluation, in this instance up to five years after the original surgery. We also do not know the ovulatory status of these patients and there was no assessment for coagulopathy, factors that may impact outcome.

A single-institutional RCT from the Netherlands also compared Thermachoice with rollerball ablation in 137 patients who appear to have HMB-E [47] (Class I-2). At 24 months the reduction in bleeding was greater with balloon ablation but success and satisfaction rates (REA 75%; Thermachoice 80%) were equivalent.

Complications in these two studies were lower in the balloon ablation groups; in the US trial there were very few minor complications with balloon ablation, while with REA both uterine perforation and fluid overload were far more common.

There is a relative paucity of information regarding the performance of the Thermachoice device in women with abnormal endometrial cavities, particularly those distorted by leiomyomas, but one RCT demonstrated equivalence in patients with type II myomas (< 50% of diameter within the endometrial cavity) that were up to 3 cm in diameter [48] (Class I-2).

Hyperthermic free fluid (Hydro ThermAblator®, BEI Medical/Boston Scientific, Natick, MA, USA) (Video 15.5): To date, only one trial has been published comparing the Hydro ThermAblator (HTA®) to REA [49, 50] (Class I-2). Despite the potential for this device to treat women with submucosal myomas and other abnormally configured cavities, those enrolled in the trial all had a normal endometrial cavity. At 3 years, satisfaction was high for the patients in both groups (98% HTA; 97% REA) and hysterectomy was performed in 16 (9%) of the HTA group and 5 (6%) of the REA patients. There were 3 repeat ablations in each group – 2% of the HTA patients and 4% of the REA group. Complications seemed to be limited to those involving the cervix and vagina where leaking heated fluid can be associated with burns that are generally minor.

Cryotherapy (Her Option®, American Medical Systems Inc, Minnetonka, MN, USA) (Video 15.6): Published data regarding the device has been limited to a single RCT on 279 subjects (193 allocated to cryoablation) with endometrial cavities that were normal and which sounded to 10 cm or less. At 12 months, 84.6% of the cryoablation patients had a successful outcome, similar to those undergoing REA (88.9%) [51] (Class I-2). Evaluation of the two-year outcomes is difficult as amenorrhea rates are not reported. However, the investigators reported that 7.0% of the cryoablation group and 8.1% of the REA group underwent hysterectomy in the followup period, while repeat ablations were performed on 8.1% and 1.2% respectively [52]. These 2-year outcomes must also be considered in the context of a relatively high attrition rate, with less than 50% of the original cohort available for followup at 2 years.

Microwave endometrial ablation (MEA®, Microsulis Medical Ltd, Pompano Beach, FL, USA) (Video 15.8): A number of high quality RCTs have compared MEA to endometrial resection with outcomes published at one [53], two [54], and five years [55] (Class I-2). At 5 years, for 236 of the original 263 women available for follow up, bleeding and pain scores both were significantly reduced and amenorrhea rates were similar (MEA 65%; REA 69%), but those assigned MEA were more likely to be satisfied with therapy than those who underwent REA (86% vs 74%). Another high quality RCT performed in North America compared microwave ablation to REA and showed similar one-year results [56].

These trials allowed subjects with submucus myomas up to 3 cm in diameter provided that they did not interfere with the positioning of the probe; analysis of this subgroup suggested that, success, amenorrhea, and patient satisfaction rates did not differ from those experienced by women with normally configured endometrial cavities.

Radiofrequency bipolar (NovaSure®, Cytyc Surgical Division of Hologic Inc, Marlborough, MA, USA) (Video 15.4): The NovaSure device has been subjected to prospective observational studies [57, 58] and RCTs, comparing the device with REA [59] and other NREA techniques [60] (Class I-2). Success rates, as defined by the study (PBAC scores ≤ 75) are experienced, at least in the short term, by 90% of patients, but there are relatively few studies beyond 1 year.

Comparisons of one NREA device to another

Although there are abundant trials comparing REA to NREA techniques, there are only a few comparative studies involving two or more NREA devices. Cavaterm® (PNN Medical A/S, Kvistgard, Denmark) has been compared to NovaSure in 57 women; at 1 year, NovaSure was associated with a higher amenorrhea rate (43% to 11%) and, paradoxically, an increased failure rate (13% to 0%) [61] (Class I-2). The authors note that there were problems with the generator unit in three of the five women undergoing NovaSure ablation who went on to have hysterectomy. There were no hysterectomies in the followup period in the Cavaterm group.

Another RCT compared NovaSure and the original Thermachoice device in 126 subjects in a trial also plagued by a NovaSure generator problem discovered mid-study. The rate of amenorrhea in the entire cohort in the NovaSure group was 43% (34/83) and for those assigned to Thermachoice 6% (3/43). When the patients treated prior to changing the generator were excluded, 56% of those treated with NovaSure experienced amenorrhea, a proportion that is consistent with the results obtained in other RCTs [60] (Class I-2).

Comparisons of NREA and LNG-IUS

There are now a number of RCTs comparing NREA to the LNG-IUS in women with HMB-E that show outcomes to be quite similar. When Thermachoice was the NREA, 12-month followup showed that both interventions were successful, although post-treatment bleeding volume was 5% of baseline for REA and 13% of baseline for the LNG-IUS. Quality of life scores were not quite as high in the LNG-IUS group in some sections of the assessment but similar in most suggesting that women were generally equally happy with both interventions [18] (Class I-2). A New Zealand study that randomized 79 women to the LNG-IUS or Thermachoice found that the 24-month bleeding scores were lower in the LNG-IUS group and the amenorrhea rates were higher, but that there were no differences in patient satisfaction and health-related quality of life scales [62].

Microwave endometrial ablation was compared to the LNG-IUS in a retrospective study of 62 patients published in 2002 [19] (Class II-2). Both interventions were effective with an average followup of 14 months, and there were no differences in quality of life outcomes.

A recent modified Cochrane Systematic Review has compared the randomized trials involving oral medical therapy, the LNG-IUS, REA, and hysterectomy [63] (Class I-1). Aside from noting that oral therapy suits only a minority of women long term, the LNG-IUS, REA, and hysterectomy were all equivalent with respect to satisfaction and quality of life outcomes.

It is evident that the LNG-IUS is a compelling competitor for both REA and NREA. Convenience and cost are but two important factors. The device can almost always be inserted in a relatively brief office visit rather than in the context of an operating room, such as is the case for REA. It is less expensive than a NREA device, but, because each device lasts only five years, repeated insertions would erode cost advantages to a degree.

Hysterectomy

Approximately 550, 000 hysterectomies are performed each year in the United States, making it the second most common surgery performed. The proportion of hysterectomies estimated to be for HMB-E and AUB-O has been reported at 4.5–40%, a range that reflects differences in such diverse factors such as procedure coding and patterns of practice. Indeed, there is evidence that a large proportion of hysterectomies may be done inappropriately, or at least without adequate investigation or attempts at medical therapy or less invasive surgical options [64]. Discussion of the various hysterectomy techniques and the potential advantages and disadvantages of each is found in Chapter 17.

Summary for HMB-E and HMB/AUB-O

Medical therapy has the potential to improve symptoms in the short or long term for a number of women; however, it is clear that it is not for everyone. For many women the treatments simply do not work, or do not work adequately well enough to justify continuing their use. Nevertheless, most women deserve the opportunity to at least attempt medical therapy before they commit themselves to a surgical approach that removes the opportunity for future pregnancy. An important option to consider for such women is the use of the LNG-IUS, which seems to demonstrate roughly equivalent efficacy and satisfaction to EA without the loss of reproductive function at least in women with HMB-E, and possibly for those with HMB-O.

Available evidence suggests that EA significantly reduces menstrual blood flow and, in most instances, decreases secondary dysmenorrhea. However, it is clear that while most women are likely satisfied with their choice of EA, many women subsequently choose or require either additional EA or hysterectomy. There are many factors that may influence ultimate patient satisfaction. If her goal is amenorrhea, and she has other symptoms that are less likely reduced by EA, then it is possible that she will be happier with a hysterectomy. Although women under 45 will likely be satisfied with EA, they are less likely to be so than women who have the procedure after their 45th birthday.

References

1. Auerbach M, Ballard H, Glaspy J. Clinical update: intravenous iron for anaemia. *Lancet.* 2007;**369**(9572):1502–4.

2. Cooke I, Lethaby A, Farquhar C. Antifibrinolytics for heavy menstrual bleeding. *Cochrane Database Syst Rev.* 2000;**2**:CD000249.

3. Lindoff C, Rybo G, Astedt B. Treatment with tranexamic acid during pregnancy, and the risk of thrombo-embolic complications. *Thromb Haemost.* 1993;**70**(2):238–40.

4. Rees MC, DiMarzo V, Tippins JR, Morris HR, Turnbull AC. Leukotriene release by endometrium and myometrium throughout the menstrual cycle in dysmenorrhoea and menorrhagia. *J Endocrinol.* 1987;**113**(2):291–5.

5. Rees MC, Canete-Soler R, Lopez Bernal A, Turnbull AC. Effect of fenamates on prostaglandin E receptor binding. *Lancet.* 1988;**2**(8610):541–2.

6. Lethaby A, Augood C, Duckitt K. Nonsteroidal anti-inflammatory drugs for heavy menstrual bleeding. *Cochrane Database Syst Rev.* 2002;**1**:CD000400.

7. Cameron IT, Leask R, Kelly RW, Baird DT. The effects of danazol, mefenamic acid, norethisterone and a progesterone-impregnated coil on endometrial prostaglandin concentrations in women with menorrhagia. *Prostaglandins.* 1987;**34**(1):99–110.

8. Andersch B, Milsom I, Rybo G. An objective evaluation of flurbiprofen and tranexamic acid in the treatment of idiopathic menorrhagia. *Acta Obstet Gynecol Scand.* 1988;**67**(7):645–8.

9. Fraser IS. Treatment of ovulatory and anovulatory dysfunctional uterine bleeding with oral progestogens. *Aust N Z J Obstet Gynaecol.* 1990;**30**(4):353–6.

10. Preston JT, Cameron IT, Adams EJ, Smith SK. Comparative study of tranexamic acid and norethisterone in the treatment of ovulatory menorrhagia. *Br J Obstet Gynaecol.* 1995;**102**(5):401–6.

11. Higham JM, Shaw RW. A comparative study of danazol, a regimen of decreasing doses of danazol, and norethindrone in the treatment of objectively proven unexplained menorrhagia. *Am J Obstet Gynecol.* 1993;**169**(5):1134–9.

12. Lethaby A, Irvine G, Cameron I. Cyclical progestogens for heavy menstrual bleeding. *Cochrane Database Syst Rev.* 2008;**1**: CD001016.

13. Irvine GA, Campbell-Brown MB, Lumsden MA, Heikkila A, Walker JJ, Cameron IT. Randomised comparative trial of the levonorgestrel intrauterine system and norethisterone for treatment of idiopathic menorrhagia. *Br J Obstet Gynaecol.* 1998;**105**(6):592–8.

14. Andersson JK, Rybo G. Levonorgestrel-releasing intrauterine device in the treatment of menorrhagia. *Br J Obstet Gynaecol.* 1990;**97**(8):690–4.

15. Milsom I, Andersson K, Andersch B, Rybo G. A comparison of flurbiprofen, tranexamic acid, and a levonorgestrel-releasing intrauterine contraceptive device in the treatment of idiopathic menorrhagia. *Am J Obstet Gynecol.* 1991;**164**(3):879–83.

16. Crosignani PG, Vercellini P, Mosconi P, Oldani S, Cortesi I, De Giorgi O. Levonorgestrel-releasing intrauterine device versus hysteroscopic endometrial resection in the treatment of dysfunctional uterine bleeding. *Obstet Gynecol.* 1997; **90**(2):257–63.

17. Rauramo I, Elo I, Istre O. Long-term treatment of menorrhagia with levonorgestrel intrauterine system versus endometrial resection. *Obstet Gynecol.* 2004;**104**(6):1314–21.

18. Soysal M, Soysal S, Ozer S. A randomized controlled trial of levonorgestrel releasing IUD and thermal balloon ablation in the treatment of menorrhagia. *Zentralbl Gynakol.* 2002;**124**(4):213–19.

19. Henshaw R, Coyle C, Low S, Barry C. A retrospective cohort study comparing microwave endometrial ablation with levonorgestrel-releasing intrauterine device in the management of heavy menstrual bleeding. *Aust N Z J Obstet Gynaecol.* 2002;**42**(2):205–9.

20. Lahteenmaki P, Haukkamaa M, Puolakka J, Riikonen U, Sainio S, Suvisaari J, et al. Open randomised study of use of levonorgestrel releasing intrauterine system as alternative to hysterectomy. *BMJ.* 1998;**316**(7138):1122–6.

21. Hurskainen R, Teperi J, Rissanen P, Aalto AM, Grenman S, Kivela A, et al. Clinical outcomes and costs with the levonorgestrel-releasing intrauterine system or hysterectomy for treatment of menorrhagia: randomized trial 5-year follow-up. *JAMA*. 2004; **291**(12):1456–63.

22. Bahamondes L, Petta CA, Fernandes A, Monteiro I. Use of the levonorgestrel-releasing intrauterine system in women with endometriosis, chronic pelvic pain and dysmenorrhea. *Contraception*. 2007; 75(6 Suppl):S134–9.

23. Fraser IS, McCarron G. Randomized trial of two hormonal and two prostaglandin-inhibiting agents in women with a complaint of menorrhagia. *Aust N Z J Obstet Gynaecol*. 1991;**31**(1):66–70.

24. Davis A, Godwin A, Lippman J, Olson W, Kafrissen M. Triphasic norgestimate-ethinyl estradiol for treating dysfunctional uterine bleeding. *Obstet Gynecol*. 2000; **96**(6):913–20.

25. Shrader SP, Dickerson LM. Extended- and continuous-cycle oral contraceptives. *Pharmacotherapy*. 2008;**28**(8):1033–40.

26. Dockeray CJ, Sheppard BL, Bonnar J. Comparison between mefenamic acid and danazol in the treatment of established menorrhagia. *Br J Obstet Gynaecol*. 1989; **96**(7):840–4.

27. Chimbira TH, Anderson AB, Naish C, Cope E, Turnbull AC. Reduction of menstrual blood loss by danazol in unexplained menorrhagia: lack of effect of placebo. *Br J Obstet Gynaecol*. 1980;**87** (12):1152–8.

28. Bonduelle M, Walker JJ, Calder AA. A comparative study of danazol and norethisterone in dysfunctional uterine bleeding presenting as menorrhagia. *Postgrad Med J*. 1991;**67**(791):833–6.

29. Srivastava A, Mansel RE, Arvind N, Prasad K, Dhar A, Chabra A. Evidence-based management of Mastalgia: a meta-analysis of randomised trials. *Breast*. 2007; **16**(5):503–12.

30. Mais V, Cossu E, Angioni S, Piras B, Floris L, Melis GB. Abnormal uterine bleeding: medical treatment with vaginal danazol and five-year follow-up. *J Am Assoc Gynecol Laparosc*. 2004;**11**(3):340–3.

31. Thomas EJ. Add-back therapy for long-term use in dysfunctional uterine bleeding and uterine fibroids. *Br J Obstet Gynaecol*. 1996;**103**(Suppl 14):18–21.

32. Anderson RT, Aaronson NK, Bullinger M, McBee WL. A review of the progress towards developing health-related quality-of-life instruments for international clinical studies and outcomes research. *Pharmacoeconomics*. 1996;**10**(4):336–55.

33. Cooper KG, Parkin DE, Garratt AM, Grant AM. A randomised comparison of medical and hysteroscopic management in women consulting a gynaecologist for treatment of heavy menstrual loss. *Br J Obstet Gynaecol*. 1997;**104**(12):1360–6.

34. Fritsch HI. Uterusvapokauterisation, tod durch septische peritonitis nach spontaner sekundarer perforation. *Centralblatt fur Gynakologie*. 1898;**52**:1409–18.

35. Bardenheuer F. Elektrokoagulation der Uterusschleimhaut zur Behandlungklimakterischer Blutungen. *Zentralblatt fur Gynakologie*. 1937;**4**: 209–11.

36. Gannon DM, Lombardi AV, Jr., Mallory TH, Vaughn BK, Finney CR, Niemcryk S. An evaluation of the efficacy of postoperative blood salvage after total joint arthroplasty. A prospective randomized trial. *J Arthroplasty*. 1991;**6**(2):109–14.

37. Dwyer N, Hutton J, Stirrat GM. Randomised controlled trial comparing endometrial resection with abdominal hysterectomy for the surgical treatment of menorrhagia. *Br J Obstet Gynaecol*. 1993;**100**(3):237–43.

38. Pinion SB, Parkin DE, Abramovich DR, Naji A, Alexander DA, Russell IT, et al. Randomised trial of hysterectomy, endometrial laser ablation, and transcervical endometrial resection for dysfunctional uterine bleeding. *BMJ*. 1994;**309**(6960):979–83.

39. O'Connor H, Broadbent JA, Magos AL, McPherson K. Medical Research Council randomised trial of endometrial resection versus hysterectomy in management of menorrhagia. *Lancet*. 1997;**349**(9056):897–901.

40. Crosignani PG, Vercellini P, Apolone G, De Giorgi O, Cortesi I, Meschia M. Endometrial resection versus vaginal

hysterectomy for menorrhagia: long-term clinical and quality-of-life outcomes. *Am J Obstet Gynecol.* 1997;**177**(1):95–101.

41. Dickersin K, Munro MG, Clark M, Langenberg P, Scherer R, Frick K, et al. Hysterectomy compared with endometrial ablation for dysfunctional uterine bleeding: a randomized controlled trial. *Obstet Gynecol.* 2007;**110**(6):1279–89.

42. Lethaby A, Hickey M, Garry R. Endometrial destruction techniques for heavy menstrual bleeding. *Cochrane Database Syst Rev.* 2005;**4**:CD001501.

43. Sculpher M. The cost-effectiveness of preference-based treatment allocation: the case of hysterectomy versus endometrial resection in the treatment of menorrhagia. *Health Econ.* 1998;**7**(2):129–42.

44. Aberdeen Endometrial Ablation Trials Group. A randomised trial of endometrial ablation versus hysterectomy for the treatment of dysfunctional uterine bleeding: outcome at four years. *Br J Obstet Gynaecol.* 1999;**106**(4):360–6.

45. Meyer WR, Walsh BW, Grainger DA, Peacock LM, Loffer FD, Steege JF. Thermal balloon and rollerball ablation to treat menorrhagia: a multicenter comparison. *Obstet Gynecol.* 1998;**92**(1):98–103.

46. Loffer FD, Grainger D. Five-year follow-up of patients participating in a randomized trial of uterine balloon therapy versus rollerball ablation for treatment of menorrhagia. *J Am Assoc Gynecol Laparosc.* 2002;**9**(4):429–35.

47. Van Zon-Rabelink IA, Vleugels MP, Merkus HM, De Graaf R. Efficacy and satisfaction rate comparing endometrial ablation by rollerball electrocoagulation to uterine balloon thermal ablation in a randomised controlled trial. *Eur J Obstet Gynecol Reprod Biol.* 2004;**114**(1):97–103.

48. Soysal ME, Soysal SK, Vicdan K. Thermal balloon ablation in myoma-induced menorrhagia under local anesthesia. *Gynecol Obstet Invest.* 2001;**51**(2):128–33.

49. Corson SL. A multicenter evaluation of endometrial ablation by Hydro ThermAblator and rollerball for treatment of menorrhagia. *J Am Assoc Gynecol Laparosc.* 2001;**8**(3):359–67.

50. Goldrath MH. Evaluation of Hydro ThermAblator and rollerball endometrial

ablation for menorrhagia three years after treatment. *J Am Assoc Gynecol Laparosc.* 2003;**10**(4):505–11.

51. Duleba AJ, Heppard MC, Soderstrom RM, Townsend DE. A randomized study comparing endometrial cryoablation and rollerball electroablation for treatment of dysfunctional uterine bleeding. *J Am Assoc Gynecol Laparosc.* 2003;**10**(1):17–26.

52. Townsend DE, Duleba AJ, Wilkes MM. Durability of treatment effects after endometrial cryoablation versus rollerball electroablation for abnormal uterine bleeding: two-year results of a multicenter randomized trial. *Am J Obstet Gynecol.* 2003;**188**(3):699–701.

53. Cooper KG, Bain C, Parkin DE. Comparison of microwave endometrial ablation and transcervical resection of the endometrium for treatment of heavy menstrual loss: a randomised trial. *Lancet.* 1999;**354**(9193):1859–63.

54. Bain C, Cooper KG, Parkin DE. Microwave endometrial ablation versus endometrial resection: a randomized controlled trial. *Obstet Gynecol.* 2002;**99**(6):983–7.

55. Cooper KG, Bain C, Lawrie L, Parkin DE. A randomised comparison of microwave endometrial ablation with transcervical resection of the endometrium; follow up at a minimum of five years. *BJOG.* 2005;**112**(4):470–5.

56. Cooper JM, Anderson TL, Fortin CA, Jack SA, Plentl MB. Microwave endometrial ablation vs. rollerball electroablation for menorrhagia: a multicenter randomized trial. *J Am Assoc Gynecol Laparosc.* 2004;**11**(3):394–403.

57. Gallinat A, Nugent W. NovaSure impedance-controlled system for endometrial ablation. *J Am Assoc Gynecol Laparosc.* 2002;**9**(3):283–9.

58. Baskett TF, Clough H, Scott TA. NovaSure bipolar radiofrequency endometrial ablation: report of 200 cases. *J Obstet Gynaecol Can.* 2005;**27**(5):473–6.

59. Cooper J, Gimpelson R, Laberge P, Galen D, Garza-Leal JG, Scott J, et al. A randomized, multicenter trial of safety and efficacy of the NovaSure system in the treatment of menorrhagia. *J Am Assoc Gynecol Laparosc.* 2002;**9**(4):418–28.

87

60. Bongers MY, Bourdrez P, Mol BW, Heintz AP, Brolmann HA. Randomised controlled trial of bipolar radio-frequency endometrial ablation and balloon endometrial ablation. *BJOG*. 2004;**111**(10):1095–102.

61. Abbott J, Hawe J, Hunter D, Garry R. A double-blind randomized trial comparing the Cavaterm and the NovaSure endometrial ablation systems for the treatment of dysfunctional uterine bleeding. *Fertil Steril*. 2003;**80**(1):203–8.

62. Busfield RA, Farquhar CM, Sowter MC, Lethaby A, Sprecher M, Yu Y, et al. A randomised trial comparing the levonorgestrel intrauterine system and thermal balloon ablation for heavy menstrual bleeding. *BJOG*. 2006; **113**(3):257–63.

63. Marjoribanks J, Lethaby A, Farquhar C. Surgery versus medical therapy for heavy menstrual bleeding. *Cochrane Database Syst Rev*. 2006;**2**:CD003855.

64. Broder MS, Goodwin S, Chen G, Tang LJ, Costantino MM, Nguyen MH, et al. Comparison of long-term outcomes of myomectomy and uterine artery embolization. *Obstet Gynecol*. 2002; **100**(5 Pt 1):864–8.

Therapy: structural abnormalities (AUB-P, -A, -L)

Chapter summary

- It is important for the clinician to attempt to distinguish between structural lesions that contribute to the AUB and those that are asymptomatic, particularly adenomyosis and leiomyomas that do not involve the endometrial cavity.
- When AUB exists in the presence of asymptomatic structural lesions, interventions effective for other causes of AUB, such as AUB-E and -O should be considered.
- There are a number of evolving medical interventions for leiomyomas that include aromatase inhibitors and selective progesterone receptor modulators.
- Surgery for leiomyomas is not justified by the risk of leiomyosarcoma, which is present in less than 0.1% of cases of myomectomy or hysterectomy.
- When feasible as determined by size and involvement of the myometrium, resectoscopic myomectomy is an intervention with long-term clinical effectiveness.
- There are a number of targeted surgical interventions for leiomyomas, but, excepting myomectomy, none have undergone extensive clinical investigation.

Introduction

When the cause of chronic AUB is determined to be a structural abnormality (AUB-P, -A, -L), a number of factors must be considered when developing the menu of options for the patient. Typically, AUB related to structural pathology is treated with surgery, but in recent years the value of temporary and even prolonged medical therapy has become more widely appreciated. Indeed, it is now thought that at least some affected women, particularly those in the late reproductive years, will potentially benefit from the long-term use of medical therapy, as an alternative to surgery.

Medical management

Leiomyomas

The use of medical therapy for AUB-L has expanded due to new information regarding the factors that affect myoma growth, the availability of new therapeutic agents, and to a more reasoned understanding of the relationship of leiomyomas to bleeding. In Chapter 5 we learned that while myomas frequently cause or contribute to the genesis of AUB, the majority is asymptomatic. Consequently, AUB from other causes (e.g., AUB-E, -O, and/ or -C) can coexist with these asymptomatic leiomyomas, making it important for the clinician to evaluate the endometrial cavity with sonography, SIS, and/or hysteroscopy. Most agree that myomas which involve the endometrial cavity (AUB-Ls) can cause bleeding, while those that are not submucosal (AUB-Lo) are unlikely to be actual causes of AUB (Chapter 5).

Gonadotropin releasing hormone agonists

The role that GnRH has in the regulation of pituitary gonadotropin release, and ovarian steroidogenesis and ovulation, has been discussed in Chapter 3. Following delineation of the molecular structure of GnRH, a number of synthetic analogs (gonadotropin releasing hormone agonists, or GnRHa) of the decapeptide were produced in the 1980s. When GnRHa are administered in a continuous fashion (unlike the physiological pulsatile release found in vivo) the result is initially a "flare" of FSH and LH that travels to the ovary elevating serum levels of 17-β estradiol, a circumstance that frequently contributes to an episode of iatrogenic HUB. Following the initial flare, pituitary GnRH receptors are downregulated, and there is a resulting drop in the levels of both FSH and LH that is quickly followed by a corresponding reduction in circulating levels of 17-β estradiol. Absent ovulation, progesterone levels are low as well. The end result is a medically induced hypogonadotrophic or menopausal state that can be exploited for the purposes of therapy for women with AUB, especially those with leiomyomas.

Gonadotropin releasing hormone agonists may be applied in a number of strategic fashions, ranging from short-term courses in preparation for surgery, to longer term use that may even preempt the need for operative intervention. In addition to amenorrhea, GnRHa results in a reduction of both leiomyoma and total uterine volume by a mean of about 50% by 12 weeks. This is a temporary outcome, however, as the volume of both the uterus and myoma return to baseline levels within a few months of discontinuation of therapy. Although GnRHa causes typical side effects of hypoestrogenemia, including vasomotor symptoms and vaginal atrophy, the only concerning adverse outcome is that of osteopenia and osteoporosis which may be significant if therapy is prolonged more than six months [1]. This reduction in bone density can be mitigated with the use of so-called "add-back" therapy with an estrogen, selected types of progestins, or estrogen-progestin combination therapy [2] (Class I-2) (Table 9.1).

Table 9.1 Add-back regimens for prolonged gonadotropin releasing hormone agonist (GnRHa) therapy. These approaches are options for symptomatic (e.g., vasomotor, dry vagina) women who use GnRHa for up to six months, but it is possible that progestin-containing regimens might reduce the impact of the agonist on myoma and uterine volume. For the selected women who use GnRHa for more than six months, one of these regimens is recommended for maintenance of bone density.

Type	Agent(s)	Route	Dose
Estrogen only	CEE	Oral	0.625–1.25 mg/day
	Estradiol	Oral	0.5–1.0 mg/day
	Estradiol	Transdermal	50–100 µg/day
Progestin only	Norethindrone	Oral	5 mg/day
	Norethindrone acetate	Oral	5 mg/day
Estrogen + progestin	CEE + cyclic MPA	Oral	CEE: 0.625–1.25 mg/day
			MPA: 10 mg × 14 days q 1–3 months

CEE, conjugated equine estrogen; MPA, medroxyprogesterone acetate.

There has been some concern regarding the most appropriate add-back regimen for women with AUB-L. Estrogens have the potential for exacerbating the bleeding process, while progestins may impede or negate the volume reduction effect of GnRHa. High quality evidence shows that low dose estradiol (estradiol valerate 2 mg/day) and cyclical norethisterone (equivalent to norethindrone) prevented this bone loss [3] (Class I-2). However, progestin-only regimens have been associated with a lack of reduction in uterine volume [4, 5], or even increase in volume [6], apparently confirming the influence of progestins on myoma growth (each Class I-2). In the other long-term study of GnRHa therapy, Maheux et al. found that total uterine volume reduced by 49.3% in the first 3 months, and then remained stable for the next 9 months despite being on an estrogen-progestin-based add-back regimen [7].

Facilitate correction of anemia

Short-term use (two to three months) of GnRHa provides an opportunity for the anemic woman to reconstitute her circulating hemoglobin levels and at least start replenishing iron stores without resorting to either blood transfusion or emergency surgery [8, 9] (Class I-2). By ameliorating fatigue, the woman has the opportunity to select long-term medical or surgical therapy in a less stressed environment. For the women who have decided on an operative intervention, GnRHa-induced amenorrhea is a way to defer surgery to a more convenient time. For example, a teacher who might otherwise require surgery in February could use GnRH analogs to avert loss of teaching time until July, when school was out.

Typically, patients are given a dose of sustained releasing GnRHa that lasts for 3 months, such as leuprolide acetate 11.25 mg intramuscularly. Although data in the literature are lacking, we administer (or continue) a progestin-based compound for the first three weeks after the first depot GnRHa injection to ameliorate the flare-associated bleeding; potential agents include progestins such as oral MPA (10–20 mg po bid), norethindrone, or norethindrone acetate (5 mg bid to tid), or any of the combination estrogen-progestin contraception products in oral, transdermal, or transvaginal contraceptive formulations.

There may be a lasting impact of GnRHa therapy on women with HMB-L. A study on women who had completed six months GnRHa randomized the subjects to either placebo or MPA and found that a majority (about 55%) of each group experienced an improvement in their bleeding for months following discontinuation of agonist [10] (Class I-2). This evidence suggests that prolonged GnRHa may have prolonged therapeutic benefit in women with HMB-L, making the use of intermittent courses a potential nonsurgical strategy for women in the late reproductive years.

Reduction in uterine and myoma volume

Using GnRHa to reduce uterine volume may facilitate the performance of some surgical procedures in selected patients. Stovall et al. found that 80% of women scheduled for hysterectomy with uteri greater than 14-weeks size were able to undergo vaginal hysterectomy if GnRHa was administered for the three months immediately prior to surgery [11] (Class II-1). Such an approach may also have merit in facilitating laparoscopic hysterectomy and even laparoscopic supracervical hysterectomy, the latter by reducing the time for laparoscopically-directed morcellation, although there have been no clinical trials evaluating this hypothesis.

Long-term GnRHa may be valuable for women unsuitable for surgery for medical reasons, or because there have been multiple previous pelvic surgical procedures that substantially elevate the risk of surgery. For some of these women, and particularly those who are near the time of menopause, prolonged use of GnRHa may justify the expense.

Reduced surgical complications

There is evidence that preoperative GnRHa may reduce the duration and risks of resectoscopic removal of submucosal leiomyomas. Systemic intravasation of the uterine distention medial is less, surgical time is reduced, and surgeons characterize the procedures as being easier to perform [12, 13] (Class II-2, I-2). There also exists data that shows reduced blood loss associated with abdominal myomectomy; however, the absence of a difference in the incidence of blood transfusions makes the use of GnRHa in this setting of questionable value [4].

Progestins

There is no currently available evidence regarding the use of systemic progestins for women with AUB-Ls, but there is evidence that the LNG-IUS may be effective in selected patients. A prospective but nonrandomized clinical trial included women with AUB-Ls with a sonographically determined uterine volume less than 380 mL but at least one type II submucosal leiomyoma 5 cm or less, and no type 0 or type I lesions greater than 3 cm [14] (Class III). The reduction in menstrual blood loss at 3, 6, and 12 months post insertion reached 90%, comparable with that of a group of women treated in the same center using a thermal balloon, and expulsion rates were about 5%.

Another group evaluated the impact of the LNG-IUS on women with leiomyomas without determining the relationship of those myomas to the endometrial cavity, and showed high efficacy, but, given the absence of endometrial cavity evaluation it is likely that this study included many with HMB-E [15].

Further study is required, but it would seem that the LNG-IUS is a reasonable option for women with modestly enlarged uteri and at least selected type II leiomyomas. However, for very enlarged cavities the clinical impression remains that therapeutic efficacy is less and spontaneous expulsion more common.

Antiprogestins

In Chapter 5 the critical role of progesterone in the growth and development of leiomyomas was discussed [16–18]. The selective progesterone receptor modulator (SPRM) mifepristone, 5 mg/day, is capable of dramatically reducing or eliminating bleeding while reducing the volume of leiomyomas by about 50%, with few side effects [19–21] (Class I-2). Endometrial hyperplasia was an occasional complication with higher doses of mifepristone, but seems uncommon at the 5 mg dose. Larger scale clinical trials will be necessary to further elucidate the cost effectiveness of this approach. It is anticipated that other antiprogestins will be available within the next few years that will have similar effects on myomas and bleeding related or unrelated, with little incidence of endometrial hyperplasia.

Aromatase inhibitors

Aromatase inhibitors reduce the conversion of androgens to estrogens in the ovary and in peripheral tissues. As a result of this reduced systemic estrogenic activity, the potential uses for these agents include therapy of AUB-L. Indeed, early evidence suggests that aromatase inhibitors reduce myoma volume in the range of 50% [22, 23] (Class II-3). A RCT from Iran showed that the aromatase inhibitor letrozole was superior to GnRHa in reducing myoma volume, without vasomotor symptoms [24] (Class I-2). The fact that these agents have undergone large scale, long-term clinical trials as adjuvant therapy for women diagnosed with breast cancer makes them interesting options for selected patients at least.

Larger scale trials of aromatase inhibitors and associafed their utility in the treatment of AUB-L and associated bulk symptoms are anticipated.

Adenomyosis

The enigmatic nature of adenomyosis and its variable relationship to the genesis of AUB was discussed in Chapter 5, while diagnosis of the disorder was a topic of Chapter 6. There is now a substantial amount of data demonstrating the utility of the LNG-IUS for the treatment of adenomyosis-associated symptoms of dysmenorrhea and HMB [25] (Class II-3). Multiple studies have shown that a large majority of women with ultrasound and/or MRI-demonstrated adenomyosis establish amenorrhea, oligomenorrhea, spotting, or normal menses. Indeed, there also exists evidence that disease volume, as measured by MRI, reduces proportional to symptoms [25] (Class III).

Inflammation

In Chapter 5 the lack of a known relationship between chronic AUB and inflammatory conditions was discussed. Should *Chlamydia trachomatis* be identified in an individual with AUB, it is, of course, appropriate to treat the patient (and sexual partner) for the sexually transmitted disease and determine if such therapy results in a clinical impact on the AUB. However, the presence of "chronic inflammation" on a pathology report from uterine aspirates or curettings should not translate into a justification for antibiotic therapy.

Procedural interventions

General considerations

Some procedural alternatives preserve or enhance fertility while others impair fertility or render the woman unable to conceive or carry a pregnancy. As with all interventions for disorders that affect lifestyle, the patient's desires are critical components in the process of identifying the correct procedure. Furthermore, it must be recognized that not all clinicians are skilled at, or even able to provide the intervention that may be best for the patient, so a team approach to care is important. The decision-making process for surgical treatment of HMB/AUB secondary to structural pathology is summarized in Figure 9.1.

Polypectomy

Removal of exocervical polyps can be achieved using forceps that either excise or twist off the lesion, usually with relative ease (Chapter 21).

Although there is some controversy regarding the need for removal of asymptomatic endometrial polyps, the rate of malignancy in polyps that are associated with abnormal bleeding ranges from 0.5 to 4.7%, a frequency that clearly justifies routine excision [26, 27]. Such lesions, following identification using SIS or hysteroscopy, can be blindly removed with suitable polyp forceps. However, complete excision is difficult and there is evidence that, with this blind technique, the incidence of recurrence is relatively high [28] (Class II-3) and that it is preferable to remove the lesions under direct hysteroscopic visualization with one or a combination of hysteroscopic scissors (Video 21.1), biopsy forceps, a snare (Video 21.2), or an electrosurgical cutting loop (Video 21.3). Blind removal with grasping forceps was associated with a 15% incidence of recurrence compared to the other techniques at 0–4% [29] (Class II-3).

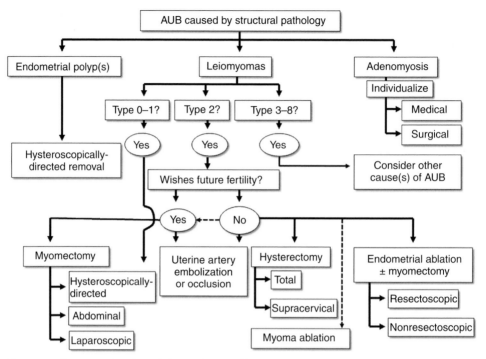

Figure 9.1 Treatment algorithm of abnormal uterine bleeding caused by structural pathology (AUB-P, -A, and -L). Following identification by uterine imaging techniques, the patient is categorized by the type and, if applicable, subtype of lesion(s) identified. Endometrial polyps should be removed by hysteroscopic techniques to reduce the risk of recurrence. Type 0 and most type 1 leiomyomas can be removed resectoscopically. Type 2 leiomyomas require more surgical skill and risk to remove resectoscopically, and more commonly require more than one procedure. In some instances they traverse the myometrium making them most suitable for laparoscopic or laparotomic (abdominal) myomectomy. The impact of uterine artery embolization or occlusion on fertility has yet to be determined, and so, in most instances, this approach should be reserved for women who do not wish for future fertility. Myoma ablation remains an investigational procedure. Endometrial ablation may be useful for selected women with HMB-Ls depending on the size of the endometrial cavity and the size, number, and type of the myoma(s).

Leiomyomas

Myomectomy

Removal of leiomyomas via laparotomy (abdominal myomectomy) was first reported by Atlee in 1845 [30]. The advent of operative endoscopy started with the introduction of hysteroscopically-directed resection of submucosal myomas by Neuwirth and Amin in 1976 [31]. Although Semm and Mettler first described laparoscopic myomectomy [32], Dubuisson et al. published the first series of laparoscopically-directed myomectomies as a potentially less morbid alternative to a laparotomy-based approach [33]. The techniques of myomectomy including abdominal, laparoscopic (Video 20.4), and resectoscopic (Video 20.1, 20.2, 20.3) are discussed and demonstrated in Chapter 20.

Patient selection for myomectomy

As discussed in Chapter 5, the mechanisms by which leiomyomas cause chronic AUB are unknown, but presumed to most often be related to diminished local endometrial hemostasis, likely secondary to one or a combination of alterations in the endometrial vasculature and the local biosynthesis of vasoactive and antifibrinolytic substances. It is perceived, but not proven, that most leiomyomas that cause bleeding do so in the context of distortion of the endometrial cavity (AUB-Ls). Consequently, the clinician should seek to evaluate the endometrial cavity for leiomyomas or other focal lesions using SIS or hysteroscopy, both to confirm that the leiomyoma(s) is/are the likely cause of the bleeding, and to, at least, begin the assessment of the most appropriate approach for removal of the lesions.

Risk of leiomyosarcoma

Many, if not most women are concerned about the risk of malignancy in a leiomyoma, and their perceptions of this risk can have a profound impact on their decisions regarding therapy. Leiomyosarcoma is extremely rare, particularly in premenopausal women, even in the context of rapid enlargement [34, 35]. Leiomyosarcoma likely represents a de novo neoplasm, not a result of malignant transformation of a benign tumor, and is more frequently encountered in the sixth or seventh decade of life where it has been reported to occur in 1.4–1.7% of women undergoing hysterectomy [35].

Understanding that a myoma is almost certainly benign should give confidence to both the patient and her physician that expectant or medical approaches, if effective, are appropriate alternatives to surgery. Furthermore, the use of preoperative GnRHa in selected women who require surgery can be justified. Rapid growth of apparent myomas in post-menopausal women is likely a contraindication to conservative surgical procedures like myomectomy.

Uterine artery embolization or occlusion

Uterine artery embolization (UAE) is the use of interventional radiology to occlude both uterine arteries with polyvinyl alcohol (PVA) microspheres, or similar particles, positioned by a catheter passed through the right femoral artery [36] (Figure 22.1) (Video 22.1). The procedure is generally performed under conscious sedation over a time that typically ranges from 30 to 90 minutes. Immediate post-procedure pain is generally substantial, requiring institutional admission at least overnight, typically with a requirement for narcotic analgesia. In some instances, this pain is experienced in conjunction with fever, nausea, and vomiting – a constellation of symptoms that has been termed *post-embolization syndrome.* Complications are relatively infrequent but include, in addition to the post-embolization syndrome, misembolization of tissues that include the ovary, ureter, and other structures, and infection which has been associated with severe sepsis and, rarely, death. Randomized trials with short-term outcomes do demonstrate that UAE is likely less morbid than hysterectomy, but patients should expect the side effects mentioned above and a readmission rate of 5–10% [37, 38] (Class I-2).

There is evidence that UAE is an effective, long-term solution for most women who select it. In a relatively large study of 200 patients, HMB was substantially reduced in 87% of patients at 3 months and 90% at 12 months of followup [39] (Class II-3). In this same group of patients, the total uterine volume reduced by 27 and 38% at 3 and 12 months respectively. By five years, 73% had continued symptom control with 13.7 and 4.4% undergoing hysterectomy and myomectomy respectively [40]. Another US registry that includes more than 2100 women has reported high degrees of satisfaction with the procedure and 3-year post-procedure hysterectomy and myomectomy rates of 9.8% and 2.8% respectively [41].

Perhaps the most extensive review of UAE has been published in 2004 by the Royal College of Obstetricians and Gynaecologists in the United Kingdom (Class I-1). In this analysis of 32 papers representing 25 series of cases, mean uterine volume and dominant fibroid volume reduced 26–50% and 40–75% respectively at 6 months following the procedure, and marked improvement in bleeding was experienced by 60–90% of those treated [42]. Finally, a Cochrane Review of the three RCTs concluded that UAE offers an alternative option to hysterectomy, and, in some instances, myomectomy; that it is associated with reduced institutional stay and faster return to normal activities; and that overall satisfaction was equal to that of hysterectomy, but unscheduled visits related to pain, fever, and discharge were more common [43].

The issue of fertility following UAE is still under investigation. It is clear that conception and successful term delivery can occur following UAE, but what is not clear is the incidence of infertility and of myoma-related pregnancy complications. The literature is mixed regarding the impact of UAE on fertility and subsequent pregnancy; it is likely that the impact is minimal in this population that already has an increased incidence of infertility (Chapter 22).

In summary, bilateral UAE seems to offer an option to women with AUB-L that may provide long-term resolution of symptoms without the need for traditional surgical interventions. The role of this procedure in women who wish to conceive is unclear and requires further study. Clearly, myomectomy is the more traditional approach, and for those with intracavitary lesions is the most appropriate procedure [44].

Localized uterine artery occlusion (UAO) using laparoscopically-directed techniques, has also been described. The uterine vessels are occluded with electrodesiccation or clips without the need for embolization. A number of series have been published with results similar to those available for UAE [44] (Class II-2) [45] (Class III). Two prospective comparative trials have demonstrated that clinical results may be similar and that patients undergoing UAO seem to experience much less pain than the patients who are treated with embolization [46, 47] (Class II-1). In a double-blind RCT from our institution, procedure-related outcomes of localized UAO using coils deposited in the uterine arteries by a fluoroscopically-guided catheter were superior to traditional UAE with microspheres [48] (Class I-2). The UAO patients had little procedure-related pain and could be discharged home the same day. Longer term studies are needed, however, to evaluate the comparative clinical outcomes of the two techniques.

Hysterectomy

Of the approximately 550, 000 hysterectomies performed each year in the United States, up to one half are performed for leiomyomas of the uterus [49]. The technical aspects of hysterectomy are discussed in Chapter 17. However, in this chapter, some of the issues specific to AUB-L and hysterectomy will be discussed.

It is clear that if total hysterectomy is to be performed, and if it can be accomplished vaginally, vaginal hysterectomy is the preferred route from the perspective of cost, morbidity, and cosmetic result. The problem arises when vaginal hysterectomy is not feasible or is beyond the skill set of the operating surgeon. In such circumstances, and with the advent of electromechanical laparoscopic morcellators and vaginal morcellating techniques, laparoscopic total Video 17.1 and supracervical hysterectomy Video 17.2 may be the only practical alternative to TAH for management of AUB in association with very large leiomyomas. Appropriate selection of patients excludes those without known or suspected preinvasive or invasive cervical and endometrial neoplasia.

Investigative surgical approaches

Leiomyoma ablation or myolysis

A number of ablative techniques have been developed or proposed as an alternative to myoma excision. The term "myolysis" has been coined to describe the use of cryotherapy (Figure 19.1), or laser, ultrasound (Figure 19.2), or electrical energy to ablate the tumors by image or endoscopically-directed means, leaving the uterus otherwise intact. Myolysis, or myoma ablation, remains a procedure under development. The impact on current or future fertility and pregnancy outcome makes current techniques frequently inappropriate for women who wish pregnancy in the future. Myoma ablation is discussed in detail in Chapter 19.

Adenomyosis

At this point, hysterectomy remains the most effective surgical procedure for AUB-A, but there are efforts to identify less radical interventions. The use of UAE for the treatment of adenomyosis was reported in a small series of 15 women with 12 reporting significant reduction in symptoms at 12-months post procedure [50] (Class II-3). Recently, in a larger cohort study a Korean group evaluated UAE in 43 patients with adenomyosis, in most instances with both dysmenorrhea and "menorrhagia," and found that at 12 months 95.2% reported improvement in dysmenorrhea and 95% improvement in HMB [51] (Class II-3).

References

1. Waibel-Treber S, Minne HW, Scharla SH, Bremen T, Ziegler R, Leyendecker G. Reversible bone loss in women treated with GnRH-agonists for endometriosis and uterine leiomyoma. *Hum Reprod.* 1989;**4**(4):384–8.

2. Surrey ES, Hornstein MD. Prolonged GnRH agonist and add-back therapy for symptomatic endometriosis: long-term follow-up. *Obstet Gynecol.* 2002;**99**(5 Pt 1):709–19.

3. Leather AT, Studd JW, Watson NR, Holland EF. The prevention of bone loss in young women treated with GnRH analogues with "add-back" estrogen therapy. *Obstet Gynecol.* 1993;**81**(1):104–7.

4. Friedman AJ, Rein MS, Harrison-Atlas D, Garfield JM, Doubilet PM. A randomized, placebo-controlled, double-blind study evaluating leuprolide acetate depot treatment before myomectomy. *Fertil Steril.* 1989; **52**(5):728–33.

5. Carr BR, Marshburn PB, Weatherall PT, Bradshaw KD, Breslau NA, Byrd W, et al. An evaluation of the effect of gonadotropin-releasing hormone analogs and medroxyprogesterone acetate on uterine leiomyomata volume by magnetic resonance imaging: a prospective, randomized, double blind, placebo-controlled, crossover trial. *J Clin Endocrinol Metab.* 1993;**76**(5):1217–23.

6. Thomas EJ. Add-back therapy for long-term use in dysfunctional uterine bleeding and uterine fibroids. *Br J Obstet Gynaecol.* 1996;**103**(Suppl 14):18–21.

7. Maheux R, Lemay A, Blanchet P, Friede J, Pratt X. Maintained reduction of uterine leiomyoma following addition of hormonal replacement therapy to a monthly luteinizing hormone-releasing hormone agonist implant: a pilot study. *Hum Reprod.* 1991;**6**(4):500–5.

8. Stovall TG, Muneyyirci-Delale O, Summitt RL, Jr., Scialli AR. GnRH agonist and iron versus placebo and iron in the anemic patient before surgery for leiomyomas: a randomized controlled trial. Leuprolide Acetate Study Group. *Obstet Gynecol.* 1995;**86**(1):65–71.

9. Benagiano G, Kivinen ST, Fadini R, Cronje H, Klintorp S, van der Spuy ZM. Zoladex (goserelin acetate) and the anemic patient: results of a multicenter fibroid study. *Fertil Steril.* 1996;**66**(2):223–9.

10. Scialli AR, Jestila KJ. Sustained benefits of leuprolide acetate with or without

subsequent medroxyprogesterone acetate in the nonsurgical management of leiomyomata uteri. *Fertil Steril.* 1995;**64**(2):313–20.

11. Stovall TG, Ling FW, Henry LC, Woodruff MR. A randomized trial evaluating leuprolide acetate before hysterectomy as treatment for leiomyomas. *Am J Obstet Gynecol.* 1991;**164**(6 Pt 1):1420–3; discussion 3–5.

12. Perino A, Chianchiano N, Petronio M, Cittadini E. Role of leuprolide acetate depot in hysteroscopic surgery: a controlled study. *Fertil Steril.* 1993;**59**(3):507–10.

13. Phillips DR, Nathanson HG, Milim SJ, Haselkorn JS. The effect of dilute vasopressin solution on the force needed for cervical dilatation: a randomized controlled trial. *Obstet Gynecol.* 1997;**89**(4):507–11.

14. Soysal S, Soysal ME. The efficacy of levonorgestrel-releasing intrauterine device in selected cases of myoma-related menorrhagia: a prospective controlled trial. *Gynecol Obstet Invest.* 2005;**59**(1):29–35.

15. Grigorieva V, Chen-Mok M, Tarasova M, Mikhailov A. Use of a levonorgestrel-releasing intrauterine system to treat bleeding related to uterine leiomyomas. *Fertil Steril.* 2003;**79**(5):1194–8.

16. Rein MS, Barbieri RL, Friedman AJ. Progesterone: a critical role in the pathogenesis of uterine myomas. *Am J Obstet Gynecol.* 1995;**172**(1 Pt 1):14–18.

17. Rein MS. Advances in uterine leiomyoma research: the progesterone hypothesis. *Environ Health Perspect.* 2000;**108**(Suppl 5):791–3.

18. Zhao K, Kuperman L, Geimonen E, Andersen J. Progestin represses human connexin43 gene expression similarly in primary cultures of myometrial and uterine leiomyoma cells. *Biol Reprod.* 1996;**54**(3):607–15.

19. Eisinger SH, Bonfiglio T, Fiscella K, Meldrum S, Guzick DS. Twelve-month safety and efficacy of low-dose mifepristone for uterine myomas. *J Minim Invasive Gynecol.* 2005;**12**(3):227–33.

20. Fiscella K, Eisinger SH, Meldrum S, Feng C, Fisher SG, Guzick DS. Effect of mifepristone for symptomatic leiomyomata on quality of life and uterine size: a randomized controlled trial. *Obstet Gynecol.* 2006;**108**(6):1381–7.

21. Carbonell Esteve JL, Acosta R, Heredia B, Perez Y, Castaneda MC, Hernandez AV. Mifepristone for the treatment of uterine leiomyomas: a randomized controlled trial. *Obstet Gynecol.* 2008;**112**(5):1029–36.

22. Varelas FK, Papanicolaou AN, Vavatsi-Christaki N, Makedos GA, Vlassis GD. The effect of anastrazole on symptomatic uterine leiomyomata. *Obstet Gynecol.* 2007;**110**(3):643–9.

23. Gurates B, Parmaksiz C, Kilic G, Celik H, Kumru S, Simsek M. Treatment of symptomatic uterine leiomyoma with letrozole. *Reprod Biomed Online.* 2008; **17**(4):569–74.

24. Parsanezhad ME, Azmoon M, Alborzi S, Rajaeefard A, Zarei A, Kazerooni T, et al. A randomized, controlled clinical trial comparing the effects of aromatase inhibitor (letrozole) and gonadotropin-releasing hormone agonist (triptorelin) on uterine leiomyoma volume and hormonal status. *Fertil Steril.* 2009 Jan 8 [epub.].

25. Bragheto AM, Caserta N, Bahamondes L, Petta CA. Effectiveness of the levonorgestrel-releasing intrauterine system in the treatment of adenomyosis diagnosed and monitored by magnetic resonance imaging. *Contraception.* 2007; **76**(3):195–9.

26. Anastasiadis PG, Koutlaki NG, Skaphida PG, Galazios GC, Tsikouras PN, Liberis VA. Endometrial polyps: prevalence, detection, and malignant potential in women with abnormal uterine bleeding. *Eur J Gynaecol Oncol.* 2000;**21**(2):180–3.

27. Shushan A, Revel A, Rojansky N. How often are endometrial polyps malignant? *Gynecol Obstet Invest.* 2004;**58**(4):212–15.

28. Liberis V, Dafopoulos K, Tsikouras P, Galazios G, Koutlaki N, Anastasiadis P, et al. Removal of endometrial polyps by use of grasping forceps and curettage after diagnostic hysteroscopy. *Clin Exp Obstet Gynecol.* 2003;**30**(1):29–31.

29. Preutthipan S, Herabutya Y. Hysteroscopic polypectomy in 240 premenopausal and postmenopausal women. *Fertil Steril.* 2005;**83**(3):705–9.

30. Atlee WL. Case of successful extirpation of a fibrous tumor of the peritoneal surface of

the uterus by the large peritoneal section. *Am J Med Sci.* 1845;**9**:309–35.

31. Neuwirth RS, Amin HK. Excision of submucus fibroids with hysteroscopic control. *Am J Obstet Gynecol.* 1976;**126** (1):95–9.

32. Semm K, Mettler L. Technical progress in pelvic surgery via operative laparoscopy. *Am J Obstet Gynecol.* 1980;**138**(2):121–7.

33. Dubuisson JB, Lecuru F, Foulot H, Mandelbrot L, Aubriot FX, Mouly M. Myomectomy by laparoscopy: a preliminary report of 43 cases. *Fertil Steril.* 1991;**56**(5):827–30.

34. Parker WH, Fu YS, Berek JS. Uterine sarcoma in patients operated on for presumed leiomyoma and rapidly growing leiomyoma. *Obstet Gynecol.* 1994;**83** (3):414–18.

35. Leibsohn S, d'Ablaing G, Mishell DR, Jr., Schlaerth JB. Leiomyosarcoma in a series of hysterectomies performed for presumed uterine leiomyomas. *Am J Obstet Gynecol.* 1990;**162**(4):968–74; discussion 74–6.

36. Ravina JH, Merland JJ, Ciraru-Vigneron N, Bouret JM, Herbreteau D, Houdart E, et al. [Arterial embolization: a new treatment of menorrhagia in uterine fibroma]. *Presse Med.* 1995;**24**(37):1754.

37. Pinto I, Chimeno P, Romo A, Paul L, Haya J, de la Cal MA, et al. Uterine fibroids: uterine artery embolization versus abdominal hysterectomy for treatment – a prospective, randomized, and controlled clinical trial. *Radiology.* 2003;**226**(2):425–31.

38. Hehenkamp WJ, Volkers NA, Donderwinkel PF, de Blok S, Birnie E, Ankum WM, et al. Uterine artery embolization versus hysterectomy in the treatment of symptomatic uterine fibroids (EMMY trial): peri- and postprocedural results from a randomized controlled trial. *Am J Obstet Gynecol.* 2005;**193**(5):1618–29.

39. Spies JB, Ascher SA, Roth AR, Kim J, Levy EB, Gomez-Jorge J. Uterine artery embolization for leiomyomata. *Obstet Gynecol.* 2001;**98**(1):29–34.

40. Spies JB, Bruno J, Czeyda-Pommersheim F, Magee ST, Ascher SA, Jha RC. Long-term outcome of uterine artery embolization of leiomyomata. *Obstet Gynecol.* 2005; **106**(5 Pt 1):933–9.

41. Goodwin SC, Spies JB, Worthington-Kirsch R, Peterson E, Pron G, Li S, et al. Uterine artery embolization for treatment of leiomyomata: long-term outcomes from the FIBROID Registry. *Obstet Gynecol.* 2008;**111**(1):22–33.

42. Coleman P. *Systematic Review of the Efficacy and Safety of Uterine Artery Embolixation in the Treatment of Fibroids.* Sheffield: National Institute for Clinical Excellence; 2004.

43. Gupta JK, Sinha AS, Lumsden MA, Hickey M. Uterine artery embolization for symptomatic uterine fibroids. *Cochrane Database Syst Rev.* 2006;**1**: CD005073.

44. Liu WM, Ng HT, Wu YC, Yen YK, Yuan CC. Laparoscopic bipolar coagulation of uterine vessels: a new method for treating symptomatic fibroids. *Fertil Steril.* 2001;**75** (2):417–22.

45. Lichtinger M, Hallson L, Calvo P, Adeboyejo G. Laparoscopic uterine artery occlusion for symptomatic leiomyomas. *J Am Assoc Gynecol Laparosc.* 2002;**9**(2):191–8.

46. Park KH, Kim JY, Shin JS, Kwon JY, Koo JS, Jeong KA, et al. Treatment outcomes of uterine artery embolization and laparoscopic uterine artery ligation for uterine myoma. *Yonsei Med J.* 2003; **44**(4):694–702.

47. Hald K, Klow NE, Qvigstad E, Istre O. Laparoscopic occlusion compared with embolization of uterine vessels: a randomized controlled trial. *Obstet Gynecol.* 2007;**109**(1):20–7.

48. Cunningham E, Barreda L, Ngo M, Terasaki K, Munro MG. Uterine artery embolization versus occlusion for uterine leiomyomas: a pilot randomized clinical trial. *J Minim Invasive Gynecol.* 2008; **15**(3):301–7.

49. Farquhar CM, Steiner CA. Hysterectomy rates in the United States 1990–1997. *Obstet Gynecol.* 2002;**99**(2):229–34.

50. Siskin GP, Tublin ME, Stainken BF, Dowling K, Dolen EG. Uterine artery embolization for the treatment of adenomyosis: clinical response and evaluation with MR imaging. *AJR Am J Roentgenol.* 2001;**177**(2): 297–302.

51. Kim MD, Won JW, Lee DY, Ahn CS. Uterine artery embolization for adenomyosis without fibroids. *Clin Radiol.* 2004;**59**(6):520–6.

Chapter 1

Acute uterine bleeding

Chapter summary

- Acute uterine bleeding is nongestational bleeding that, in the opinion of the clinician, requires urgent or emergent medical or surgical management.
- There exist a number of systemic and orally administered medical interventions for acute uterine bleeding that have been determined to be clinically effective.
- A number of emergent procedures may be considered including intrauterine tamponade, uterine artery embolization, and, in selected instances, endometrial ablation and hysterectomy.
- Since acute uterine bleeding often occurs in the context of chronic AUB, it is important to investigate the patient appropriately following the successful treatment of the acute episode.

Introduction

Acute uterine bleeding was defined in Chapter 4 as heavy flow not associated with pregnancy but of sufficient volume to require urgent or emergent medical intervention. The management of acute AUB frequently requires utilization of urgent care, emergency, and/ or operating room resources to control the bleeding. Fortunately, there exist a number of nonsurgical approaches that may control the acute problem without the need for operative intervention. Once the acute episode is successfully managed, the patient should be evaluated for underlying chronic conditions that could increase the risk of repeat episodes.

Pathogenesis of acute uterine bleeding

For a given patient, the exact mechanism of an instance of acute uterine bleeding is not always clear. In some instances, the episode may be related to a localized lesion such as a submucosal leiomyoma, while in others, acute bleeding may occur in the context of a structurally normal endometrial cavity.

It is the general clinical impression that acute bleeding occurs more commonly in women with disorders of ovulation (AUB-O), perhaps because, in such individuals, there is a lack of progesterone-dependent endometrial biosynthesis of factors important for endometrial hemostasis, such as $PGF_{2\alpha}$ and endothelin-1 [1, 2] (Chapter 3). The pathogenesis of AUB-O, discussed in Chapter 5, is systemic in nature, and ranges from immaturity of the hypothalamic-pituitary-ovarian axis, frequently seen in perimenarcheal girls, to a number of entities that are known or suspected to impact on the normal function of the hypothalamic-pituitary-ovarian axis, including medical disorders like polycystic ovarian syndrome, hyperprolactinemia, and hypothyroidism, and pharmacologic agents that affect dopamine metabolism. Other common causes of anovulation are thought to include psychological stress, rapid changes in weight, and excessive exercise.

Acute uterine bleeding, particularly when it occurs in perimenarcheal girls, may be associated with an inherited systemic disorder of hemostasis, most often von Willebrand disease, which can be found in 13% of women with "menorrhagia" [3] (Chapter 5). Such disorders may amplify the heavy uterine bleeding associated with disorders of ovulation that frequently occur in the early months following menarche, that itself is characterized by reduced local hemostasis as described above.

The causes of heavy bleeding associated with leiomyomas (HMB-L) have not been clearly elucidated, but it is clear that the majority of leiomyomas are asymptomatic, and it is generally accepted that those situated near or adjacent to the endometrium cause the bleeding (Chapter 5). Consequently, when women with acute uterine bleeding present with myomas that do not involve the endometrial cavity, it is likely that the bleeding is *not* caused by the myomas.

Arteriovenous malformations are rare entities that contribute to enigmatic AUB, but should be included in the differential diagnosis of women who present with acute HMB.

Initial management and clinical investigation

Acute uterine bleeding ranges from modestly heavy bleeding at one end of the spectrum to excessive HMB associated with hypovolemic shock at the other, so it is important to have a well-planned method of initial evaluation and triage (Figure 10.1).

If the patient is hemodynamically unstable, all efforts should be directed at establishing appropriate intravenous lines and infusion of isotonic fluid. Blood should be taken for a hemoglobin level, a serum pregnancy test, other tests as appropriate, and for cross matching of blood should transfusion be deemed necessary based upon the patient's clinical condition. These steps are followed by, or performed simultaneously with, obtaining enough history and performing a sufficient pelvic examination to confirm that the bleeding indeed is emanating from the uterus and to appropriately and safely manage the acute clinical situation. Although a careful bimanual examination of the pelvis should be performed seeking evidence of leiomyoma and pregnancy, including findings suggestive of an ectopic gestation, the clinician should be cautioned that the manual pelvic examination is usually of limited value, for lesions such as subserosal leiomyomas generally do not cause bleeding, while submucosal fibroids that may contribute to AUB, are not detectable with such an assessment.

In most instances the patient is hemodynamically stable, eliminating the need for intravenous fluid, and allowing for a more circumspect investigation. If the patient has a positive screen for an inherited disorder of hemostasis (Chapter 12), suitable laboratory investigation for the detection of such disorders should be obtained. For those women using anticoagulants, INR, and other appropriate measures of coagulation function should be measured as well.

Both histological evaluation of the endometrium and sonographic and hysteroscopic evaluation of the structure of the endometrial cavity may be suboptimal due to the influence of intrauterine blood and clot. If endometrial biopsy is necessary, a sample may be obtained using a catheter-based technique (Chapter 16). However, if the specimen is deemed inadequate by the pathologist, repeat sampling would be necessary following the resolution of the acute phase (presuming that D&C is not part of the treatment plan). A similar approach may be considered for sonographic imaging. Absent pregnancy, the value of transvaginal

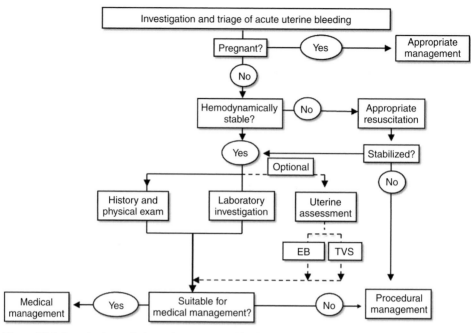

Figure 10.1 Investigation and triage of acute uterine bleeding. First the patient is evaluated for pregnancy and hypovolemia and, if necessary, stabilized with appropriate resuscitative measures. If these are unsuccessful, management in the operating room setting may be necessary. Hemodynamically stable patients are evaluated with appropriate history and laboratory investigation, including measurement of hemoglobin and hematocrit; endometrial biopsy, and ultrasound should be considered, but may be less easy to interpret in the context of heavy bleeding. At this point patients are categorized into those who may be medically managed and those who require procedures to arrest the bleeding.

sonography in the acute situation is questionable, but it may be performed if deemed appropriate by the clinical condition, remembering that interpretation of endometrial findings may be impeded by clot and blood in the cavity.

If hysteroscopy is part of the acute evaluation, it may be facilitated with a continuous flow system that allows efficient evacuation of intrauterine blood [4].

When bleeding does not respond to usual measures, arteriovenous malformation should be considered. If such suspicion exists, color Doppler or MRI seem to be the most appropriate diagnostic techniques [5, 6].

Therapy

Medical options for the management of acute uterine bleeding

Medical management of nongestational acute AUB should be considered before surgical approaches, unless bleeding is suspected to emanate from lesions such as aborting submucous leiomyomas (Figure 10.2).

Estrogens

A very useful approach for acute uterine bleeding is parenteral conjugated estrogens. Following placement of an intravenous line, 25 mg of conjugated equine estrogens (CEE, Premarin ® Wyeth-Arest Pharmaceuticals, Philadelphia PA, USA) are administered

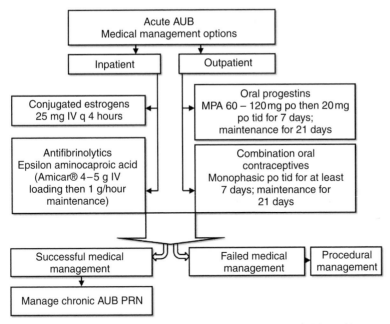

Figure 10.2 Medical management options. Inpatient options are administered intravenously. Outpatient options should likely be reserved for those with moderately heavy bleeding in women with a hemoglobin of at least 8 g/dL who have no impediment to returning for care should the bleeding not promptly stop.

as a bolus. This dose is repeated every 4 hours for up to 24 hours or until there is cessation of bleeding. When the bleeding stops, patients are generally converted to either a mono-phasic multidose oral contraceptive or a moderate to high dose progestin regimen, similar to those described below. If the bleeding does not slow down or stop, a procedural approach must be considered. Even if the volume of bleeding suggests that surgical intervention may be needed, the use of intravenous CEE may still be attempted while waiting for the oper-ating room – if the bleeding stops in the interim, surgery can be postponed or cancelled.

The mechanism of action of CEE is unclear, and may not be specific to the endomet-rium itself, as similar approaches have been successfully reported in the gastrointestinal and otolaryngology literature [7, 8]. Limited but high quality evidence comes from a RCT that demonstrated bleeding to cease within 5 hours in 72% of the cases compared to 38% for those who received a placebo. Aside from excluding pregnancy, there was no detailed evaluation of cause [9] (Class I-2). There have been no studies evaluating the added benefit of continued dosing, and there are no trials describing or comparing the various approaches described above for management of the woman after bleeding stops with the unopposed CEE.

Estrogens plus progestins

For less severe acute bleeding, administration of high dose, combination oral contraceptives may be considered. Virtually nothing is known about the relative value of one preparation versus another, but most would consider that a monophasic formulation makes the most sense. There is also relatively little known about the ideal administration regimen as clinicians use a number of ad hoc protocols that initiate therapy with, for example, three times or four times per day administration with gradual reduction ("tapering") of the dose once bleeding stops.

Until recently, only textbooks supported this approach [10] but a clinical trial performed at our institution evaluated one multidose monophasic regimen in the context of a RCT [11] (Class I-2). In this relatively modestly sized trial, product with 35 µg of ethinyl estradiol and 1 mg of norethindrone was shown to be equivalent to a progestin-only regimen, as bleeding resolved in a median of three days when the estrogen-progestin formulation was administered three times daily for a week and then daily for three weeks (Table 10.1).

Progestins

Another approach to the treatment of moderately severe acute uterine bleeding is orally administered progestins. Only two studies have evaluated this approach with, one using oral MPA in a total dose of 60–120 mg during the first day and 20 mg/day for the following 10 days [12] (Class III). A reduction in blood loss was reported in all the individuals; 25% stopped bleeding in the first 24 hours; while the remainder ceased bleeding by the 4th day. In the RCT from our institution, 60 mg of MPA was administered in three divided doses for the first week after which the dose was reduced to 20 mg/day for 3 weeks [11] (Class I-2). With this approach bleeding stopped, on average, on day three of the regimen, and patients were generally satisfied with both the treatment and the results (Table 10.1).

Other agents

There are no published studies specifically evaluating the use of antifibrinolytics for the treatment of acute HMB, but there may be a role. I have used epsilon aminocaproic acid (Amicar) 1 g/hour, following a 4–5 g loading dose (Class III).

There are no published data evaluating the role of GnRHa in the management of women with acute AUB but the clinician should be careful when administering GnRHa to anemic women for the gonadotropin "flare" (Chapter 9) frequently causes heavy bleeding in the second post-injection week. Consequently, if GnRHa are used, they should be "covered" by three weeks of a progestin-containing formulation such as MPA (10–20 mg twice daily) or a combination oral, transdermal, or transvaginal contraceptive for the same period of time.

Procedures for acute abnormal uterine bleeding

Surgical therapy is generally considered second line therapy for acute AUB, but may be the first choice for hemodynamically unstable patients or known intracavitary lesions such as aborting myomas (Figure 10.3).

Intracavitary tamponade

Tamponade using an inflated intracavitary Foley catheter balloon has been shown effective in a number of case reports and one series of 20 patients where 17 were successfully treated [13] (Class III). The balloon is inflated to 30–50 mL and left inflated for 2–48 hours, depending upon a number of factors including the perceived cause of the bleeding.

Dilation and curettage (with hysteroscopy)

The effectiveness of dilation and curettage (D&C) for the treatment of acute uterine bleeding is generally accepted but little investigated. It should be remembered that, for

Table 10.1 Outpatient medical therapy for acute abnormal uterine bleeding.

A. Combination oral contraceptives

1. Formulation

a. Monophasic estrogen-progestin

b. Estrogen: 30–35 µg ethinyl estradiol

c. Progestin: Potent progestins such as norethindrone or norethindrone acetate (≥ 1 mg); or norgestrel (≥ 1 mg 150 µg)

d. Examples

i. Norinyl 1/35 ® (also sold as Ortho 1/35 ®, Necon ®, and Norethin ®)

ii. Levlen ®, Nordette ®, and Lo/Ovral ®

2. Dosing

a. Three or four times daily until bleeding stops for at least 2 days

b. Then daily for 3–6 weeks (eliminating placebo pills)

3. Precautions

a. Use with caution in those at high risk for thromboembolic disease

b. May experience nausea; consider antiemetic

c. Return for reassessment if bleeding not adequately resolved in 48–72 hours

d. Will require followup with gynecologist if underlying history of chronic AUB

B. Oral progestins

1. Formulation

a. MPA (Provera ®)

b. NA (Aygestin ®)

2. Dosing

a. MPA

i. 60–120 mg MPA daily until bleeding stops for at least 2 days

ii. 20–40 mg MPA daily to follow for 3–6 weeks

b. NA

i. 5–15 mg NA daily until bleeding stops for at least 2 days

ii. 5–10 mg NA daily to follow for 3–6 weeks

3. Precautions

a. MPA is preferable in those at higher risk for thromboembolic disease

b. Return for reassessment if bleeding not adequately resolved in 48–72 hours

c. Will require followup with gynecologist if underlying history of chronic AUB

AUB, abnormal uterine bleeding; MPA, medroxyprogesterone acetate; NA, norethindrone acetate.

women with chronic AUB, the cycles that follow a successful D&C will resume to be similar to those that were present prior to curettage [14]. Because D&C frequently misses lesions that may contribute to or be the cause of the acute bleeding, concomitant hysteroscopy should be performed.

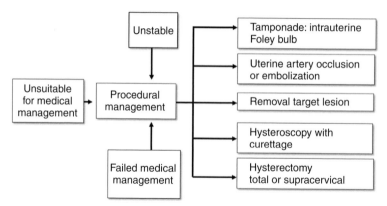

Figure 10.3 Procedural management options. These patients are either unstable, have failed medical management, or are unsuitable for medical management because of, for example, a contraindication to parenteral estrogens. If the intrauterine Foley catheter is selected, the balloon should be one designed for 30 mL although inflation to 50 mL is acceptable.

Endometrial ablation

Endometrial ablation performed under direct vision with a resectoscope, also called resectoscopic endometrial ablation (REA), has been described in a number of case reports or short series [15]. Similarly, nonresectoscopic endometrial ablation (NREA) with a thermal balloon has been described for the treatment of acute HMB.

Uterine artery occlusion

Transcatheter uterine artery embolization (UAE), described in Chapter 22 (Video 22.1), has been used frequently for treatment of obstetrical hemorrhage, cervical ectopic pregnancies, and postoperative bleeding. Although there are very few reports in the literature using UAE for acute uterine bleeding [16], the approach should be considered, at least, for women who have failed medical management, and who may not tolerate surgical therapy or who require/desire preservation of their uterus.

Anecdotal reports of compression of the uterine arteries vaginally with ring forceps have led to the development of a Doppler-guided clamp, which may be available soon, that assists the clinician by targeting the uterine artery flow and then confirming that the vessel is compressed when flow ceases.

Hysterectomy

Total or supracervical hysterectomy is generally seen as a last resort in the management of women with acute uterine bleeding. The procedure can be performed via laparotomy, vaginally, or under laparoscopic direction.

Summary

Acute uterine bleeding in nonpregnant girls and women of reproductive age is a clinical entity that challenges the clinician, and consumes health care resources. When interventions successfully result in cessation of the acute phase, the clinician must ensure that, if a chronic AUB process exists, the patient is sufficiently evaluated to allow the development of an appropriate treatment plan. Clearly, well-designed clinical trials will be necessary to better elucidate the causes and appropriate therapy for women with nongestational acute AUB.

References

1. Word RA, Kamm KE, Casey ML. Contractile effects of prostaglandins, oxytocin, and endothelin-1 in human myometrium in vitro: refractoriness of myometrial tissue of pregnant women to prostaglandins E2 and F2 alpha. *J Clin Endocrinol Metab*. 1992; **75**(4):1027–32.

2. Livingstone M, Fraser IS. Mechanisms of abnormal uterine bleeding. *Hum Reprod Update*. 2002;**8**(1):60–7.

3. Shankar M, Lee CA, Sabin CA, Economides DL, Kadir RA. Von Willebrand disease in women with menorrhagia: a systematic review. *BJOG*. 2004;**111**(7):734–40.

4. Crescini C, Artuso A, Repetti F, Reale D, Pezzica E. [Hysteroscopic diagnosis in patients with abnormal uterine hemorrhage and previous endometrial curettage.] *Minerva Ginecol*. 1992;**44**(5):233–5.

5. Timmerman D, Van den Bosch T, Peeraer K, Debrouwere E, Van Schoubroeck D, Stockx L, et al. Vascular malformations in the uterus: ultrasonographic diagnosis and conservative management. *Eur J Obstet Gynecol Reprod Biol*. 2000;**92**(1):171–8.

6. Huang MW, Muradali D, Thurston WA, Burns PN, Wilson SR. Uterine arteriovenous malformations: gray-scale and Doppler US features with MR imaging correlation. *Radiology*. 1998;**206**(1):115–23.

7. Daniell HW. Estrogen prevention of recurrent epistaxis. *Arch Otolaryngol Head Neck Surg*. 1995;**121**(3):354.

8. Marshall JK, Hunt RH. Hormonal therapy for bleeding gastrointestinal mucosal vascular abnormalities: a promising alternative. *Eur J Gastroenterol Hepatol*. 1997;**9**(5):521–5.

9. DeVore GR, Owens O, Kase N. Use of intravenous Premarin in the treatment of dysfunctional uterine bleeding – a double-blind randomized control study. *Obstet Gynecol*. 1982; **59**(3):285–91.

10. Chuong CJ, Brenner PF. Management of abnormal uterine bleeding. *Am J Obstet Gynecol*. 1996;**175**(3 Pt 2):787–92.

11. Munro MG, Mainor N, Basu R, Brisinger M, Barreda L. Oral medroxyprogesterone acetate and combination oral contraceptives for acute uterine bleeding: a randomized controlled trial. *Obstet Gynecol*. 2006;**108**(4):924–9.

12. Aksu F, Madazli R, Budak E, Cepni I, Benian A. High-dose medroxyprogesterone acetate for the treatment of dysfunctional uterine bleeding in 24 adolescents. *Aust N Z J Obstet Gynaecol*. 1997; **37**(2):228–31.

13. Goldrath MH. Uterine tamponade for the control of acute uterine bleeding. *Am J Obstet Gynecol*. 1983; **147**(8):869–72.

14. Nilsson L, Rybo G. Treatment of menorrhagia. *Am J Obstet Gynecol*. 1971;**110**(5):713–20.

15. Richards SR. Endometrial ablation for life-threatening abnormal uterine bleeding. A report of two cases. *J Reprod Med*. 1994; **39**(9):741–2.

16. Phelan JT, 2nd, Broder J, Kouides PA. Near-fatal uterine hemorrhage during induction chemotherapy for acute myeloid leukemia: a case report of bilateral uterine artery embolization. *Am J Hematol*. 2004;**77**(2):151–5.

Breakthrough bleeding (AUB-I)

Chapter summary

- Breakthrough bleeding is unanticipated bleeding that occurs in women using estrogen, progestin, estrogen and progestin, or any other gonadal steroidal therapy.
- Bleeding induced by gonadal steroid withdrawal in the context of, for example, cyclically administered hormonal contraceptive agents or postmenopausal hormone replacement regimens with a cyclical progestin should not be considered breakthrough bleeding.
- A common cause of breakthrough bleeding is poor patient compliance.
- There are a number of potential interventions for breakthrough bleeding but none that are predictably successful. Often the problem diminishes with time on the therapeutic regimen.

Introduction

Unscheduled endometrial bleeding that occurs during the use of gonadal steroid therapy is termed "breakthrough bleeding," or BTB, the major component of the AUB-I classification. Breakthrough bleeding is a common reason for discontinuing hormonal contraception or postmenopausal HRT. For the clinician faced with patients experiencing unscheduled vaginal bleeding while using gonadal steroid therapy, it is important first to ensure that the bleeding is coming from the endometrium, and then be properly equipped to counsel and, if necessary, treat the patient appropriately.

Pathogenesis of breakthrough bleeding

Bleeding with combined estrogen-progestin/progestin contraceptive preparations

It is likely that many, if not most episodes of BTB are related to reduced circulating gonadal steroid levels secondary to compliance issues such as missed, delayed, or erratic use of pills, transdermal patches, or vaginal rings. With the reduced suppression of FSH production, and resultant development of follicles that produce endogenous estradiol, additional and irregular stimulation of the endometrium may result in BTB. In one pooled study of seven trials, 35% of women with large follicles had BTB [1]. As a result, it should not be surprising that preparations with lower amounts of ethinyl estradiol are associated with an increased risk of BTB [2]. It is also likely that the type and dose of progestin is related to BTB – one trial demonstrated that pills with 100 μg of levonorgestrel were associated with less BTB than 0.5 mg of norethindrone in preparations with the same type and dose of estrogen [3].

There are other factors that can impact the circulating concentrations of gonadal steroids. Individuals with malabsorption syndromes or episodes of diarrhea may have reduced absorption of orally administered contraceptives. There exist a number of agents that can induce the cytochrome P-450 (CYP-450) system in the liver which, in turn, can increase the metabolism of estrogens and progestins. Examples include anticonvulsants, the antituberculosis agent rifampin, antifungals such as griseofulvin, and the active agent in the herbal preparation "St. John's Wort" [4]. Cigarette smoking can reduce levels of contraceptive steroids because of enhanced hepatic metabolism, an observation that may explain the relatively high incidence of BTB in smokers [5].

Lower quality evidence suggests that the use of some broad spectrum antibiotics such as penicillins and tetracycline may reduce the enterohepatic circulation of the therapeutic estrogen and, consequently, may be associated with reduced systemic and local levels [6].

Many cases of BTB with combined estrogen-progestin compounds have no apparent cause; these mechanisms are yet to be determined but may be similar to those with progestin-only contraceptive agents.

Breakthrough bleeding with progestin-only contraceptive preparations

Progestin-only contraceptive agents may be administered orally, by intramuscular injection or subdermal implant, and with an intrauterine progestin releasing device. Worldwide, it would appear that injection with depot medroxyprogesterone acetate (DMPA; Depo-Provera®, Pharmacia & Upjohn, Puurs, Belguim) and the levonorgestrel-releasing intra-uterine system (LNG-IUS; Mirena®, Bayer Schering Pharma AG, Berlin, Germany) are the two most commonly employed preparations, although the subdermal implant etonogestrel (Implanon®, Organon BioSciences NV, Oss, the Netherlands) is used by an increasing number of individuals. Oral norethindrone is relatively widely used, particularly in the breast-feeding population, or in women who have a desire for oral contraception but who cannot or should not use estrogen-containing preparations. What all of these agents have in common is the creation of an endometrial environment that is continuously exposed to progestagen with relatively low levels of estrogen. This is a situation that is recognized to frequently result in BTB, particularly early in the therapeutic course. While the exact mechanisms of the breakthrough are still being worked out, superficial blood vessel fragility is the leading candidate, with other mechanisms such as changes in endometrial steroid response, alterations of the structural integrity of the microanatomy of the endometrium, and variations in tissue perfusion that seem to contribute as well.

Morphologically, with continuous exposure to a progestin, the endometrium becomes thinner and may ultimately appear completely atrophic. Using hysteroscopy to evaluate women using a subdermal implant called Norplant® (Wyeth-Ayerst, Philadelphia, PA, USA), investigators have demonstrated irregular surface breakdown and abnormal angio-genesis manifesting in the development of new, variable sized, and unusually fragile vessels over the endometrial surface [7]. At a microscopic level the increased vascular fragility is associated with deficiencies in both basement membrane formation and the cells (pericytes) that surround the endometrial arteries [8].

At a cellular and molecular level, the endometrium of women exposed to continuous progestagens is associated with reduced estradiol and progesterone receptors, increased levels of MMP [9]; endothelial cell dysfunction [10], VEGF [11]; reduced cytokeratin expression [12], increased TF [13], alterations in endometrial leukocytes [14], and other abnormal angiogenic factors.

While there are differences among the various progestin-only contraceptive agents with respect to the specifics of morphologic and local molecular changes, there is evidence that many of these alterations are reduced over time, in parallel with the development of endometrial atrophy, an observation that may explain the frequent evolution of amenorrhea in women using DMPA or the LNG-IUS.

Postmenopausal hormone replacement therapy

Compared to contraceptive steroids, much less has been done to elucidate the mechanisms involved with BTB in women using postmenopausal estrogens with or without progestins.

In general, systemic postmenopausal HRT can comprise either estrogen alone, or an estrogen combined with a progestin, the approach generally used in women with a uterus to reduce the acknowledged increased risk of endometrial carcinoma associated with unopposed estrogen use. While the estrogenic component is generally used continuously, the progestin can be used either continuously, or cyclically, with cycles ranging from monthly to every six months in some studies.

With cyclical progestin use, the woman will generally experience a withdrawal bleed lasting a few days – this is *not* BTB. On the other hand, for women using continuous progestins, the incidence of BTB is 40–70% in the first month but typically declines substantially over the ensuing months of continued use [15].

The limited investigation of the potential BTB mechanisms for women using HRT suggests that there may be similarities to those for steroid contraception. For women whose menopausal status is uncertain, episodes of follicular function may be associated with the endogenous production of estradiol and resulting BTB. From an endometrial perspective, the formation of abnormal and fragile capillaries may be related to local alterations in angiogenic factors such as VEGF and thrombospondin-1. Also, alterations in the concentrations of MMPs responsible for extracellular matrix breakdown may be involved [16]. There is also evidence that uterine natural killer cells are increased in women using progestin containing HRT formulations – these cells produce cytokines that could disrupt the integrity of the capillary bed [17]. Further research is needed to more clearly characterize these mechanisms.

Clinical evaluation

To make the diagnoses of BTB, the clinician is required to evaluate the patient to seek other causes of the bleeding (Table 11.1 [1]). If baseline clinical assessment has demonstrated an entirely normal exam prior to the initiation of therapy, particularly with formulations containing a continuous progestin, the patient with spotting or light bleeding can be counseled that further evaluation can be deferred for a few months, as most such episodes resolve with time.

For those on continuous progestins with bleeding that persists beyond six months, or which starts after a well-established period of amenorrhea, clinical evaluation is important. When the progestin is administered cyclically, bleeding unrelated to withdrawal should be investigated. A careful search should be undertaken for focal lesions of the gastrointestinal or urinary tracts, the perineum and perianal region, and the lower genital tract including the cervix, vagina, or vulva. If bleeding comes from a friable cervix, neoplasia should be considered as well as infection with *Chlamydia trachomatis*, which is known to cause bleeding from the cervix or endometrium. In one study, nearly 30% of women with BTB

Table 11.1 Differential diagnosis of breakthrough bleeding.

- Poor compliance
- Poor gastrointestinal absorption (for oral preparations)
- Drug interactions
- Coagulation defects
- Liver disease
- Gynecological disorders, including but not limited to endometrial cancer, endometrial polyps, and cervical or vaginal lesions
- Nonreproductive tract origins

  a. urinary tract

  b. gastrointestinal tract

who had been taking combined OCs for at least months had a positive test for *C. trachomatis* [18].

If it is determined that the bleeding is coming from the uterine cavity, it is prudent to evaluate the endometrium if this has not been done recently. Such an assessment can be performed with one or a combination of TVS and endometrial sampling (Chapter 13).

Management

Breakthrough bleeding with combined estrogen-progestin contraceptive steroids

Women initiating contraceptive steroids should be counseled that BTB is relatively common in the first months of therapy, and that it will likely settle with continued compliant use [19]. For orally administered agents, preinitiation counseling should also emphasize consistent ingestion, where the pills are taken at the same time every day – erratic ingestion will result in equally unstable systemic levels and potentiate the risk of BTB. If the patient is a smoker, every effort should be made to have her stop smoking, not only to reduce the chance of BTB, but for the other obvious health reasons as well. Certainly the clinician should resist the temptation to change formulations in the first four months of use, but, if the bleeding persists beyond that time, a change in formulation could be considered.

There is no quality, evidence-based rationale for the selection of alternative formulations for the treatment of women with persistent BTB. For those whose lifestyle may preclude consistent ingestion of oral agents, a transdermal or transvaginal patch or ring may be a useful alternative. There is some evidence that formulations with low amounts of ethinyl estradiol (< 30 μg/day) may be associated with an increased incidence of BTB; consequently, one approach for women taking such agents might be to move the patient to a product with 30–35 μg of ethinyl estradiol. For those using phasic compounds, with varying doses of estrogen and/or progestin, a monophasic agent could be considered. If they already are using monophasic preparations, then one could consider changing from an estrane to a 13-ethylgonane, as there could be more consistent impact on the endometrium with such agents. A classification of progestins is found in Table 11.2 [20].

Table 11.2 Classification of progestins.

I. Natural
i. Progesterone
II. Synthetic
A. Structurally related to progesterone
1. Pregnane derivatives
a. Acetylated
i. Medroxyprogesterone acetate
ii. Megesterol acetate
iii. Cyproterone acetate
b. Nonacetylated
i. Dydrogesterone
ii. Medrogestone
2. 19-Norpregnane derivatives
a. Acetylated
i. Normegestrol acetate
ii. Nesterone
b. Nonacetylated
i. Demegestone
ii. Promegestone
iii. Trimegestone
B. Structurally related to testosterone
1. Ethinylated
a. Estranes
i. Norethindrone
ii. Norethindrone acetate
iii. Ethynodiol diacetate
iv. Norethynodrel
v. Lynestrenol
vi. Tibolone
b. 13-Ethylgonanes
i. Levonorgestrel
ii. Desogestrel
iii. Norgestimate
iv. Gestodene
2. Nonethinylated
a. Dienogest
b. Drospirenone

From Endrikat et al. [1]

Breakthrough bleeding and progestin-only contraceptive regimens

Levonorgestrel-releasing intrauterine system

Up to 55% of women using the LNG-IUS can be expected to experience BTB in the first 6 months of therapy [21] (Class I). After that time, the incidence of this side effect reduces to about 15–20%, and about 20% become amenorrheic by the end of the 2nd year, rising to 50% by year 5. It is my experience that most women will accept expectant management, particularly if they are using the LNG-IUS for HMB, where overall, their major problem is typically successfully treated, even at the time of the first post-insertion menses.

While there are no studies evaluating available treatments for such BTB, there may be a relative deficit of local endometrial estradiol in the first six months of treatment with the LNG-IUS. This effect seems to be secondary to temporarily increased local levels of 17-β hydroxysteroid dehydrogenase which converts E_2 to the less potent E_1 (Figure 11.1). Consequently, administration of very low levels of oral or transdermal estradiol may theoretically have value in the treatment of LNG-IUS-related AUB-I.

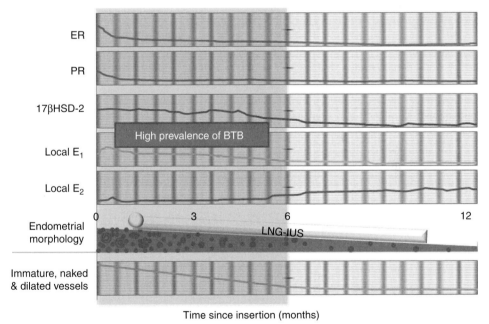

Time since insertion (months)

Figure 11.1 Endometrial impact of the levonorgestrel-releasing intrauterine system (LNG-IUS). This graphical depiction demonstrates the impact of LNG on the local endometrial levels of estrogen (ER) and progestin receptors (PR), 17-β hydroxysteroid dehydrogenase (17βHSD-2), estrone (E_1), and 17-β estradiol (E_2). The E_2 is converted to the less potent E_1 by 17βHSD-2, and in the initial months the progestin seems to increase the local levels of 17βHSD-2 thereby reducing the amount of local E_2 and creating, in essence, a hypoestrogenic state. Simultaneously, there are a great number of so-called "naked" immature and otherwise fragile vessels in the endometrium, a circumstance that likely creates the intermenstrual spotting. With time, the levels of 17βHSD-2 diminish, there is less conversion of E_1 to E_2, local estrogenic activity increases, and the number of abnormal and fragile vessels also reduces as breakthrough bleeding typically stops.

113

Progestin-only oral contraceptives

There has been a single study evaluating therapeutic approaches for AUB-I associated with oral progestin contraceptive agents. A medication available in Europe named Cyclo 3 Fort is a proprietary formulation of ruscus aculeatus, ascorbic acid, hesperidin, and methyl chalcone, and is called a "venotonic." In a randomized trial, use of four capsules per day was associated with a significant reduction in bleeding days [22]. Other studies evaluating the use of oral estrogens on progestin-only pill BTB have been inconclusive.

Depot medroxyprogesterone acetate

Episodes of DMPA-associated AUB-I may be reduced with the use of orally administered ethinyl estradiol at a dose of 50 μg/day for 14 days; in a RCT this effect persisted somewhat for 3 months [23] (Class I-2). Studies evaluating the use of prophylactic estrogens, including transdermal estradiol, have failed to produce any consistent therapeutic value, a finding which suggests that only women who experience the DMPA-associated BTB should be offered therapy [22]. The 50-μg dose described above seems quite high, so one would be tempted to use a much lower dose of ethinyl estradiol – perhaps 30 μg/day, although the relative efficacy of this dose is unknown.

Nonsteroidal anti-inflammatory agents have been evaluated for the treatment of DMPA-related BTB in high quality RCTs. Both mefenamic acid, 500 mg twice daily for 5 days [24] (Class I-2) and the COX-2 inhibitor valdecoxib 40 mg daily [25] (Class I-2) were associated with significant reductions in BTB.

The use of antiprogestational agents has been seen as a theoretically sound approach to the treatment of AUB-I associated with progestin-only contraceptive agents. One high quality study demonstrated that a single 50 mg mifepristone pill taken orally every 14 days significantly reduces BTB frequency and severity [26] (Class I-2).

Implantables: Norplant® and Implanon®

Given the use of subdermal levonorgestrel (Norplant®, Wyeth-Ayerst, Philadelphia, PA, USA) for about two decades, it is not surprising that the vast majority of studies relate to its use; relatively few studies apply specifically to the more recently approved etonogestrel-containing Implanon® implant (Organon BioSciences NV, Oss, the Netherlands). How the results of studies of one can be translated to the other is not known.

There is evidence from two high quality RCTs that the use of a combined estrogen and progestin (oral ethinyl estradiol and levonorgestrel) oral contraceptive agent for 21 days is effective at reducing BTB associated with subdermal levonorgestrel implants [27, 28] (Class I-2). Another small randomized trial demonstrated that just adding a progestin, in this case 60 μg of oral levonorgestrel for 20 days, can have sustained benefit as well [29] (Class I-2).

Antiprogestins have also been investigated in the treatment of Norplant-associated BTB. There may be a sustained impact of monthly oral mifepristone, 50 mg, in reducing the number of bleeding days, but it is not clear that this is clinically significant for the patient, either when used prophylactically [30] (Class I-2), or therapeutically [31] (Class I-2).

Nonsteroidal anti-inflammatory agents have been shown effective at reducing BTB. Both oral ibuprofen 800 mg three times per day for 5 days [29] (Class I-2) and mefenamic acid 500 mg twice daily [32] (Class I-2), also for 5 days, were effective at reducing the amount of BTB and the incidence of requests to have the implant removed.

The antifibrinolytic tranexamic acid (TA) has been evaluated for the treatment of Norplant-related BTB in a RCT using TA 500 mg twice daily for 5 days [33]. The results are somewhat discrepant as short-term BTB was reduced while four weeks later there was less bleeding in the placebo group.

Other agents have been evaluated for Norplant-associated BTB. Vitamin E, 200 mg/day for 10 days has been associated with improved BTB in one RCT and no measurable effect in another. Finally, there has been some work using the selective estrogen receptor modulator tamoxifen that has demonstrated reduction in BTB and increased treatment-related satisfaction rates [34]. The authors used 10 mg of tamoxifen twice daily for 10 days, comparing the results to women blindly assigned to placebo.

In Chapter 3 the role of MMPs in the initiation of ECM breakdown and the onset of menstrual flow was discussed. Doxycycline, an antibiotic, and a potent inhibitor of MMP-related matrix degradation, administered at a dose of 200 mg/day, for 5 days, was associated with an increased chance (over placebo) of stopping an episode of Implanon-related BTB [35] (Class I-2).

Breakthrough bleeding associated with hormone replacement therapy

As discussed previously, the potential causes of HRT-related AUB-I are similar to those for women taking contraceptive steroids. However, endometrial hyperplasia and carcinoma are much more common in this age group, a circumstance that requires evaluation that could include one or a combination of transvaginal ultrasound and endometrial biopsy (Chapter 13).

For patient counseling, both prior to initiation of HRT and should BTB occur, there are a number of points that can be made. First of all, withdrawal bleeding associated with cyclical progestin therapy is entirely normal, and is to be expected. Such bleeding may onset shortly after the discontinuation of the progestin, or may start late in the progestin-containing component of the regimen. Bleeding that occurs outside this time-frame is considered abnormal, and clearly should incite evaluation of the endometrial cavity.

When BTB is associated with continuous progestin-containing persists beyond six months, or should bleeding or spotting begin after a period of amenorrhea using the regimen, investigation of the endometrial cavity is mandatory.

If a diagnosis of HRT-associated BTB is made, there is currently no evidenced-based approach for therapy. As a result, options must be based on opinion and common sense. For some, changing to a cyclical progestin is a viable alternative, that may provide other benefits.[1] If the BTB is occurring with a cyclical progestin regimen, or if the woman wishes to continue with a continuous progestin approach, reducing the amount of estrogen in the formulation may beneficially impact the bleeding, an approach that is likely associated with reduced estrogen receptors. Alternatively, and perhaps paradoxically, increasing the amount of progestin may have a therapeutic effect as well, again, perhaps by reduction of both estrogen and progesterone receptors.

---

[1] It is my opinion that there are logical advantages to the use of cyclical progestins in postmenopausal replacement regimens. Such approaches may minimize or avoid risks of continuous progestins, which could include loss or reduction of some of the known benefits of postmenopausal estrogen.

References

1. Endrikat J, Gerlinger C, Plettig K, Wessel J, Schmidt W, Grubb G, et al. A meta-analysis on the correlation between ovarian activity and the incidence of intermenstrual bleeding during low-dose oral contraceptive use. *Gynecol Endocrinol.* 2003;**17**(2):107–14.

2. Akerlund M, Rode A, Westergaard J. Comparative profiles of reliability, cycle control and side effects of two oral contraceptive formulations containing 150 micrograms desogestrel and either 30 micrograms or 20 micrograms ethinyl oestradiol. *Br J Obstet Gynaecol.* 1993; **100**(9):832–8.

3. Endrikat J, Hite R, Bannemerschult R, Gerlinger C, Schmidt W. Multicenter, comparative study of cycle control, efficacy and tolerability of two low-dose oral contraceptives containing 20 microg ethinylestradiol/100 microg levonorgestrel and 20 microg ethinylestradiol/500 microg norethisterone. *Contraception.* 2001;**64**(1):3–10.

4. Murphy PA, Kern SE, Stanczyk FZ, Westhoff CL. Interaction of St. John's Wort with oral contraceptives: effects on the pharmacokinetics of norethindrone and ethinyl estradiol, ovarian activity and breakthrough bleeding. *Contraception.* 2005;**71**(6):402–8.

5. Rosenberg MJ, Waugh MS, Stevens CM. Smoking and cycle control among oral contraceptive users. *Am J Obstet Gynecol.* 1996;**174**(2):628–32.

6. Dickinson BD, Altman RD, Nielsen NH, Sterling ML; Council on Scientific Affairs, American Medical Association. Drug interactions between oral contraceptives and antibiotics. *Obstet Gynecol.* 2001;**98** (5 Pt 1):853–60.

7. Hickey M, Lau TM, Russell P, Fraser IS, Rogers PA. Microvascular density in conditions of endometrial atrophy. *Hum Reprod.* 1996;**11**(9):2009–13.

8. Murphy AA, Zhou MH, Malkapuram S, Santanam N, Parthasarathy S, Sidell N. RU486-induced growth inhibition of human endometrial cells. *Fertil Steril.* 2000;**74**(5):1014–19.

9. Vincent AJ, Salamonsen LA. The role of matrix metalloproteinases and leukocytes in abnormal uterine bleeding associated with progestin-only contraceptives. *Hum Reprod.* 2000;**15**(Suppl 3):135–43.

10. Rodriguez-Manzaneque JC, Graubert M, Iruela-Arispe ML. Endothelial cell dysfunction following prolonged activation of progesterone receptor. *Hum Reprod.* 2000;**15**(Suppl 3):39–47.

11. Charnock-Jones DS, Macpherson AM, Archer DF, Leslie S, Makkink WK, Sharkey AM, et al. The effect of progestins on vascular endothelial growth factor, oestrogen receptor and progesterone receptor immunoreactivity and endothelial cell density in human endometrium. *Hum Reprod.* 2000; **15**(Suppl 3):85–95.

12. Wonodirekso S, Affandi B, Siregar B, Barasila AC, Damayanti L, Rogers PA. Endometrial epithelial integrity and subepithelial reticular fibre expression in progestin contraceptive acceptors. *Hum Reprod.* 2000;**15**(Suppl 3):189–96.

13. Lockwood CJ, Runic R, Wan L, Krikun G, Demopolous R, Schatz F. The role of tissue factor in regulating endometrial haemostasis: implications for progestin-only contraception. *Hum Reprod.* 2000; **15**(Suppl 3):144–51.

14. Song JY, Fraser IS. Effects of progestogens on human endometrium. *Obstet Gynecol Surv.* 1995;**50**(5):385–94.

15. Archer DF. Endometrial bleeding during hormone therapy: the effect of progestogens. *Maturitas.* 2007;**57**(1):71–6.

16. Hickey M, Crewe J, Mahoney LA, Doherty DA, Fraser IS, Salamonsen LA. Mechanisms of irregular bleeding with hormone therapy: the role of matrix metalloproteinases and their tissue inhibitors. *J Clin Endocrinol Metab.* 2006; **91**(8):3189–98.

17. Hickey M, Goodridge JP, Witt CS, Fraser IS, Doherty D, Christiansen FT, et al. Menopausal hormone therapy and irregular endometrial bleeding: a potential role for uterine natural killer cells? *J Clin Endocrinol Metab.* 2005;**90**(10):5528–35.

18. Krettek JE, Arkin SI, Chaisilwattana P, Monif GR. Chlamydia trachomatis in patients who used oral contraceptives and had intermenstrual spotting. *Obstet Gynecol.* 1993;**81**(5 Pt 1):728–31.

19. Darney PD. OC practice guidelines: minimizing side effects. *Int J Fertil Womens Med.* 1997;(Suppl 1):158–69.

20. Stanczyk FZ. All progestins are not created equal. *Steroids.* 2003;**68**(10–13):879–90.

21. Irvine GA, Campbell-Brown MB, Lumsden MA, Heikkilä A, Walker JJ, Cameron IT. Randomised comparative trial of the levonorgestrel intrauterine system and norethisterone for treatment of idiopathic menorrhagia. *Br J Obstet Gynaecol.* 1998;**105**(6):592–8.

22. Abdel-Aleem H, d'Arcangues C, Vogelsong KM, Gülmezoglu AM. Treatment of vaginal bleeding irregularities induced by progestin only contraceptives. *Cochrane Database Syst Rev.* 2007;**4**:CD003449.

23. Said S, Omar K, Koetsawang S, Kiriwat O, Srisatayapan Y, Kazi A, et al. A multicentered phase III comparative clinical trial of depot medroxyprogesterone acetate given three-monthly at doses of 100 mg or 150 mg: II. The comparison of bleeding patterns. World Health Organization. Task Force on Long-Acting Systemic Agents for Fertility Regulation Special Programme of Research, Development and Research Training in Human Reproduction. *Contraception.* 1987;**35**(6):591–610.

24. Tantiwattanakul P, Taneepanichskul S. Effect of mefenamic acid on controlling irregular uterine bleeding in DMPA users. *Contraception.* 2004;**70**(4):277–9.

25. Nathirojanakun P, Taneepanichskul S, Sappakitkumjorn N. Efficacy of a selective COX-2 inhibitor for controlling irregular uterine bleeding in DMPA users. *Contraception.* 2006;**73**(6):584–7.

26. Jain JK, Nicosia AF, Nucatola DL, Lu JJ, Kuo J, Felix JC. Mifepristone for the prevention of breakthrough bleeding in new starters of depo-medroxyprogesterone acetate. *Steroids.* 2003;**68**(10–13):1115–9.

27. Alvarez-Sanchez F, Brache V, Thevenin F, Cochon L, Faundes A. Hormonal treatment for bleeding irregularities in Norplant implant users. *Am J Obstet Gynecol.* 1996;**174**(3):919–22.

28. Witjaksono J, Lau TM, Affandi B, Rogers PA. Oestrogen treatment for increased bleeding in Norplant users: preliminary results. *Hum Reprod.* 1996;**11**(Suppl 2):109–14.

29. Diaz S, Croxatto HB, Pavez M, Belhadj H, Stern J, Sivin I. Clinical assessment of treatments for prolonged bleeding in users of Norplant implants. *Contraception.* 1990;**42**(1):97–109.

30. Massai MR, Pavez M, Fuentealba B, Croxatto HB, d'Arcangues C. Effect of intermittent treatment with mifepristone on bleeding patterns in Norplant implant users. *Contraception.* 2004;**70**(1):47–54.

31. Cheng L, Zhu H, Wang A, Ren F, Chen J, Glasier A. Once a month administration of mifepristone improves bleeding patterns in women using subdermal contraceptive implants releasing levonorgestrel. *Hum Reprod.* 2000;**15**(9):1969–72.

32. Kaewrudee S, Taneepanichskul S, Jaisamraun U, Reinprayoon D. The effect of mefenamic acid on controlling irregular uterine bleeding secondary to Norplant use. *Contraception.* 1999;**60**(1):25–30.

33. Phupong V, Sophonsritsuk A, Taneepanichskul S. The effect of tranexamic acid for treatment of irregular uterine bleeding secondary to Norplant use. *Contraception.* 2006;**73**(3):253–6.

34. Abdel-Aleem H, Shaaban OM, Amin AF, Abdel-Aleem AM. Tamoxifen treatment of bleeding irregularities associated with Norplant use. *Contraception.* 2005;**72**(6):432–7.

35. Weisberg E, Hickey M, Palmer D, O'Connor V, Salamonsen LA, Findlay JK, et al. A pilot study to assess the effect of three short-term treatments on frequent and/or prolonged bleeding compared to placebo in women using Implanon. *Hum Reprod.* 2006; **21**(1):295–302.

117

Premenarcheal bleeding

Chapter summary

- Premenarcheal bleeding must always be considered abnormal and it requires investigation.
- It is important for the examiner to be experienced in the gynecological evaluation of the pediatric patient using techniques that minimizes both physical and emotional trauma.
- The most common causes of such bleeding are inflammation and infections of the vulva and perineum.
- Sexual abuse has to be considered, and the evaluation and management done in a way that is consistent with local customs and legal considerations.

Introduction

Uterovaginal bleeding that occurs prior to menarche must always be considered abnormal. The symptom can also be a source of fear and concern for both the girl and her family, and often may be suppressed or ignored because of some combination of psychological and social barriers. In such instances, and particularly if the bleeding is not profuse, presentation may not occur until development of significant anemia. Indeed, it may be at this time that otherwise occult disorders of hemostasis may manifest. As a result, the young patient with premenarcheal bleeding requires careful evaluation in the context of a comprehensive and structured approach that considers the psyche of the individuals involved and the spectrum of potential causes.

What defines premenarcheal bleeding?

Generally speaking, uterovaginal bleeding that occurs prior to the age of 10 is considered abnormal; after that time, such bleeding is usually considered physiological. However, there is a range of normal, and indeed careful judgment which must be exercised, as physiological bleeding may occur before the age of 10, and bleeding from pathological causes may present at a later age.

Causes of premenarcheal bleeding

There exists a multitude of potential causes of bleeding in the premenarcheal child, many of which are not from the reproductive tract. The most common contributor is infections and inflammation of the vulva and vagina, which comprise more than one half, with foreign bodies, trauma (including sexual abuse), ovarian, and vaginal tumors, and exogenous estrogens comprising less commonly encountered [1]. In older girls, idiopathic precocious menstruation is commonly encountered (Table 12.1).

Table 12.1 The categorization and causes of premenarcheal bleeding.

Classification	Subclassification	Causes
Hormonal	Endogenous	Neonatal estrogen withdrawal
		Precocious puberty
		Sex steroid-producing tumors
	Exogenous	Combination contraceptives
		Estrogens for postmenopausal use
Inflammatory	STDs	*Chlamydia*, gonorrhea, etc.
	Parasites	Amebiasis, fungal, *Enterobius vermicularis*
	Bacterial	*Staphylococcus aureus*, Beta-Hemolytic streptococcus
	Chemical	Soaps, cosmetics
	Hygiene	Poor hygiene
	HPV	"Condyloma"
Dermatologic		Lichen sclerosus
		Lichen simplex
Foreign body		
Trauma		Sexual abuse
		Physical activity
		Instrumentation
Urologic		Urethral prolapse
		Hematuria
		Neoplasm
		Infection
Neoplasm	Ovarian	Granulosa-thecal, embryonal, other
	Vaginal/cervical	Adenocarcinoma, rhabdomyosarcoma
	Polyps	
Idiopathic		

HPV, human papillomavirus; STDs, sexually transmitted diseases.

General principles of evaluation

Gynecological evaluation of the prepubertal child must be approached carefully, in the proper context, and with the close collaboration of the child and her parents or an/other family representative(s). Without such a reassuring environment, the lack of trust will likely inhibit the process and limit the information to be gained as apprehensive young girls may well become uncooperative.

Getting the history

The source of the history will vary greatly with the age and maturity of the child and it may be best to interview the parent separately. Information that is typically of value includes the volume and frequency of the bleeding as well as the duration of symptoms. There should be an enquiry regarding the potential availability of estrogens in the home, the presence or absence of known trauma, and any other historical information that might suggest a cause for the bleeding.

Preparing the patient

It is useful to spend time, using age appropriate terms, explaining why examination of the genital tract is needed and how the examination will be performed, including what instruments, if any, will be used. If possible, the provider should convey the notion that the child has at least some control of the environment allowing, for example, the opportunity to select the gown that she will wear and to view the light source or other instruments to be used.

The goal of the examination is to obtain information without traumatizing the child. At all times, the child and her guardian or parent should be reassured that the examination will be stopped if there is a level of discomfort that is unacceptable. The older girl can be asked to climb onto the examining table but for younger patients, examination may be more successful while sitting in a parent's or guardian's lap.

Positioning for vulvar examination can be done with the child lying supine with the legs in a "frog-leg" or "butterfly" position (Figure 12.1). For visualization of the vagina, the "knee-chest" position may be best (Figure 12.2). Should an adequate examination not be feasible in the office or institutional outpatient setting, examination under anesthesia may be required. Typically, this is performed in an outpatient ambulatory surgical center or procedure room with mask general anesthesia or intravenous conscious sedation [2].

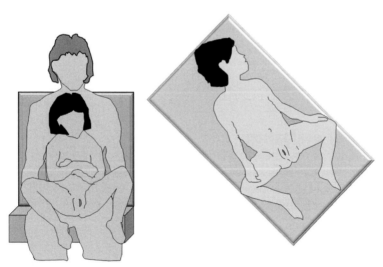

Figure 12.1 The frog-leg position. This position facilitates evaluation of the perineum and introitus. The infant or young girl may feel more comfortable if she assumes this position while sitting on her parent or guardian's lap (left).

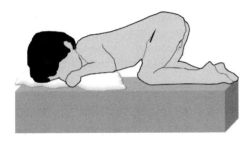

Figure 12.2 The knee-chest position. This position is an alternative to the frog-leg position and may allow for limited evaluation of the vagina with a nasal speculum or hysteroscope.

The examination

General examination

Vital signs are important, particularly if there is a concern about heavy bleeding. The older child in particular should have Tanner staging of both breast and pubic hair development as early menarche is a relatively common cause of physiological "premenarcheal" bleeding. In addition, breast development without adrenarche may indicate that there is an abnormal endogenous or exogenous source of estrogenic activity. The clinician should also note evidence of bruising, not only considering physical abuse, but also the possibility of a bleeding disorder; the family history may not be adequate in this regard. Finally, observation of the child's interactions with the parent or guardian is an important component of the overall assessment.

Vulva and hymen

Examination of the vulva in the child may be facilitated by using a colposcope, especially in cases of sexual abuse. The colposcope magnifies the area being examined and allows photography of areas of interest. However, magnification with an otoscope, hand lens, or 35 mm camera with macro-lens can also be used.

Examination of the hymen may be important, particularly in circumstances where sexual abuse is suspected. The examiner must be able to distinguish the spectrum of appearances of the normal hymen from the acutely or chronically traumatized hymeneal opening. However, it is important to note that 80–90% of girls who are known victims of sexual abuse have a normal genital examination [3]. The appearance of the hymen changes with the age of the child. The newborn typically has a redundant, thick, elastic hymen, reflecting intrauterine estrogenization, often with a prominent ridge located posteriorly in the midline. Estrogenic stimulation also contributes to cervical mucus production that may appear at the hymeneal orifice. On the other hand, the hymen of prepubertal girls is thin, and in addition to the typical annular configuration has a range of appearances [2]. Girls who are pubertal tend to have thicker elastic, hymens, reflecting systemic estrogenic activity. There may also be some mucus and/or a white discharge each of which are a reflection of estrogenic activity.

Cervix and vagina

Visual inspection of the upper vagina and cervix can often be performed in the office setting, or, if necessary, in a procedure or operating room under anesthesia. The vulva is examined directly, and the clinician should also consider potential nongenital tract sources of bleeding located in the periurethral or perianal regions.

For the vagina, a lighted Killian nasal speculum may be used, or for larger children, some clinicians use a pediatric laryngoscope. My preference is to perform vaginoscopy using a rigid or fiberoptic hysteroscope which can be passed into most pediatric vaginas with relative comfort. Liquid distention media such as saline or dextrose in water can be used once appropriate specimens are obtained.

Evaluation of the contours of the uterus and adnexae can be achieved through examination using a finger placed rectally and the other hand abdominally with the patient lying supine. If a mass is suspected or cannot be excluded, then an abdominal pelvic ultrasound or MRI can be obtained.

Trauma

Accidental trauma

Genital tract bleeding secondary to vulvar trauma is somewhat seasonal, as children may be more likely to encounter trauma in the summer months, related to bicycle riding or other physical activity. Falling on sharp objects usually impacts the labia majora and/or the perineum. With blunt trauma, external bleeding is usually limited, but deep tears involving the bulbocavernosus muscle of the labia majora may be associated with the formation of a hematoma.

The evaluation must be thorough considering the possibility of associated or contiguous rectal or bladder injury. To be comprehensive, it is frequently necessary to perform the examination under general anesthesia. If urination is limited by hematoma or pain, catheterization may be required. Expectant management, hemodynamic monitoring, and observation of hematoma size are usually sufficient. However, if bleeding continues as witnessed by expanding hematoma, or falling serial hematocrits, transfusion and procedural intervention may be required. Options may include exploration or, in some instances, management by interventional radiological catheter-based techniques.

Sexual abuse

Sexual abuse is defined as any sexual activity that a child cannot comprehend or give consent to, or that violates the law [2]. There is evidence that, at least in the United States, 12–25% of girls are victims of sexual abuse by the age of 18 [4]. As stated previously, most often, children who are victims of sexual abuse have normal examinations of the reproductive tract. Local laws will dictate the responsibility of the physician or other care provider when there is suspicion of sexual abuse, and the reader is encouraged to become familiar with local standards and regulations in this regard. Consequently, there may be a need to obtain forensic specimens, and document findings, including appropriate photographic evidence, all collected in a structured fashion.

Examination of the genitalia in the prepubertal age group is probably best performed in the frog-leg position, on an examining table or the lap of a parent or guardian, or in the prone knee-chest position. The latter is particularly useful for identification of posterior hymeneal trauma or lesions [5].

Although most female child victims of sexual abuse have no visible findings, nonspecific findings include labial adhesions, vaginal discharge, vulvar, introital, or anal erythema, anal fissures, and anal dilatation. Notches or clefts in the anterior or posterior hymen, and hymeneal tags are nonspecific signs, but clear evidence of penetrating trauma is demonstrated by acute lacerations or ecchymoses, absence of the posterior hymen, healed hymenal transections, and deep anal lacerations. Not all of these findings will be directly associated with premenarcheal bleeding, but the examiner should be aware and document appropriately.

If sexual abuse is suspected, particularly within the previous 72 hours, it is likely that there is mandatory collection of evidence. Specimens may include any or a combination of blood, semen, sperm, hair, or skin fragments as well as samples for sexually transmitted diseases, such as *Chlamydia trachomatis* or gonorrhea. *Chlamydia trachomatis* and gonorrhea may require delayed testing in about two weeks, particularly if prophylactic antibiotic therapy has not been administered. Other tests that may not be positive initially include syphilis, human immunodeficiency virus, and hepatitis B, which should be obtained at 6, 12, and 24 weeks following any suspected exposure.

Foreign body

If a foreign body is present in the vagina for a prolonged period of time, the skin and vaginal epithelium may become excoriated and result in a purulent, foul-smelling, and sometimes bloody discharge. Foreign bodies have been found in as many as 50% of preteenage girls with vaginal bleeding without concomitant discharge [6]. Toilet paper wads or remnants are the most commonly encountered foreign bodies but other examples include pen tops, fruit pits, small toys, and coins [1]. These objects are usually located in the lower third of the vagina and can be removed with bayonet forceps or even with warm saline irrigation. When there is suspicion that the object is in the upper vagina, vaginoscopy with a hysteroscope is a useful approach.

Infection and inflammation

Inflammation with or without infection of the vulva and/or vagina may be the most common cause of urogenital bleeding in the premenarcheal population [1, 7]. Inflammation includes irritative reactions to agents such as soaps, bubble bath oil, cosmetics, and clothing. Infection with parasites may manifest with bleeding. If evidence of *C. trachomatis*, genital herpes, or exophytic human papillomavirus ("warts") is found, sexual abuse is a strong possibility.

Dermatologic lesions

Lichen sclerosus may be found in the pediatric age group, as young as six months of age, with the typical thin, white, cigarette-paper appearance and areas of excoriation that are the reason for the bleeding. Typically the young patient presents with associated pruritis and dysuria [8].

Urinary tract disorders

In children, bleeding from the urinary tract may be confused with genital tract bleeding making it necessary, in many instances, to evaluate for urinary tract sources. Cystitis may result in hematuria, so appropriate clean catch or catheter-based specimens should be obtained as deemed appropriate. Unusual urinary tract infections such as schistosomiasis can be encountered in individuals who have traveled to countries where the disease is endemic. Upper urinary tract sources of hematuria should also be considered including those of both glomerular and nonglomerular origin.

Urethral prolapse is an external eversion of the transitional epithelium through the urethral meatus. The lesion is often perceived as a soft circular mass arising from the vagina and, consequently, may be misdiagnosed as a vaginal tumor. The etiology of such prolapse is unknown but may be related to previous trauma or conditions associated with increased intra-abdominal pressure. Medical treatments include antibiotics and local estrogens. Surgical procedures include excision, ligation, or cryosurgical ablation, but such interventions are reserved for large necrotic lesions and when there is urinary retention.

Tumors

Genital tract bleeding related to neoplasms may be caused directly by lower tract lesions, or indirectly if tumor-related estrogenic activity results in endometrial stimulation. Most of the vaginal neoplasms are benign, such as hemangiomas and vaginal polyps, but malignant lesions such as rhabdomyosarcoma (sarcoma botyroides) and vaginal adenocarcinoma must be considered.

Systemic hyperestrogenemia related to estrogen producing structures can lead to isosexual precocious puberty generally defined when thelarche and adrenarche have reached Tanner stage 4. So where do these estrogens come from?

Approximately one third of all space-occupying lesions found on the ovary are later shown to be nonneoplastic; most commonly follicular and corpus luteal cysts. Follicular cysts are relatively common in prepubertal girls, a consequence of the early stimulation by FSH. The vast majority of the other two thirds of the ovarian lesions are benign neoplasms. Any ovarian neoplasm that has a functioning layer of granulosa cells can produce enough estradiol to result in sexual precosity and uterovaginal bleeding. The neoplasm most likely to produce estradiol is the granulosa tumor, but these are still quite rare before the onset of puberty. Nevertheless, serum estradiol may be an important assay to perform when presented with premenarcheal bleeding, especially if there are other indicators of premature estrogenic activity such as breast development.

Another rarely encountered group of neoplasms that can be found in the ovary and contribute to estrogen-related endometrial stimulation are the malignant germ cell tumors such as endodermal sinus tumors, embryonal cell carcinomas, and nongestational choriocarcinoma. These solid and very malignant tumors also tend to manufacture measurable markers such as human chorionic gonadotropin (HCG, choriocarcinoma, embryonal cell carcinomas) and α-fetoprotein (endodermal sinus tumor). As a result, if clinical assessment suggests that such tumors may be present, assays for these markers should be performed.

Exogenous hormonal

Exogenous estrogens may result in vaginal bleeding. Many families have in bathrooms, purses, and bedrooms, estrogens in the form of hormonal contraception or postmenopausal hormone replacement products, including both systemic and topical agents. A careful history from the parent should seek to identify any potential access to such estrogen-containing compounds.

References

1. Sanfilippo JS, Wakim NG. Bleeding and vulvovaginitis in the pediatric age group. *Clin Obstet Gynecol.* 1987; 30(3):653–61.
2. Lahoti SL, McClain N, Girardet R, McNeese M, Cheung K. Evaluating the child for sexual abuse. *Am Fam Physician.* 2001;63 (5):883–92.
3. McCann J, Voris J, Simon M, Wells R. Comparison of genital examination techniques in prepubertal girls. *Pediatrics.* 1990;85(2):182–7.
4. Hymel KP, Jenny C. Child sexual abuse. *Del Med J.* 1997;69(8):415–29.

5. Bays J, Chadwick D. Medical diagnosis of the sexually abused child. *Child Abuse Negl.* 1993;**17**(1):91–110.

6. Paradise JE, Willis ED. Probability of vaginal foreign body in girls with genital complaints. *Am J Dis Child.* 1985; **139**(5):472–6.

7. Fishman A, Paldi E. Vaginal bleeding in premenarchal girls: a review. *Obstet Gynecol Surv.* 1991;**46**(7):457–60.

8. Poindexter G, Morrell DS. Anogenital pruritus: lichen sclerosus in children. *Pediatr Ann.* 2007;**36**(12):785–91.

Chapter 13

Postmenopausal bleeding

Chapter summary

- Postmenopausal uterine bleeding (PMB) may be either spontaneous or associated with the use of HRT.
- The risk of endometrial malignancy increases with increasing age of the individual with spontaneous PMB.
- Evaluation of the endometrium may be initiated with either transvaginal ultrasound or endometrial sampling.
- If PMB persists despite a negative endometrial biopsy or transvaginal scan, the endometrial cavity should be evaluated, preferably with hysteroscopy, and appropriate directed samples obtained.

Introduction

Virtually all providers of gynecologic care encounter the problem of PMB. The clinician is faced with the possibility that there exists an underlying malignancy, while knowing that, in most instances, the bleeding comes from a benign source. In years past, the "gold standard" of clinical investigation of PMB thought to emanate from the uterus was the institution-based D&C, but there now exist a number of office-based methods for the evaluation of women with this complaint.

The clinician should appreciate that while the focus of investigation of PMB is on the endometrium, bleeding in the postmenopausal woman may arise from a number of extra endometrial gynecologic and nongynecologic sites such as the cervix, vagina, and urological and gastrointestinal tracts. As a result, it is important to consider all of these possibilities when evaluating a patient with PMB.

What constitutes postmenopausal bleeding?

The World Health Organization defines menopause as the permanent cessation of menstruation resulting from the loss of ovarian follicular activity [1]. Because disturbances of ovulation and resulting irregular bleeding (AUB-O) and/or episodes of multimonth amenorrhea frequently precede menopause, there is no consensus regarding the appropriate interval of amenorrhea preceding an episode of bleeding that would allow for a clinical definition of PMB. Furthermore, while most endometrial cancer occurs in postmenopausal women, perhaps 25% is found in women prior to menopause. Consequently, the clinician should not rigidly adhere to a preconceived period of amenorrhea before determining that an episode of AUB in a perimenopausal woman deserves evaluation of the endometrium. If there is doubt about the ovarian function in a given woman with AUB, serum levels of 17-β estradiol and/or FSH should be obtained.

What is the risk of endometrial cancer?

For women with PMB who do not use HRT, the incidence of endometrial cancer ranges from 5.7 to 11.5% [2–4]. There are a number of factors that impact the risk including age, family history, and the use of tamoxifen and gonadal steroids.

Age

The Scottish national data suggest that the incidence of endometrial carcinoma is about 6–8/100000 women per year after the age of 50 [5]. If only women over the age of 60 with PMB are considered, 13% have endometrial cancer [2]. The incidence of endometrial cancer is low below the age of 50, and especially prior to age 40 (Class II-2). Swedish data demonstrate that the incidence of PMB declines with succeeding years after menopause, and that the incidence of endometrial carcinoma is increased as the age of the patient with PMB increases [3] (Class II-2).

Hormone replacement therapy

The relative risk of developing endometrial cancer using unopposed estrogen preparations in historically typical doses is about five times that for nonusers [6] (Class II-2). This increased risk is almost, if not totally, eliminated if appropriate cyclic or continuous progestins are added to the regimen [6, 7] (Class I-2, II-2). However, the addition of a progestin to an estrogen-based HRT regimen is frequently associated with bleeding that is generally predictable with cyclic progestins and unpredictable for women taking continuous progestin preparations as discussed in Chapter 12 [8, 9]. As a result, the proportion of women having underlying endometrial carcinoma can be expected to be much lower in women using combined HRT regimens than it is for those using estrogen alone, and is even lower than that for those taking no HRT at all [10] (Class II-2). There is relatively recent evidence that ultra low doses of unopposed estrogen may not increase the incidence of endometrial carcinoma but these preparations are not yet in widespread use [11] (Class II-1).

So how much progestin is necessary to minimize the risk of endometrial hyperplasia and carcinoma? Continuous progestins seem to maximally reduce the incidence of endometrial hyperplasia while cyclical dosing is to some extent dependent upon the duration and timing of exposure [7]. The minimum cycle duration has generally been considered to be 1 month; however, there is fair evidence that quarterly or even semiannual [12–14] cycling for 14 days of MPA, 10 mg/day, is adequate to prevent the vast majority of cases of endometrial hyperplasia or carcinoma, at least with CEE, or equivalent, doses up to 0.625 mg/day (Class I-2, II-2).

Tamoxifen

Tamoxifen is a nonsteroidal compound that is one of the family of selective estrogen receptor modulators (SERMs) typically used as adjuvant therapy for selected women with breast cancer [14]. For such women, the weak estrogenic activity contributes to a three to six times increase in the incidence of endometrial carcinoma with an overall risk of about 10% [15–18] (Class II-2). This risk is proportional both to the dose of the drug and the duration of therapy, with those women treated for five or more years experiencing a fourfold risk [19, 20] (Class II-2). There exists some evidence that, for women developing endometrial carcinoma following prolonged tamoxifen use, both the grade and stage of the tumor may be higher, thereby potentially compromising survival [21] (Class III).

Formerly, routine endometrial sampling was thought by some to be necessary for women using tamoxifen; however, current evidence suggests that such an approach consumes resources without improving survival rates [22, 23] (Class II-2). Consequently, and at least for the present, only women on tamoxifen who experience AUB should be investigated.

Nonpolyposis colonic cancer

Hereditary nonpolyposis colonic cancer is a relatively common, autosomal dominant cancer family syndrome. Endometrial cancer is the most common extracolonic cancer found in women with this syndrome. The estimated lifetime risk of endometrial cancer in women with the gene is from 42 to 60% [24, 25] and, unlike spontaneous endometrial cancer, these malignancies often present in the premenopausal years [26] (Class II-2).

Other risk factors

The evidence linking other risk factors to the development of endometrial cancer is relatively weak but worth considering. These include obesity, hypertension, and a past history of either endogenous or exogenous hyperestrogenism [27] (Class II-1).

Clinical investigation

Examination of women with PMB is done to confirm that the bleeding is indeed coming from the uterus, or, in the absence of active bleeding, that there are no discernible lesions in the urinary, gastrointestinal, or lower genital tract (Chapter 7). If there is uncertainty, this evaluation may require one or a combination of urinalysis, stool for occult blood, and endoscopy of the urinary and gastrointestinal tracts.

Evaluation of the endometrium for postmenopausal bleeding

Assessment of the endometrium has traditionally been based upon obtaining endometrial tissue via D&C, and then using office-based techniques. More recently it has become apparent that there is an important role for transvaginal ultrasound and ultrasound in the contemporary evaluation of women with PMB.

Histological assessment

Sampling of the endometrium can be accomplished by devices designed for office use (Video 16.1), by D&C (Video 16.3), or under hysteroscopic direction Video 16.2, with any method missing a proportion of endometrial cancers [28–31] (Chapter 16).

Comparison of office-based endometrial sampling with the Pipelle® device (Prodimed, Neuilly en Thelle, France) with combined curettage and hysteroscopy reveals that each blind procedure is an excellent screening tool but they do miss usually benign lesions such as endometrial polyps [30]. However, it is not completely clear that D&C is equivalent to catheter-based endometrial sampling as one group of investigators from Sweden demonstrated that D&C was slightly superior to the Endorette® (Medscand AB, Malmö, Sweden), a suction catheter device similar to the Pipelle for diagnosing endometrial cancer when the EEC was 7 mm or more [32] (Class I-2) [33, 34].

Office-based sampling of the endometrium is associated with a procedure failure rate of approximately 10% and a tissue yield failure rate that is historically approximately 10% [10, 28, 35]. There may be useful alternatives to the catheter-based techniques. In a randomized trial from Scotland, the Tao Brush™ (Cook Medical Inc., Bloomington, IN, USA) was found to be superior to the Pipelle catheter in obtaining a satisfactory endometrial sample (72% to 43%) [34] (Class I-2) (Chapter 16).

Transvaginal sonography

As described in Chapter 23 (Figure 23.3) Video 23.1, the endometrium is measured sonographically by calculating the thickness of the juxtaposed double layer in a sagittal, an image that is called the endometrial echo complex (EEC). If there is fluid in the endometrial cavity, which is generally an unconcerning finding, each layer is measured separately and the sum of the two measurements comprises the EEC. The morphology should be uniform and, if there are irregularities, investigation with endometrial sampling is generally warranted, and imaging using saline infusion sonography and/or hysteroscopy should be considered.

There are a number of EEC thickness thresholds that have been published, above which further investigation with endometrial sampling is recommended. The thinner the threshold, the fewer cases of hyperplasia and cancer missed, but the more additional procedures must be performed. Using the largest metaanalysis to date, with just over 9000 patients, an EEC of 3 mm or less would provide a post-test probability of 0.4% for endometrial cancer, a 4 mm threshold 1.2%, and a 5 mm threshold 2.3%. In this study, the best quality evidence was that for the 5 mm threshold [36] (Class I-1). In the other large metaanalysis of nearly 6000 women, an EEC of 5 mm or less was associated with a 4% chance of endometrial cancer. This sensitivity did not vary in women using HRT [37] (Class I-1). Thicker EECs are also associated with a greater likelihood of other intracavitary pathology, including endometrial polyps and hyperplasia [38] (Class II-2).

What all this means is that the reliability of transvaginal ultrasound (TVS) allows the clinician to identify a group of women with PMB who have a thin endometrium and thus a very low likelihood of hyperplasia or neoplasia. Unless there is a recurrence of bleeding, this group of women with PMB and a thin EEC generally require no more investigation [37] (Class I-1) [28, 39, 40].

Saline infusion sonography

Transcervical instillation of saline into the endometrial cavity allows for contrast enhanced sonographic evaluation that can provide diagnostic utility for lesions involving the endometrial cavity such as polyps or submucous myomas (Chapter 23) (Figure 23.2) (Video 23.2). It can be successfully performed in more than 85% of postmenopausal women in an office setting [41] (Class II-2).

Saline infusion sonography (SIS) seems superior to TVS in defining intrauterine lesions in women with PMB and a measured EEC greater than 5 mm, particularly for the delineation of endometrial polyps where it seems as accurate as hysteroscopy [42] (Class II-2). While there is no current evidence suggesting that SIS enhances the diagnosis of malignancy, the utility at identifying endometrial polyps facilitates diagnosis, targeted removal, and resolution of symptoms, thereby reducing resource utilization and improving patient satisfaction with the overall process of evaluating and managing PMB.

Hysteroscopy with curettage

Hysteroscopy is an endoscopic technique that allows direct visualization of the endometrial cavity, and is described in Chapter 23 (Video 23.4). One inherent advantage of hysteroscopy is that endoscopically-guided removal of lesions may be performed immediately after diagnosis, during the same procedure, and in an office setting. Despite the seemingly obvious advantages of the technique, the data supporting the use of hysteroscopy for management of women with PMB is relatively sparse and generally of relatively poor quality.

Hysteroscopy does have good diagnostic accuracy for benign structural lesions, such as polyps and myomas, that frequently contribute to the genesis of PMB [29, 43] (Class I-1).

However, hysteroscopic visualization alone is relatively inaccurate for the diagnosis of atypical hyperplasia and carcinoma [44] (Class II-2). Consequently, hysteroscopy should not be performed on women with PMB without antecedent endometrial sampling, or concurrent endometrial sampling by suction or sharp curettage.

Sequencing investigations

The exact sequencing of investigations for women with PMB will necessarily vary somewhat depending upon the local resources and expertise, the judgment of the clinician and patient preference.

Primary assessment of spontaneous postmenopausal bleeding

For postmenopausal women with spontaneous uterine bleeding, the endometrium can be primarily assessed by either TVS or office-based endometrial biopsy. Should TVS be selected, those who have an EEC greater than 5 mm, localized thickening, or an indistinct or nonvisible EEC, should undergo endometrial sampling as the next step (Figure 13.1). If

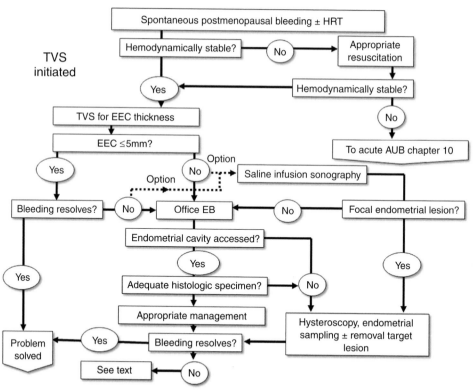

Figure 13.1 Investigation of postmenopausal bleeding initiated by transvaginal ultrasound (TVS). Provided the patient is hemodynamically stable, and there is no convincing evidence of another site of bleeding, evaluation may begin with TVS. If the endometrial echo complex (EEC) is uniform and less than or equal to 5 mm, the patient may be handled expectantly, but if bleeding continues endometrial sampling is indicated. Women with an EEC greater than 5 mm should have the cavity evaluated, at least histologically, with endometrial sampling, and in many instances with saline infusion sonography or hysteroscopy to detect focal lesions, most commonly polyps.

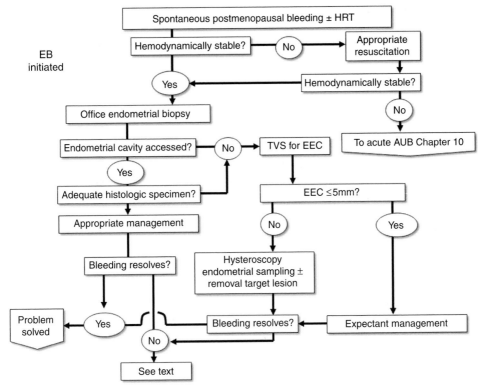

Figure 13.2 Investigation of postmenopausal bleeding initiated by endometrial biopsy. An alternative to transvaginal ultrasound (TVS) is to go straight to endometrial sampling with an office-based technique (Chapter 16). If there is difficulty accessing the cavity or otherwise obtaining a good specimen, TVS can be utilized. If the endometrial echo complex (EEC) is greater than 5 mm operative evaluation that includes hysteroscopy is justified.

the EEC is homogenous and 5 mm or less the patient may be handled expectantly, understanding that recurrent episodes of PMB will dictate endometrial sampling. Alternatively, the clinician may wish to start the process with endometrial biopsy, liberally using local anesthesia, and, if there is difficulty in sampling the cavity, remembering that TVS may be an appropriate alternative (Figure 13.2).

Primary assessment of HRT-related postmenopausal bleeding

The increased risk of endometrial cancer for women on unopposed estrogen requires assessment in all circumstances. For women with PMB while on combined estrogen and progestin-based regimens, the approach depends on a number of factors. Certainly, the withdrawal bleeding induced by cyclically administered progestins requires no investigation unless there is a substantial change in bleeding volume. In addition, those women who use estrogen and continuous progestin regimens will frequently experience breakthrough bleeding in the first six months of therapy and generally require no investigation. However, those women on cyclic progestin regimens with bleeding outside the scheduled time, or for those on continuous progestins who have breakthrough bleeding beyond six months, and, especially following a period of amenorrhea, the endometrium should be assessed.

Available evidence suggests that either endometrial biopsy or TVS can be used, with EEC thresholds for endometrial sampling similar to those for spontaneous bleeding (Class I-1). To limit the number of false positive results in women on cyclical progestin regimens, it is probably best to measure EEC late in the progestagenic portion of the regimen or very early in the estrogenic phase when the thickness should be at its lowest.

Recurrent spontaneous or breakthrough bleeding

Spontaneous or HRT-related PMB may occur despite a negative primary assessment, but there is no current evidence supporting any specific recommendations for reinvestigation. Considering the false negative rates associated with either a TVS or biopsy-initiated approach, the indications for reassessment should be rather liberal considering one or a combination of repeat TVS, repeat endometrial biopsy, and SIS or hysteroscopy [28, 39, 45, 46] (Class III). Determination of the specific order and combinations of these investigations will depend upon the clinical judgment of, and resources available to, the clinician.

Tamoxifen-related bleeding

Any woman who presents with bleeding while on tamoxifen should undergo office-based endometrial sampling if possible. If not feasible, such patients should undergo hysteroscopy and curettage (Figure 13.3).

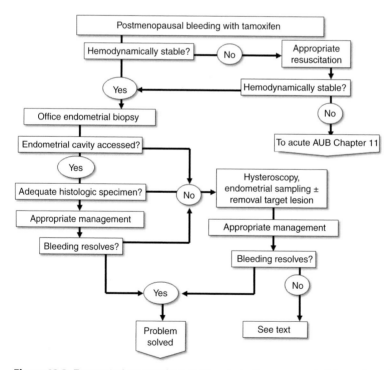

Figure 13.3 Transvaginal sonography is inadequate for the assessment of the endometrium in women on tamoxifen with bleeding. Consequently, endometrial sampling with office-based techniques is usually the first diagnostic step.

The tamoxifen-induced impact on the endometrium frequently if not usually creates a thickened EEC, often with diffuse cystic change that is in no way indicative of endometrial hyperplasia or malignancy. As a result, transvaginal scanning for EEC thickness is not useful in the evaluation of tamoxifen-related postmenopausal bleeding.

Many patients with tamoxifen-related bleeding have endometrial polyps. Consequently, if bleeding persists, direct evaluation of the endometrial cavity is indicated, generally with hysteroscopy, with hysteroscopically-guided excision of any identified polyps and curettage for reassessment of the endometrium. Saline infusion sonography may also be useful in this regard; however, there is evidence that SIS is inferior to hysteroscopy in detecting focal lesions in these patients [47] (Class II-1).

For patients who are on tamoxifen, who have persisting episodes of PMB, despite a negative evaluation, annual repeat sampling is indicated (Class IV).

References

1. Research on the menopause in the 1990s. Report of a WHO Scientific Group. *World Health Organ Tech Rep Ser.* 1996;**866**:1–107.
2. Ferrazzi E, Torri V, Trio D, Zannoni E, Filiberto S, Dordoni D. Sonographic endometrial thickness: a useful test to predict atrophy in patients with postmenopausal bleeding. An Italian multicenter study. *Ultrasound Obstet Gynecol.* 1996;**7**(5): 315–21.
3. Gredmark T, Kvint S, Havel G, Mattsson LA. Histopathological findings in women with postmenopausal bleeding. *Br J Obstet Gynaecol.* 1995;**102**(2):133–6.
4. Lidor A, Ismajovich B, Confino E, David MP. Histopathological findings in 226 women with post-menopausal uterine bleeding. *Acta Obstet Gynecol Scand.* 1986; **65**(1):41–3.
5. Harris V, Sandridge AL, Black RJ, Brewster DH, Gould A. *Cancer Registration Statistics Scotland 1986–1995.* Edinburgh: ISD Scotland Publications; 1998.
6. Weiderpass E, Adami HO, Baron JA, Magnusson C, Bergstrom R, Lindgren A, et al. Risk of endometrial cancer following estrogen replacement with and without progestins. *J Natl Cancer Inst.* 1999; **91**(13):1131–7.
7. Lethaby A, Suckling J, Barlow D, Farquhar CM, Jepson RG, Roberts H. Hormone replacement therapy in postmenopausal women: endometrial hyperplasia and irregular bleeding. *Cochrane Database Syst Rev.* 2004;**3**:CD000402.
8. Barret-Connor E. Hormone replacement. *Am J Geriatr Cardiol.* 1993;**2**(5):36–7.
9. Archer DF, Pickar JH, Bottiglioni F. Bleeding patterns in postmenopausal women taking continuous combined or sequential regimens of conjugated estrogens with medroxyprogesterone acetate. Menopause Study Group. *Obstet Gynecol.* 1994;**83**(5 Pt 1):686–92.
10. Nagele F, O'Connor H, Baskett TF, Davies A, Mohammed H, Magos AL. Hysteroscopy in women with abnormal uterine bleeding on hormone replacement therapy: a comparison with postmenopausal bleeding. *Fertil Steril.* 1996;**65**(6):1145–50.
11. Ettinger B, Ensrud KE, Wallace R, Johnson KC, Cummings SR, Yankov V, et al. Effects of ultra low-dose transdermal estradiol on bone mineral density: a randomized clinical trial. *Obstet Gynecol.* 2004;**104**(3):443–51.
12. Williams DB, Voigt BJ, Fu YS, Schoenfeld MJ, Judd HL. Assessment of less than monthly progestin therapy in postmenopausal women given estrogen replacement. *Obstet Gynecol.* 1994; **84**(5):787–93.
13. Ettinger B, Li DK, Klein R. Unexpected vaginal bleeding and associated gynecologic care in postmenopausal women using hormone replacement therapy: comparison of cyclic versus continuous combined schedules. *Fertil Steril.* 1998;**69**(5):865–9.
14. Ettinger B, Pressman A, Van Gessel A. Low-dosage esterified estrogens opposed by progestin at 6-month intervals. *Obstet Gynecol.* 2001;**98**(2):205–11.

15. Rutqvist LE, Johansson H, Signomklao T, Johansson U, Fornander T, Wilking N. Adjuvant tamoxifen therapy for early stage breast cancer and second primary malignancies. Stockholm Breast Cancer Study Group. *J Natl Cancer Inst*. 1995; **87**(9):645–51.

16. Fisher B, Costantino JP, Wickerham DL, Redmond CK, Kavanah M, Cronin WM, et al. Tamoxifen for prevention of breast cancer: report of the National Surgical Adjuvant Breast and Bowel Project P-1 Study. *J Natl Cancer Inst*. 1998; **90**(18):1371–88.

17. Fornander T, Rutqvist LE, Cedermark B, Glas U, Mattsson A, Silfversward C, et al. Adjuvant tamoxifen in early breast cancer: occurrence of new primary cancers. *Lancet*. 1989;**1**(8630):117–20.

18. Curtis RE, Boice JD, Jr., Shriner DA, Hankey BF, Fraumeni JF, Jr. Second cancers after adjuvant tamoxifen therapy for breast cancer. *J Natl Cancer Inst*. 1996;**88**(12):832–4.

19. Bernstein L, Deapen D, Cerhan JR, Schwartz SM, Liff J, McGann-Maloney E, et al. Tamoxifen therapy for breast cancer and endometrial cancer risk. *J Natl Cancer Inst*. 1999;**91**(19):1654–62.

20. Van Leeuwen FE, Benraadt J, Coebergh JW, Kiemeney LA, Gimbrere CH, Otter R, et al. Risk of endometrial cancer after tamoxifen treatment of breast cancer. *Lancet*. 1994;**343**(8895):448–52.

21. Bergman L, Beelen ML, Gallee MP, Hollema H, Benraadt J, van Leeuwen FE. Risk and prognosis of endometrial cancer after tamoxifen for breast cancer. Comprehensive Cancer Centres' ALERT Group. Assessment of liver and endometrial cancer risk following tamoxifen. *Lancet*. 2000;**356**(9233):881–7.

22. Markovitch O, Tepper R, Aviram R, Fishman A, Shapira J, Cohen I. The value of sonohysterography in the prediction of endometrial pathologies in asymptomatic postmenopausal breast cancer tamoxifen-treated patients. *Gynecol Oncol*. 2004;**94** (3):754–9.

23. Love CD, Muir BB, Scrimgeour JB, Leonard RC, Dillon P, Dixon JM. Investigation of endometrial abnormalities in asymptomatic women treated with tamoxifen and an evaluation of the role of endometrial screening. *J Clin Oncol*. 1999;**17**(7):2050–4.

24. Aarnio M, Sankila R, Pukkala E, Salovaara R, Aaltonen LA, de la Chapelle A, et al. Cancer risk in mutation carriers of DNA-mismatch-repair genes. *Int J Cancer*. 1999;**81**(2):214–18.

25. Dunlop MG, Farrington SM, Carothers AD, Wyllie AH, Sharp L, Burn J, et al. Cancer risk associated with germline DNA mismatch repair gene mutations. *Hum Mol Genet*. 1997;**6**(1):105–10.

26. Vasen HF, Wijnen JT, Menko FH, Kleibeuker JH, Taal BG, Griffioen G, et al. Cancer risk in families with hereditary nonpolyposis colorectal cancer diagnosed by mutation analysis. *Gastroenterology*. 1996;**110**(4):1020–7.

27. Feldman S, Cook EF, Harlow BL, Berkowitz RS. Predicting endometrial cancer among older women who present with abnormal vaginal bleeding. *Gynecol Oncol*. 1995; **56**(3):376–81.

28. Gordon SJ, Westgate J. The incidence and management of failed Pipelle sampling in a general outpatient clinic. *Aust N Z J Obstet Gynaecol*. 1999;**39**(1):115–18.

29. Tahir MM, Bigrigg MA, Browning JJ, Brookes ST, Smith PA. A randomised controlled trial comparing transvaginal ultrasound, outpatient hysteroscopy and endometrial biopsy with inpatient hysteroscopy and curettage. *Br J Obstet Gynaecol*. 1999;**106**(12):1259–64.

30. Dijkhuizen FP, De Vries LD, Mol BW, Brolmann HA, Peters HM, Moret E, et al. Comparison of TVS and SIS for the detection of intracavitary abnormalities in premenopausal women. *Ultrasound Obstet Gynecol*. 2000;**15**(5):372–6.

31. Epstein E, Ramirez A, Skoog L, Valentin L. Dilatation and curettage fails to detect most focal lesions in the uterine cavity in women with postmenopausal bleeding. *Acta Obstet Gynecol Scand*. 2001;**80**(12):1131–6.

32. Epstein E, Skoog L, Valentin L. Comparison of Endorette and dilatation and curettage for sampling of the endometrium in women with postmenopausal bleeding. *Acta Obstet Gynecol Scand*. 2001;**80**(10):959–64.

33. Van den Bosch T, Vandendael A, Van Schoubroeck D, Wranz PA, Lombard CJ.

Combining vaginal ultrasonography and office endometrial sampling in the diagnosis of endometrial disease in postmenopausal women. *Obstet Gynecol.* 1995;**85**(3):349–52.

34. Critchley HO, Warner P, Lee AJ, Brechin S, Guise J, Graham B. Evaluation of abnormal uterine bleeding: comparison of three outpatient procedures within cohorts defined by age and menopausal status. *Health Technol Assess.* 2004;**8**(34): iii–iv, 1–139.

35. Giusa-Chiferi MG, Goncalves WJ, Baracat EC, de Albuquerque Neto LC, Bortoletto CC, de Lima GR. Transvaginal ultrasound, uterine biopsy and hysteroscopy for postmenopausal bleeding. *Int J Gynaecol Obstet.* 1996;**55**(1):39–44.

36. Gupta JK, Chien PF, Voit D, Clark TJ, Khan KS. Ultrasonographic endometrial thickness for diagnosing endometrial pathology in women with postmenopausal bleeding: a meta-analysis. *Acta Obstet Gynecol Scand.* 2002;**81**(9):799–816.

37. Smith-Bindman R, Kerlikowske K, Feldstein VA, Subak L, Scheidler J, Segal M, et al. Endovaginal ultrasound to exclude endometrial cancer and other endometrial abnormalities. *JAMA.* 1998;**280**(17):1510–17.

38. Wolman I, Amster R, Hartoov J, Gull I, Kupfermintz M, Lessing JB, et al. Reproducibility of transvaginal ultrasonographic measurements of endometrial thickness in patients with postmenopausal bleeding. *Gynecol Obstet Invest.* 1998;**46**(3):191–4.

39. Guner H, Tiras MB, Karabacak O, Sarikaya H, Erdem M, Yildirim M. Endometrial assessment by vaginal ultrasonography might reduce endometrial sampling in patients with postmenopausal bleeding: a prospective study. *Aust N Z J Obstet Gynaecol.* 1996;**36**(2):175–8.

40. Wolman I, Sagi J, Pauzner D, Yovel I, Seidman DS, David MP. Transabdominal ultrasonographic evaluation of endometrial thickness in clomiphene citrate-stimulated cycles in relation to conception. *J Clin Ultrasound.* 1994;**22**(2):109–12.

41. De Kroon CD, de Bock GH, Dieben SW, Jansen FW. Saline contrast hysterosonography in abnormal uterine bleeding: a systematic review and meta-analysis. *BJOG.* 2003; **110**(10):938–47.

42. Epstein E, Ramirez A, Skoog L, Valentin L. Transvaginal sonography, saline contrast sonohysterography and hysteroscopy for the investigation of women with postmenopausal bleeding and endometrium > 5 mm. *Ultrasound Obstet Gynecol.* 2001;**18**(2):157–62.

43. Kremer C, Duffy S, Moroney M. Patient satisfaction with outpatient hysteroscopy versus day case hysteroscopy: randomised controlled trial. *BMJ.* 2000;**320**(7230):279–82.

44. Deckardt R, Lueken RP, Gallinat A, Moller CP, Busche D, Nugent W, et al. Comparison of transvaginal ultrasound, hysteroscopy, and dilatation and curettage in the diagnosis of abnormal vaginal bleeding and intrauterine pathology in perimenopausal and postmenopausal women. *J Am Assoc Gynecol Laparosc.* 2002;**9**(3):277–82.

45. Tsuda H, Kawabata M, Umesaki N, Kawabata K, Ogita S. Endometrial assessment by transabdominal ultrasonography in postmenopausal women. *Eur J Obstet Gynecol Reprod Biol.* 1993;**52**(3):201–4.

46. Grimes DA. Diagnostic dilation and curettage: a reappraisal. *Am J Obstet Gynecol.* 1982;**142**(1):1–6.

47. Garuti G, Cellani F, Grossi F, Colonnelli M, Centinaio G, Luerti M. Saline infusion sonography and office hysteroscopy to assess endometrial morbidity associated with tamoxifen intake. *Gynecol Oncol.* 2002;**86**(3):323–9.

Procedures
Uterine anesthesia

Chapter summary
- The uterus has two distinctly different sources of innervation; the cervix is supplied by S 2–4 largely through the uterosacral ligaments, while the corpus receives sensory afferents via the T 10–L 1 roots.
- Any strategy for local anesthesia must consider both the sources of uterine innervation and the time required for maximal anesthetic effect.

Introduction
Whereas many uterine procedures should remain in the domain of standard operating rooms, with general or regional anesthesia, an increasing number can be performed in the office or procedure-room setting. Office-based procedures are attractive for women and providers alike, provided the goals of the procedure are achieved and the experience is one that is comfortable for the patient. Comfort is the product of a number of factors that include the dimensions of the instrumentation, the specifics and duration of the procedure, individual characteristics of the patient, and the judicious application of analgesia and anesthesia. It should be stated that there exists controversy over the value of local anesthesia, but, at the same time, I feel strongly that it has an important role that has not yet been adequately demonstrated in the available literature.

Background
Understanding the rationale for, and evidence regarding, the various approaches to local uterine anesthesia requires an understanding of uterine anatomy, and, in particular, the innervation of the uterus discussed in Chapter 2. A critical point to understand is that the cervix receives its innervation from S 2–4 largely via the uterosacral ligaments, while the corpus is innervated by T 10–L 1, distributed with the uterine and ovarian vasculature more cephalad in the broad ligament and above. As a result, uterine anesthesia using local anesthetic agents must consider all pathways. There is also an evolving understanding of the distribution of nerves in the uterus associated with various disease states, particularly in the endometrium, where it is evident that even the functional layer contains nerve fibers [1].

The vagina may be another source of discomfort or even pain associated with uterine procedures. One example is the postmenopausal woman with vaginal atrophy and the associated sensitivity that may play a role in the patient's experience with the placement of a vaginal speculum. Another potential source of pain is the musculature of the pelvic floor; contracted levator muscles are not consistent with comfortable vaginal manipulation involved in many uterine procedures.

The potential for a painful experience is related to a number of factors that we can call the *patient-instrumentation interface*. It seems obvious that the larger the diameter of the cervical dilator or hysteroscope sheath, the greater the possibility of pain secondary to stretched or otherwise stimulated pain fibers. From the patient perspective, the cervical canal of reproductive-aged women who have had vaginal deliveries is generally larger in caliber than that of women who have never been pregnant, those who have had only Cesarean sections, or those who are many years postmenopausal without estrogen-based HRT. The same can be said of the relative dimensions of the vagina and the speculum used to expose the cervix – an overly large speculum in a narrow vagina is likely to elicit discomfort. Finally, the nature and duration of the procedure may play an important role in the patient's unanesthetized experience. For example, a low pressure sonohysterogram using a narrow caliber catheter and lasting for one minute may be experienced very differently from a pressurized balloon containing heated fluid that is in place for nearly ten minutes.

Finally, it is important to understand some pharmacodynamic fundamentals of the local anesthetic agents that are in common use, particularly the time between application or injection and the achievement of maximal anesthesia. For local injections of some agents, anesthesia may be nearly immediate, while for topical applications, it may be 20 minutes or more until the maximum impact is reached. Understanding these issues, together with having the patience to wait the appropriate amount of time to achieve the optimal effect, is an important part of achieving the diagnostic and therapeutic goals while providing a comfortable experience. Respecting these principles, in our Uterine Procedure and Imaging Center, we are able to consistently, comfortably, and successfully perform a wide spectrum of uterine procedures, requiring dilation, application of energy, and intrauterine dissection without need for systemic anesthesia or anxiolysis.

Local anesthetic agents

Mechanism of action and metabolism

There exist a variety of local anesthetic agents, but most are either from the amino amide or amino ester class, the latter modified versions of para-aminobenzoic acid (PABA) (Figure 14.1). Such local anesthetics exert their effect by altering neuronal depolarization by blocking the sodium channels in the cell membrane, most commonly those of sensory nerves, thereby preventing transmission of the sensation of pain to the higher neurons. They are largely metabolized in the liver with a half-life that varies according to the specific agent and a number of factors discussed below, but typically is approximately 1.5–2.0 hours.

Factors affecting onset, potency, and duration

The onset of action is largely related to the pKa of the agent – the closer to local pH the greater the penetration of the nonionized particles into the lipid rich nerve membrane [2–4] (Table 14.1). There are other factors that impact onset of action; the larger the nerve diameter the slower the onset, and local inflammation may decrease local pH thereby slowing the onset of action.

Potency is impacted by a number of factors. Anesthetics with increased lipophilic properties more easily pass into the lipid nerve membrane thereby increasing the anesthetic effect. Local vasodilation promotes vascular absorption of the agent, thereby reducing the local concentration and potency. Adding epinephrine or sodium bicarbonate increases local pH which, in turn, increases the nonionized particles that are more lipid

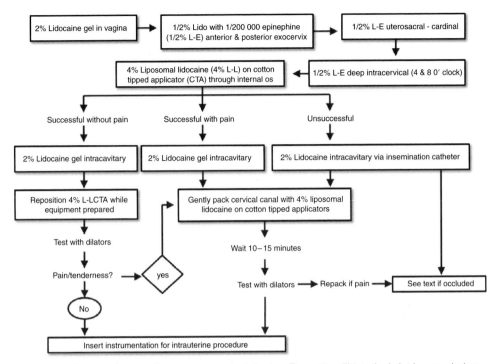

Figure 14.1 Suggested approach to uterine anesthesia in the office setting. This is the hybrid approach that I use in the office setting, which is supported by some evidence, with much to be gathered. The speculum is coated with 2% lidocaine gel, but, for selected patients, about 5 mL is self-administered gel placed in the vagina about 30–60 minutes before the procedure. Following placement of the speculum, the cervix is injected with anesthetic just below the epithelium at about 12 and 6 o'clock. The posterior cervix is then grasped with a tenaculum and the "paracervical" block is administered bilaterally aiming for the uterosacral-cardinal ligament complex, taking care not to push the spinal needle so far that the anesthetic goes into the peritoneal cavity. Typically I inject about 5–8 mL of 0.5% lidocaine with epinephrine in each side, hoping that the anesthetic will track in a way that captures both the nerves from the sacral and hypogastric plexi (Chapter 2). I also generally place about 5–8 mL of the same anesthetic into cervical stroma (intracervical block) passing the spinal needle as high as the lower uterine segment – about 4–5 cm in. The anesthetic is injected as the needle is withdrawn. I then take a sterile cotton-tipped applicator coated with 4% liposomal lidocaine and pass it through the internal os to determine comfort, patency, and the need for prolonged topical application of anesthesia. Then 2% lidocaine gel is placed in the endometrial cavity and the canal is packed with the 4% liposomal lidocaine-coated cotton-tipped applicators. After a suitable period of time, in part determined by the cotton-tipped applicator "test" and in part by the procedure to be performed, the procedure is commenced. It may take up to 20 minutes for some women to become anesthetized with the topical agent.

soluble. Of course the concentration of the anesthetic solution is an important factor – local anesthetic concentrations are generally expressed as a percentage (e.g., lidocaine 1%, bupivacaine 0.5%).[1]

The duration of action is largely determined by the amount of protein binding of the agent; a high degree of protein binding is associated with prolongation of the anesthetic effect. Increased duration can also be facilitated by use of local epinephrine which both decreases local systemic absorption and increases local pH.

---

[1] The mg/mL concentration can be calculated by moving the decimal point one place to the right (e.g., 1% lidocaine = 10 mg/mL).

Table 14.1 Types of local injectable anesthetic agents.

Amides
• Lidocaine (Xylocaine)
• Bupivacaine (Marcaine)
• Mepivacaine (Carbocaine)
• Prilocaine (Citanest)
• Etidocaine (Duranest)
Esters
• Procaine (Novocain)
• Chloroprocaine (Nesacaine)
• Tetracaine (Pontocaine)

Table 14.2 Injectable anesthetic agents.

Anesthetic	Concentration	Onset (min)	Duration (hours)	Maximal dose (mg/kg)	Maximum dose (mL/70 kg)
Lidocaine (Xylocaine)	1%, 2%	< 2	1.5–2	4 mg/kg not to exceed 280 mg	28mL (1%); 14 mL (2%)
Mepivacaine (Carbocaine)	1%	3.5	0.75–1.5	4 mg/kg not to exceed 280 mg	28 mL
Prilocaine (Citanest)	1%	< 2	> 1	7 mg/kg not to exceed 500 mg	50 mL
Lidocaine with epinephrine	Lidocaine 0.5%, 1%, 2% Epinephrine 1:100 000, 1:200 000	< 2	2–6	7 mg/kg not to exceed 500 mg	100 mL (0.5%) 50 mL (1%) 25 mL (2%)
Bupivacaine (Marcaine)	0.25%	5.8	2–4	2.5 mg/kg not to exceed 175 mg	50 mL
Etidocaine (Duranest)	0.25, 1%	4.6	2–3	4 mg/kg not to exceed 300 mg	50 mL (0.5%) 25 mL (1%)

The most effective, currently available topical anesthetic agent is lidocaine, used either alone or combined with other agents such as tetracaine and prilocaine with or without epinephrine. The dynamics of topical anesthesia are very different from those of injectable agents with most taking 20 minutes or more to achieve the maximal effect (Table 14.2). The onset, depth, and duration of action appear to depend upon a number of factors including the nature and integrity of the epithelial surface, the dose and duration of application, and the vehicle that contains the agent. For example, there is available a liposomal matrix that can be used as a vehicle for lidocaine that appears to allow the agent to work much faster, likely by facilitating absorption into the skin and neural membrane [5].

The other issue related to topical application is that of systemic absorption, which may also vary depending on the location of application and the nature, integrity, and vascularity of the epithelial surface.

Adverse events

Adverse reactions are rare with appropriate use but have been described in relationship to high plasma concentrations that are secondary to one or a combination of: (1) inadvertent intravascular injection; (2) excessive dose; and (3) delayed clearance/metabolism. The potential CNS side effects of high plasma levels include mouth tingling, tremor, dizziness, blurred vision, and seizures – and can culminate in respiratory depression and apnea. Cardiovascular side effects are those of direct myocardial depression – bradycardia and potential cardiovascular collapse – an adverse event more commonly described in association with bupivacaine. The other adverse reaction is related to the immune system, where an IgE-mediated allergic reaction can be experienced. This type of sensitization is usually associated with the ester class of anesthetics, related to the immunogenicity of PABA. Amino amide anesthetics do not contain PABA, a circumstance that has made the amides by far the most commonly used agents.

The adverse events associated with the use of injectable local anesthetic agents are virtually eliminated by screening for allergy, and with strict attention to both total dosage (in mg/kg) and injection technique, taking care to avoid intravascular injection. The use of solutions with dilute epinephrine has the benefit of reducing the chances of systemic absorption.

Topical agents can also be associated with adverse events, including systemic absorption that may be facilitated when the agent is applied to disrupted epithelial surfaces. The local effects may be limited to burning or stinging, while systemic effects mirror those associated with injectable agents, although serious and severe manifestations are extremely rare.

Anesthetic targets and techniques

Vagina

There are no available data describing the use of topical vaginal anesthesia for the uterine procedures described in this book, an approach that I came to rather lately at the suggestion of my friend and colleague Dr Alan Johns from Fort Worth, Texas. There is only one identifiable placebo-controlled RCT that evaluated topical vaginal anesthesia with a 10% spray solution in women undergoing brachytherapy for cervical cancer that demonstrated a significant decrease in the amount of pain perceived during the procedures [6] (Class I-2). Clearly some structured investigation is needed to evaluate the efficacy of this approach.

Cervix

The cervix may be anesthetized using one or a combination of intracervical, paracervical, and topical injections/applications.

Paracervical

The concept of paracervical block is to anesthetize the nerves supplying the cervix by injecting local anesthetic agents in the uterosacral and/or broad ligaments. There is a substantial difference among clinicians in the location(s) and depths of injection as well as the anesthetic agent, its concentration, and the time allowed prior to starting the procedure. Indeed, high quality RCTs evaluating paracervically administered agents at hysteroscopy or D&C have demonstrated either no difference [7, 8] or a significant difference [9–11] in pain scores (Class I-2). Unfortunately many of the studies that showed no difference allowed relatively little time between injection and uterine manipulation. This circumstance begs the question of outcomes should a longer time interval be standardized prior to uterine manipulation.

Intracervical

Intracervical block involves injecting the local anesthetic agent directly into the cervical stroma with any of a wide spectrum of techniques, some of which have not been particularly well described. In addition, the usual inconsistency in injection-procedure times and variation in the agent and dose used confounds evaluation. One relatively large series of REA for HMB was done exclusively using intracervical anesthesia with only 3 of 278 that could not be completed because of inadequate pain control [12] (Class III). In the only available placebo-controlled RCT, pain experienced during insertion of a hysteroscope was less in the lidocaine group, although the pain of injection was described to be as painful as the procedure [13] (Class I-2).

Topical

Topical anesthetics may be applied either to the exocervix or in the cervical canal using vehicles that include spray solutions, topical gels, and creams (Table 14.3). The use of topical anesthetic sprays on the exocervix has generally been shown ineffective for biopsy [14], but one well-designed placebo-controlled RCT demonstrated that there was less pain with tenaculum attachment [15] (each Class I-2).

The use of topical agents in the cervical canal has had some evaluation. One RCT demonstrated that spray anesthesia for office-based hysteroscopy using a 10% solution was not different from placebo [15], while well-designed RCTs from France (5% lidocaine gel) [16] and Italy [17] (prilocaine/lidocaine cream or lidocaine spray) showed significant reduction in procedure-related pain scores (all Class I-2).

Corpus

As reviewed previously (Chapter 2), the innervation of the corpus is largely from fibers that originate from the T 10–L 1 roots which primarily enter the uterus via Frankenhauser's plexus and the broad ligament in association with the uterine arteries. As a result, it is theoretically possible to provide uterine anesthesia via paracervical injection including injections aimed at Frankenhauser's plexus. The section above, entitled "Paracervical," dealt with the high quality studies published to date and the problems with research design that leave the ultimate value of these approaches still to be determined.

An alternate or additional strategy for the corpus is the application of topical anesthesia to the endometrial surface via agents injected into the endometrial cavity via the cervical canal. Using a double blinded RCT, investigators have demonstrated that instilling 2% lidocaine solution (5 mL) into the endometrial cavity 10 minutes prior to performing SIS significantly reduced patient-perceived pain [18] (Class I-2). For hysteroscopy and directed biopsy, a well-designed RCT that injected 2% lidocaine via the hysteroscope demonstrated near significance for the hysteroscopy and statistically significant differences for biopsy [19]. Unfortunately, only two minutes transpired between injection and the performance of the procedures. Other RCTs evaluating hysteroscopy that allowed 3–5 minutes from injection of 2% mepivacaine to the procedure demonstrated a significant reduction in pain [20, 21] and, in one study, reduction in vasovagal reactions [21]. However, even these findings are not consistent in the literature as another RCT that did allow 5 minutes

Table 14.3 Topical anesthetic agents: dermatological application.

Anesthetic formulation	Onset	Duration	Complications
0.5% Tetracaine, 1:2000 epinephrine, 11.8% cocaine (TAC)	10–30 min	Unknown	Rare severe toxicity including seizures and sudden cardiac death
4% Lidocaine, 1:2000 epinephrine, 0.5% tetracaine (LET)	20–30 min	Unknown	No severe adverse reactions reported
2.5% Lidocaine, 2.5% prilocaine (EMLA)	1 hour	0.5–2 hours	Contact dermatitis, methemoglobinemia (very rare)
4% Liposomal lidocaine	30 min	0.5–2+ hours	No severe adverse reactions reported

between placing 2% lidocaine in the endometrial cavity demonstrated no measured benefit [22]. Similar inconsistency can be found for other procedures such as endometrial biopsy, D&C, and SIS. Understanding that topical anesthetics may need substantial time to have an effect leads one to believe that optimal uterine topical anesthesia may require up to 20 minutes depending on the epithelial surface and specifics of the anesthetic agent used. Obviously proof of this concept requires the performance, or re-performance, of many of the clinical trials described above.

Systemic agents

Systemic agents can provide problems for the clinician performing office-based procedures, for the use of narcotics and anxiolytics during the procedure requires equipment and personnel for monitoring. Furthermore, post-procedure monitoring is also required and patients require an individual for transportation to their home. While there clearly are procedures or patients who require such an approach, I will not enter that discussion here, in part because we and others have been very successful in accomplishing a wide spectrum of procedures without the need for such agents.

There may be value to preprocedural administration of COX inhibitors but the only identifiable RCT (compared to placebo) evaluated a 500 mg oral dose of mefenamic acid given 1 hour before hysteroscopy. There was no difference in the pain experienced at hysteroscopy but, importantly, post-procedure pain was less in the treatment group [23].

Summary of the evidence

Evaluation of the evidence, on the surface, could lead to confusion regarding the role of local anesthesia in the performance of uterine procedures. One issue is that populations can vary substantially based on parity and other features that may make, for example, unanesthetized cervical dilation painful for some and painless for others. Indeed, a number of investigators have touted the performance of hysteroscopy without anesthesia of any sort [24, 25] (Class III); however, it is clear from the studies that a substantial number of the women, albeit a minority, experienced substantial pain. Duration of the procedure and the size of polyps seem to be factors involved in the amount of pain perceived. As a result, and pending the performance of studies that allow us to understand better the relative values of the various anesthetic techniques, we have formulated an approach that uses a combination of techniques that we feel provides predictable comfort during a wide variety of uterine procedures from endometrial biopsy and IUD insertion to hysteroscopic polypectomy and myomectomy.

Suggested regimen

Background

The suggested approach is admittedly one that "overlaps" a number of techniques described above, while keeping the total potential dose of anesthetic well within the allowable range. It should also be noted that the evidence supporting this regimen is clearly "Class III."

Essentially five separate sites are considered; injectable 0.5% lidocaine with 1/200 000 epinephrine is used intra- and paracervically, while topical 2–4% lidocaine is used in the vagina, the endocervical canal, and the endometrial cavity. I believe that, equally critical to the spectrum of techniques, is the commitment of the clinician to wait an adequate amount of time for the anesthetic agents to reach their maximum effectiveness. This particularly applies to topical agents that appear to require more time to traverse the epithelial surfaces to the desired nerve fibers.

The anesthetic regimen in Figure 14.1 (Video 14.1) represents our local anesthetic protocol in our Uterine Procedure and Imaging Center, which we use in its entirety for hysteroscopy and hysteroscopically-directed procedures. While we know that some women do not really need anesthesia, in our opinion, it is better to provide anesthesia for those who do not need it than not to provide it for those who do. With this regimen we have never had to stop a procedure because of pain and our overall mean pain score, including institution of the anesthesia, has a mean of 3.4 out of 10.

Basic technique

Preprocedure

Patients are given the option of using a COX inhibitor the evening before and two to four hours prior to the procedure. We suggest sodium naproxen (440–550 mg) or ibuprofen (400–800 mg) but have no evidence that these are better than other agents. When difficulty with cervical dilation is anticipated, an evening dose of vaginally administered misoprostol (200 mg) is provided. For women whom we know or suspect have very sensitive vaginal epithelium, I prescribe 2% lidocaine gel with an applicator and instruct the patient to place approximately 5 mL in the vagina about 1 hour prior to the procedure.

Preparing the patient

The procedure room is one with a very relaxed atmosphere, and anything that can be done to enhance this (music, paintings, color selection) is probably worthwhile. It is very important that this room is perceived to be clean and tidy.

After the patient is positioned in the modified lithotomy position, with feet in comfortable stirrups, an appropriately sized, heated metal speculum, coated with 2% lidocaine gel, is placed in the vagina to expose the cervix. While there is no initial impact beyond lubrication, I suspect that there is clinical impact by 10–15 minutes into the case.

Injectable agent

I use a dilute solution of 0.5% lidocaine with 1/200 000 epinephrine that allows a larger volume of anesthetic to be used for a given dose. Epinephrine, as described above, prolongs the anesthetic effect, reduces the amount of systemic absorption, and facilitates transfer of the anesthetic agent into the nerve fiber by increasing local pH. The effect of the epinephrine is predictable with a transient (40–60 seconds) period of palpitation that quickly disappears. For patients who are unstable enough that epinephrine is considered to be too much of a risk, alternative anesthesia and/or anesthetic environment is suggested.

Intra- and paracervical components

The agent is drawn into a syringe and a 22-gauge spinal needle is attached. The needle tip is placed by the cervical epithelium and the patient is asked to cough, a technique that appears to reduce the pain of injection [26, 27], and which pushes the cervix against the needle where it is positioned so that the bevel is just below the epithelial surface. Then 1–3 mL of the agent are injected in this fashion into the anterior (11–1 o'clock) and posterior aspects (5–7 o'clock) of the cervix.

The posterior cervix is grasped where the anesthetic agent has been injected and it is retracted anteriorly, a technique that aids in identification of the attachment of the uterosacral ligaments using an instrument such a sound or dilator. Again using the cough technique, a small amount of anesthetic agent is injected into the vaginal epithelium at the junction with the cervix; then the needle is advanced to a depth of 4–5 mm aiming to position the bevel medially on the ligament but not in the peritoneal cavity. Approximately 5–8 mL of anesthetic solution is placed in each side in this fashion, taking care to aspirate prior to injection. Then, the tenaculum is removed from the posterior cervix and affixed to the anterior lip. Exerting a slight amount of traction, an intracervical injection of about 4 mL of the 0.5% lidocaine with 1/200 000 epinephrine is placed deeply in each side of the cervix, at about 4–5 o'clock on the left side, and 7–8 o'clock on the right side, attempting to hit the area of greatest innervation.

Topical agents

After the injectable aspect of the procedure, a sterile cotton-tipped applicator soaked in 4% liposomal lidocaine cream is passed through the cervical canal and through the internal os. If this can be accomplished with relative ease, the patient's tolerance is noted, the applicator removed, and a conical-tipped syringe prefilled with 2% lidocaine gel is pushed against the exocervix. Approximately 5–8 mL of the gel is injected into the endometrial cavity. The patient's response to this is noted as well. The syringe is removed and 2–3 cotton-tipped applicators soaked in the 4% liposomal lidocaine cream are positioned in the cervical canal, from the internal to the level of the external os. The patient is then left for 5–15 or more minutes depending upon her response to the cotton-tipped applicator and intracavitary injection, and upon the procedure to be performed.

Troubleshooting

There are a few minor modifications that may come up depending upon specific features of the patient. In some instances, the external os is too narrow to accommodate even a cotton-tipped applicator or the prefilled syringe. In these cases, an insemination catheter may be used to navigate the cervical canal into the endometrial cavity and 2% lidocaine solution may be injected using a syringe.

In other instances, the cotton-tipped applicator cannot be advanced past the internal os. In these circumstances, we pack the canal with 4% liposomal lidocaine coated applicators, leave the patient for at least 10 minutes, and then use either a flexible or rigid hysteroscope of appropriate diameter to navigate the canal into the endometrial cavity dissecting aduesious, if encountered, with scissors passed through the working channel. Upon reaching the cavity, a channel of the hysteroscope system can be used to allow instillation of lidocaine solution into the endometrial cavity, taking care to wait an appropriate time before continuing further, depending on the procedure to be performed.

Summary

It is recognized that this approach may be "overkill" for many simple procedures such as endometrial biopsy and LNG-IUS insertion, where modifications may be considered, consistent with the experience of the clinician and the specific characteristics of the patient. However, in our experience, this regimen is safe and keeps dosing well within prescribed limits, even considering the unlikely event of total absorption of topically administered agents. While it is understood that many women do not require anesthesia at all, it is difficult to anticipate who those individuals are. Consequently, liberal use of local anesthesia, combined with the patience to wait an adequate amount of time, particularly for topical agents, should result in a greater number of uterine procedures being completed both successfully and comfortably in the office setting.

References

1. Tokushige N, Markham R, Russell P, Fraser IS. High density of small nerve fibres in the functional layer of the endometrium in women with endometriosis. *Hum Reprod.* 2006;**21**(3):782–7.
2. Dripps RD, Eckenhoff JE, Vandam LD. Introduction to anesthesia. In Longenecker DE, Murphy FL, eds. *Introduction to Anesthesia*, 8th edn. Philadelphia: Saunders; 1992.
3. Arca MJ, Biermann JS, Johnson TM, Chang AE. Biopsy techniques for skin, soft-tissue, and bone neoplasms. *Surg Oncol Clin N Am.* 1995;**4**(1):157–74.
4. *Drug Facts and Comparisons.* St Louis: Facts and Comparisons; 2009.
5. Koh JL, Harrison D, Myers R, Dembinski R, Turner H, McGraw T. A randomized, double-blind comparison study of EMLA and ELA-Max for topical anesthesia in children undergoing intravenous insertion. *Paediatr Anaesth.* 2004;**14**(12):977–82.
6. Chen HC, Leung SW, Wang CJ, Sun LM, Fang FM, Huang EY, et al. Local vaginal anesthesia during high-dose-rate intracavitary brachytherapy for cervical cancer. *Int J Radiat Oncol Biol Phys.* 1998;**42**(3):541–4.
7. Vercellini P, Colombo A, Mauro F, Oldani S, Bramante T, Crosignani PG. Paracervical anesthesia for outpatient hysteroscopy. *Fertil Steril.* 1994;**62**(5):1083–5.
8. Lau WC, Lo WK, Tam WH, Yuen PM. Paracervical anaesthesia in outpatient hysteroscopy: a randomised double-blind placebo-controlled trial. *Br J Obstet Gynaecol.* 1999;**106**(4):356–9.
9. Cicinelli E, Didonna T, Schonauer LM, Stragapede S, Falco N, Pansini N. Paracervical anesthesia for hysteroscopy and EB in postmenopausal women. A randomized, double-blind, placebo-controlled study. *J Reprod Med.* 1998;**43**(12):1014–18.
10. Titapant V, Chawanpaiboon S, Boonpektrakul K. Double-blind randomized comparison of xylocaine and saline in paracervical block for diagnostic fractional curettage. *J Med Assoc Thai.* 2003;**86**(2):131–5.
11. Giorda G, Scarabelli C, Franceschi S, Campagnutta E. Feasibility and pain control in outpatient hysteroscopy in postmenopausal women: a randomized trial. *Acta Obstet Gynecol Scand.* 2000;**79**(7):593–7.
12. Ferry J, Rankin L. Transcervical resection of the endometrium using intracervical block only. A review of 278 procedures. *Aust N Z J Obstet Gynaecol.* 1994;**34**(4):457–61.
13. Broadbent JA, Hill NC, Molnar BG, Rolfe KJ, Magos AL. Randomized placebo controlled trial to assess the role of intracervical lignocaine in outpatient

hysteroscopy. *Br J Obstet Gynaecol.* 1992;**99** (9):777–9.

14. Prefontaine M, Fung-Kee-Fung M, Moher D. Comparison of topical Xylocaine with placebo as a local anesthetic in colposcopic biopsies. *Can J Surg.* 1991;**34**(2):163–5.

15. Davies A, Richardson RE, O'Connor H, Baskett TF, Nagele F, Magos AL. Lignocaine aerosol spray in outpatient hysteroscopy: a randomized double-blind placebo-controlled trial. *Fertil Steril.* 1997;**67**(6):1019–23.

16. Soriano D, Ajaj S, Chuong T, Deval B, Fauconnier A, Darai E. Lidocaine spray and outpatient hysteroscopy: randomized placebo-controlled trial. *Obstet Gynecol.* 2000;**96**(5 Pt 1):661–4.

17. Zullo F, Pellicano M, Stigliano CM, Di Carlo C, Fabrizio A, Nappi C. Topical anesthesia for office hysteroscopy. A prospective, randomized study comparing two modalities. *J Reprod Med.* 1999;**44** (10):865–9.

18. Guney M, Oral B, Bayhan G, Mungan T. Intrauterine lidocaine infusion for pain relief during saline solution infusion sonohysterography: a randomized, controlled trial. *J Minim Invasive Gynecol.* 2007;**14**(3):304–10.

19. Costello M, Horowitz SD, Williamson M. A prospective randomised double-blind placebo controlled study of local anaesthetic injected through the hysteroscope for outpatient hysteroscopy and endometrial biopsy. *Gynaecol Endoscopy.* 1998;**7**:121–6.

20. Zupi E, Luciano AA, Valli E, Marconi D, Maneschi F, Romanini C. The use of topical anesthesia in diagnostic hysteroscopy and endometrial biopsy. *Fertil Steril.* 1995; **63**(2):414–16.

21. Cicinelli E, Didonna T, Ambrosi G, Schonauer LM, Fiore G, Matteo MG. Topical anaesthesia for diagnostic hysteroscopy and endometrial biopsy in postmenopausal women: a randomised placebo-controlled double-blind study. *Br J Obstet Gynaecol.* 1997;**104**(3):316–19.

22. Lau WC, Tam WH, Lo WK, Yuen PM. A randomised double-blind placebo-controlled trial of transcervical intrauterine local anaesthesia in outpatient hysteroscopy. *BJOG.* 2000;**107**(5):610–13.

23. Nagele F, Lockwood G, Magos AL. Randomised placebo controlled trial of mefenamic acid for premedication at outpatient hysteroscopy: a pilot study. *Br J Obstet Gynaecol.* 1997;**104**(7):842–4.

24. Bettocchi S, Ceci O, Nappi L, Di Venere R, Masciopinto V, Pansini V, et al. Operative office hysteroscopy without anesthesia: analysis of 4863 cases performed with mechanical instruments. *J Am Assoc Gynecol Laparosc.* 2004; **11**(1):59–61.

25. Litta P, Cosmi E, Saccardi C, Esposito C, Rui R, Ambrosini G. Outpatient operative polypectomy using a 5 mm-hysteroscope without anaesthesia and/or analgesia: advantages and limits. *Eur J Obstet Gynecol Reprod Biol.* 2008;**139**(2):210–14.

26. Usichenko TI, Pavlovic D, Foellner S, Wendt M. Reducing venipuncture pain by a cough trick: a randomized crossover volunteer study. *Anesth Analg.* 2004; **98**(2):343–5.

27. Agarwal A, Sinha PK, Tandon M, Dhiraaj S, Singh U. Evaluating the efficacy of the valsalva maneuver on venous cannulation pain: a prospective, randomized study. *Anesth Analg.* 2005;**101**(4):1230–2.

15 Endometrial ablation

Chapter summary

- Endometrial ablation (EA) is targeted destruction of the endometrium.
- Resectoscopic ablation is EA performed using a uterine resectoscope.
- Nonresectoscopic endometrial ablation (NREA) refers to a number of devices that ablate the endometrium without the use of a resectoscope.
- It is possible to perform NREA in an office setting under local anesthesia.

Introduction

Endometrial ablation is targeted destruction of the endometrium for the treatment of AUB for women who have no desire for future fertility.

Background

The concept of surgical destruction of the endometrial lining for the treatment of AUB is not new. A published report of EA with steam can be found in 1898 [1], and a monopolar radiofrequency electrosurgical probe inserted blindly into the uterus was the subject of a series published by Bardenheuer, from Germany, in 1937 [2]. However, the world seemed to forget about this approach to the clinical problem of HMB for more than 30 years when cryotherapy (freezing) of the endometrium for AUB was first introduced [3] and then subjected to clinical evaluation [4, 5]. It was more than a decade until the introduction of endoscopically-guided techniques for EA, first using a hysteroscope to direct Nd:YAG laser energy to coagulate and vaporize the endometrium [6], and then the urological resectoscope to remove endometrial tissue with a radiofrequency (RF) electrosurgical loop electrode [7]. For more than a decade, resectoscopically-directed EA was the principal method used for performing targeted removal and/or destruction of the endometrium, but, beginning in the late 1990s a number of nonresectoscopic techniques, conceptually similar to those first introduced in the 1930s and mislabeled as "second generation devices," began to appear.

Techniques

Resectoscopic endometrial ablation

Destruction of the endometrial lining under endoscopic guidance was originally described using the Nd:YAG laser via a fiber passed through the instrument channel of an operating hysteroscope [6], but was quickly replaced by the more efficient, modified urological RF resectoscope. The initial resectoscopic technique employed a loop electrode to remove endometrium (Video 15.2) [7], but was quickly followed with electrosurgical desiccation/coagulation with a ball or barrel-shaped electrode (Video 15.1) [8] and grooved or spiked electrodes that allowed the surgeon to electrosurgically vaporize the target tissue (Video 15.3) [9, 10]. Vaporization has been shown in the context of a comparative trial to be associated with markedly reduced systematic absorption of distension media [9].

Complications of REA

For REA, the most serious complications are uterine distension media overload, uterine perforation, and damage to surrounding structures such as bowel and blood vessels. Other complications include those related to anesthesia, failed access, and hemorrhage.

The largest published evaluation of adverse outcomes with hysteroscopic surgery suggests that techniques involving endometrial resection are most often associated with serious complications secondary to hemorrhage or perforation [11] (Class II-2). This study also documents that experience is an important variable as these complications were most commonly encountered in the first 100 cases of a given surgeon. As a result, the low incidence of complications found in the literature from series and trials may not reflect the risk in the population at large because of the expertise and experience of most published investigators.

The use of monopolar RF instruments makes it necessary that the distention media be electrolyte-free, so solutions such as 3% sorbitol, 1.5% glycine, 5% mannitol, and combined solutions of sorbitol and mannitol are used. These media, on occasion, can be absorbed into the systemic circulation, particularly when veins in the myometrium are breached, and if sufficient volume is intravasated, both hypoosmolar fluid overload and a dilutional hyponatremia typically results [12, 13] (Class II-3). Taken to an extreme, resulting subsequent brain edema can, in some instances, result in permanent neurological damage or death. Such outcomes may be more common in premenopausal women because of the inhibitory impact of estrogen and progesterone on the brain's sodium pump, making such women more vulnerable to cerebral edema [14].

Early detection of intravasation is enhanced by adherence to a strict fluid measurement and management protocol, which preferably includes an automated system that measures fluid inflow and captures all fluid that leaves the uterus. The development of hysteroscopic electrosurgical systems that can operate in electrolyte rich media such as normal saline has provided an opportunity to eliminate the risk of hyponatremia, [15, 16], but risks of fluid overload remain.

The volume of systemically absorbed distension media may be reduced with the pre-operative use of GnRH analogs [14, 17] (Class I-2) and/or with the immediate preoperative administration of dilute intracervical vasopressin [18] (Class I-2). There exist a number of other measures that should reduce the extent of systemic intravasation that include operating at the lowest effective intrauterine pressure and avoidance of preoperative over hydration.

The management of intraoperatively-recognized excessive intravasation varies according to the patient's baseline medical condition, her intraoperative assessment, the status of the procedure, and the amount of measured fluid intravasation. If the deficit reaches a predetermined limit, which, depending on the patient's baseline status, could range from 750 to 1500 mL, serum electrolytes are measured, and furosemide 10–40 mg is given intravenously. Should the serum sodium fall below 125 mEQ/L, or should the deficit reach 1500–2000 mL, the procedure is expeditiously terminated.

Shortly after the introduction of REA, post-ablation tubal ligation syndrome was first described as a complication of EA performed in women with previous contraceptive tubal occlusion. Patients experience cyclical pelvic pain presumably related to residual and trapped endometrium in one or both cornua. The incidence of this syndrome is unclear but has been reported to be as high as 10% [19]. Hysteroscopic decompression and laparoscopic salpingectomy are frequently not successful and hysterectomy has been described as the most effective treatment [19] (Class III).

An early concern about EA was the potential for delaying the diagnosis of a subsequent endometrial carcinoma. However, it seems clear that at least the majority of those women who have been reported to develop endometrial malignancy following EA are those who have the usual risk factors for endometrial hyperplasia [20] (Class III) and that the incidence in "low risk" populations may be similar to women who have not received EA [21] (Class III). Consequently, women who are at enhanced risk for endometrial hyperplasia because of chronic anovulation may be counseled that they will remain at greater risk than ovulatory women for developing such a disorder following EA. In such instances, it may be wise to consider the use of an intermittent progestational agent.

Factors affecting outcome of resectoscopic endometrial ablation

As is the case with most surgical procedures, clinical outcomes of REA appear to be related to a number of patient- and surgeon-specific factors. Women 45 and older appear to be less likely to have subsequent hysterectomy, and more likely than those under 45 to be amenorrheic and satisfied with their outcome [22, 23]. Surgeon experience and/or ability also seem to be important. In one study, the subsequent hysterectomy rate was 12.6% when endometrial resection was performed exclusively by the consultant surgeon, compared to 38% if all or part of the procedure was done by a trainee [22] (Class II-2).

The presence of adenomyosis has also been associated with an increased risk of REA failure [24] and has been found in up to 75% of post-EA hysterectomy specimens [25]. There is some evidence that with increasing depth of resection and ablation, the failure rate with deep resection drops to as low as 5%, a result that may reflect more complete removal of adenomyosis [26] (Class III). Although failures may be higher in women with larger uteri and correspondingly larger endometrial cavities, at least in experienced and able hands, success rates in uteri greater than 12-gestational weeks size may be equivalent to that of women with smaller sized uteri [27] (Class II-2). This is an important observation given the limitations of the currently available NREA systems to be discussed subsequently.

Nonresectoscopic endometrial ablation

As we have seen, achievement of optimal clinical outcomes with REA, including low complication rates, requires substantial skill and experience on the part of the surgeon and the use of an institutional setting (operating room or surgical center) because of the requirements for anesthesia and relatively sophisticated equipment for monitoring fluid balance. These factors created a renewed interest in, and development of, nonresectoscopic techniques and devices for performing EA with a view to reducing: (a) the required training and skill; (b) the need for an institutional setting; and (c) the complications associated with the procedure. Consequently, NREA techniques are those that are designed to destroy the endometrium without the need for a resectoscope (Figure 15.1). Unlike the case for REA, each of these devices differs in the required cervical dilation, the minimum and maximum sounded length of the uterus, and the capability for treatment of submucosal leiomyomas (Table 15.1).

Balloon ablation devices

Cavaterm

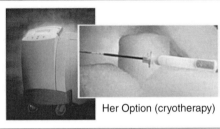

Thermachoice

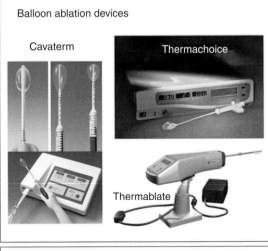

Thermablate

NovaSure
(radiofrequency
electricity)

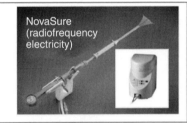

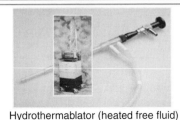

Hydrothermablator (heated free fluid)

Her Option (cryotherapy)

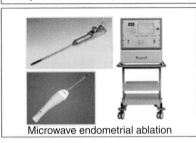

Microwave endometrial ablation

Figure 15.1 Nonresectoscopic endometrial ablation devices. *Upper left panel*. Balloon ablation devices: the Thermachoice® system is upper right and in the lower right is the portable Thermablate® system, while the Cavaterm® system is on the left. Each use heated fluid contained within a balloon deployed within the endometrial cavity. *Upper right*. The NovaSure® radiofrequency endometrial ablation device. The bipolar mesh is deployed after the probe is placed in the endometrial cavity. The procedure is automated and automatically stops when a threshold impedance of 50 Ω is reached. *Middle right*. Hydro ThermAblator® circulates and then heats free fluid in the endometrial cavity for 10 minutes to coagulate the endometrium. *Lower right*. Microwave endometrial ablation (MEA®) utilizes microwaves at the tip of the probe to coagulate the endometrium with the surgeon using temperature to control the procedure. *Lower left*. Her Option®, a hypothermic probe controlled by the surgeon who uses a combination of time and transabdominal ultrasound monitoring to determine the endpoint of the procedure.

Balloon hyperthermal NREA

For this technique a balloon-tipped catheter is placed through the cervical canal into the endometrial cavity, where it is distended with fluid, which is heated to a temperature adequate to result in destruction of the adjacent endometrium. There are now four such systems available worldwide.

The *Cavaterm*® balloon ablation device (PNN Medical A/S, Kvistgard, Denmark) has an outside diameter (OD) of 6 mm and a preshaped adjustable balloon, designed to facilitate intimate contact with the endometrial surface. The disposable balloon catheter is connected to the central control unit that heats (78°C) and circulates the fluid inside the balloon for 10 minutes at a constant pressure of 230–240 mm Hg. The procedure is limited to normal endometrial cavities that measure from 4 to 10 cm, *from the internal os to the fundus*, rather than the sounded length from the external os to the fundus, which is used as the parameter for the Thermachoice® and MenoTreat® devices discussed subsequently. The manufacturer also

Table 15.1 Patient, device, and treatment parameters of the five nonresectoscopic endometrial ablation (NREA) devices in widest use. Pretreatment refers to the requirement for thinning or removing the endometrium prior to the procedure. The OD is the outside diameter of the device and an indication of how much the cervix must be dilated prior to inserting the device. The sounded uterine lengths depict the minimum and maximum uterine length that can be treated. Some of these devices have been evaluated for the treatment of heavy menstrual bleeding in the context of submucosal leiomyomas (HMB-Ls). The quality of evidence, type, and diameter of the myoma and the status of US Federal (FDA) approval are shown.

	Pretreatment	OD (mm)	Approx treatment time (min)	Sounded uterine length (cm)		Published evidence	Treatment in the presence of submucosal leiomyomas		
				Min	Max		Type[a]	Diameter (cm)	FDA approval
Balloon (Thermachoice®)	Curettage	5.5	8	4	10	+ (Class I)	II	≤ 3	No
Cryotherapy (Her Option®)	GnRH Agonist	4.5	10–18	–	10	None	N/A	N/A	No
Free Fluid (Hydro ThermAblator®)[b]	GnRH Agonist	7.8	14	4	10.5	+ (Class II-3)	I+, II	?	No
Microwave (MEA®)	GnRH Agonist	8.5	2.5–4.5	6	14	+ (Class I)	I+, II	≤ 3	Yes
Radiofrequency (NovaSure®)	None	7.2	1.0–2.0	6	10	+ (Class II-2)	I, II	≤ 3	No

a See PALM-COEIN classification, Figure 4.1.
b There is insufficient data to determine the type and dimension of myomas treatable with Hydro ThermAblator.

contraindicates use of the device when the cervical canal is more than 6 cm in length. The largest study to date evaluating the Cavaterm device reported on 220 patients, with 83% satisfied at an average of 19 months following the procedure [28] (Class II-3). The Cavaterm study with the longest followup interval reported on 60 women of whom 58% were amenorrheic, 33% less than normal, and 9% with normal periods at 48 months following the ablation [29] (Class II-3).

Thermachoice® (Ethicon Women's Health and Urology, Sommerville, NJ, USA) is the most widely available balloon ablation system with the first experience published in 1994 [30, 31]. The system comprises a single use 5.5 mm OD balloon catheter, a connecting cable, and a dedicated controller unit that is powered from a standard alternating current wall outlet (Video 15.7). The controller activates the element and impeller contained within the balloon itself thereby heating and circulating the fluid (5% dextrose and water) that has been injected into the balloon by the surgeon. Microcircuitry is used to monitor the target temperature (87°C), the pressure (160–180 mm Hg), and the duration of treatment (8 minutes).

As clinical outcomes are likely improved if the endometrial thickness is minimized, the manufacturer recommends that patients should either be mechanically treated with intra-operative curettage or undergo preprocedural medical suppression with gonadal steroids or GnRH analogs. In the clinical trials, patients were generally given some sort of general or regional anesthesia, but local and/or neuroleptic analgesia may be all that is necessary [32, 33] (Class II-2).

There are two other hyperthermic balloon NREA devices in very limited release worldwide; the *Thermablate*® (Idoman Ltd, Dublin, Republic of Ireland) [34], and the *MenoTreat*® balloon ablation system (Atos Medical AB, Horby, Sweden) [35, 36]. The limited data suggest that these devices may achieve results similar to the more widely available systems.

Hypothermic nonresectoscopic endometrial ablation (cryotherapy)

The first clinical series describing intrauterine cryotherapy for abnormal uterine bleeding appeared almost 40 years ago [3–5]. The currently available device is called *Her Option*® (American Medical Systems Inc, Minnetonka, MN, USA) and comprises a disposable 4.5 mm OD probe attached to a dedicated controller unit (Video 15.6). The probe is passed trans-cervically into the endometrial cavity, usually with little or minimal requirement for dilation. When activated, the device creates an elliptical freeze zone up to 12 mm deep by reducing the local endomyometrial temperature to less than –90°C. Although there exists appropriate concern about the potential for such a freeze depth to involve adjacent structures such as bowel, the surgeon can monitor the depth of the freeze using transabdominal ultrasound. The required number of freeze cycles depends in part on the size and shape of the endometrial cavity, but usually numbers two, contributing to a treatment time of about 10 minutes. Published data regarding the device has been limited to endometrial cavities that are without submucosal myomas and which sound to 10 cm or less.

Hyperthermic NREA with free heated fluid

The Hydro ThermAblator® (HTA®) (BEI Medical/Boston Scientific, Natick, MA, USA) is a system based upon the instillation of free fluid into the peritoneal cavity under hystero-scopic visualization.[1] The device comprises a single use sheath (7.8 mm OD) that adapts to

---

[1]   This feature is the reason we had to categorize these devices as "nonresectoscopic" instead of "nonhysteroscopic."

any of a number of 3 mm OD standard hysteroscopes, and is connected to a proprietary controller unit (Video 15.5). The system infuses normal saline into the endometrial cavity at low pressure (< 40 cm H_2O) and then seals the system and monitors system volume, a feature that allows early detection and system shutdown should there be egress of fluid via either the cervix or fallopian tubes. The process takes approximately 3 minutes to heat the fluid to 90°C, 10 minutes to ablate the endometrium, and about 1 minute for the fluid to cool down at which time the device is removed.

In the RCT the device was evaluated in uteri that sounded from 4.0 to 10.5 cm and had normal endometrial cavities. Two retrospective studies have indicated that women with intracavitary myomas may have outcomes similar to that of women with normal cavities [37, 38] (Class III).

Microwave NREA

Microwaves occupy the part of the electromagnetic spectrum between radio and infrared waves and exert their effect first by direct heating of tissue, and then, in adjacent deeper layers, by thermal propagation. There are currently two versions of the microwave endometrial ablation (MEA) device, one reusable and one disposable (FemWave®, Microsulis Medical, Denmead, UK), and each of which comprises a 8.5 mm OD probe, calibrated to 15 cm, and attached to a dedicated controller by a reusable cable (Video 15.8). The microwave frequency is 9.2 GHz, the power output 30 Watts, and the local tissue is heated to about 90°C, achieving an aggregate depth of tissue necrosis of about 5–6 mm.

Once the cervix is dilated and hysteroscopy confirms an intact endometrial cavity, the microwave probe is inserted to the uterine fundus and the machine is activated. The surgeon moves the probe in horizontal sweeping movements, keeping the local temperature between 80 and 90°C as measured by the probe's integrated thermal coupling device. In this fashion, the entire endometrium is "covered" as the device is gradually withdrawn from the endometrial cavity. Treatment time is usually about two to four minutes. The system has the capacity to treat uteri with a sounded cavity length of up to 14 cm, but, at this time, there are limited data available for cavities that exceed 10 cm, a length that is similar to that of other devices. Patients may be treated under local anesthesia, conscious sedation, or using regional or general anesthetics [39].

Radiofrequency NREA

The NovaSure® system (Cytyc Surgical Division of Hologic Inc, Marlborough, MA, USA) is a NREA device that uses RF outputs to perform automated EA (Video 15.4). The system is based around a single use 7.2 mm OD probe that delivers a bipolar gold mesh multi-electrode array, attached to an expandable frame located at the distal end of the device. The electrode assembly also contains a cavity integrity testing system that is based on injection of a fixed volume of CO_2 following intrauterine placement of the probe. The probe is attached to a dedicated microprocessor-based electrosurgical unit (ESU).

The technique allows performance of EA without mechanical or medical endometrial preparation. Although most procedures are likely performed in operating theaters, EA with the NovaSure device has been reported under local anesthesia with conscious sedation [40, 41].

Following cervical dilation to an appropriate diameter, the system is inserted transcervically, the mesh electrode is deployed, and measurements from the device entered into the dedicated ESU. The unit is activated, and, if the uterine integrity test is passed, RF current activates the bipolar mesh while simultaneously applying suction, thereby evacuating steam and carbonized debris. The procedure is completed when the impedance exceeds 50 Ω, usually at about 90 seconds.

In the US trial, patients with leiomyomas or polyps less than 2 cm in diameter were allowed, but there was no subgroup analysis of patients with such lesions [42].

Other NREA techniques

A number of other NREA techniques appear to be in development, including those using low power Nd:YAG laser [43], photodynamic therapy [44–46], and chemoablation using 95% trichloroacetic acid, the same substance used for the topical treatment of exophytic human papillomavirus infection [47, 48]. Whether and when these techniques are released or approved by regulatory agencies is a matter for conjecture.

Complications of NREA

Complications can occur with NREA techniques but they appear to be much less frequent than is the case for REA. A review of the US Food and Drug Administration's (FDA's) Manufacturer and User Facility Device Experience (MAUDE) database found reports of uterine perforation in all of the NREA devices on the market at that time, including at least one bowel injury in three of the four [49] (Class III). Such injuries are very uncommon but they have been associated with delayed diagnosis and even death.

Medical preparation of the endometrium for endometrial ablation

Conceptually, a thin endometrium is easier to remove or destroy than one that is thickened. For REA, there exists high quality evidence described in a Cochrane Review (Class I-1) that demonstrates that either preoperative danazol or GnRHa result in shorter procedures, greater ease of surgery, a lower rate of postoperative dysmenorrhea, and a higher rate of post-surgical amenorrhea [50].

Currently, endometrial preparation of some type is part of the preprocedural preparation for all of the NREA techniques except the NovaSure device. Consequently, patients must be counseled that anticipated clinical outcomes with these devices, except for NovaSure, are based on the supposition that endometrial preparation is included in the protocol.

NREA in an office setting under local anesthesia

The per case device costs of NREA devices are substantial (approximately US $1000 in 2008), an amount that is much greater than the combination of disposable and amortized per case costs of REA. Consequently, the value of NREA devices will only be optimized when their safety and simplicity is applied in environments that are less resource intense than standard operating rooms, as evidence already exists demonstrating that local anesthesia in standard operating rooms is unlikely to reduce costs [51] (Class II-2).

The only clinical trial of "local anesthesia" has compared NovaSure to Thermachoice in a prospective, multicenter, nonrandomized evaluation of intraoperative pain in 67 patients who also received standardized intravenous sedation with fentanyl citrate [40] (Class II-1). Unfortunately there are many design flaws in this trial, including an absence of evaluation of pain associated with dilation, and sequential pain scores during the procedure. Consequently, and unfortunately, the results of this study may not reflect the total picture of pain associated with these two modalities and, consequently, notwithstanding the use of fentanyl, it is difficult to use these results to evaluate applicability to the office environment.

There are a number of published series that have reported the use of single NREA systems using local anesthesia. Office hydrothermablation has been reported in two published series each without requirement for parenteral anxiolytics or analgesics. In one study, performed in the Northern California Kaiser system, 54 patients were treated using preoperative oral agents including hydrocodone-acetaminophen and intramuscular ketorolac and atropine [37] (Class III). The procedure was then performed using intra-cervical mepivacaine. All patients were treated successfully in the office environment but no pain or satisfaction scores were provided. In the other series, from the United Kingdom, the only preoperative medication was mefenamic acid and the only procedural anesthesia provided was a 1% lidocaine with epinephrine solution injected intra- and paracervically [52] (Class III). These patients were selected based on preference and were usually parous, but all procedures were completed with maximum median pain scores of 6.4 (4.0–8.9).

Studies evaluating the use of balloon NREA (Thermachoice) have showed that the procedure may be accomplished successfully in the office setting. A series of 20 women were treated in an office setting having received a diclofenac suppository 1 hour pre-operatively and a paracervical block with 10 mL of 1% bupivacaine. One patient was nulliparous, all were successfully treated, with a median visual analog scale score of 4/10, and all left the clinic within 65 minutes of the procedure [39] (Class III). In another study of 27 women, 14 were treated without any preprocedural anesthesia, and then the sub-sequent cohort of 13 women underwent Thermachoice NREA after taking three 600-mg ibuprofen tablets at predetermined intervals before the procedure [33]. In each of these two groups of patients, one case was abandoned because of inability to dilate the cervical canal, and one woman in the nonpremedicated group terminated the procedure midway through. Nausea and vomiting following the procedure seemed to be less frequently encountered in the pretreated group.

From the studies discussed in the preceding paragraphs, it is apparent that performance of NREA in the office setting is feasible, at least for the majority of the systems in selected patients. However, it appears that at least some anesthesia is optimal and that the full potential of local anesthetics, considering the differences in innervation of the corpus and cervix, has not been fully exploited; the design of future studies should be undertaken with this in mind [53]. The use of conscious sedation is problematic for many practitioners considering use of NREA in an office setting, because of the prerequisites for appropriately trained staff and monitoring equipment.

Summary

Provided fertility is not an issue, EA is an option for women with HMB-E or -O who do not wish for future fertility and have failed, refused, or are intolerant of medical therapy. High quality evidence suggests that for appropriately selected patients, these ablative procedures typically reduce menstrual blood flow significantly, and may reduce the severity of other associated symptoms. In expert hands, both REA and NREA techniques seem to result in similar degrees of patient satisfaction and failure rates. However, it is clear from longer-term trials that while most women are initially satisfied, many subsequently choose or require either repeat EA or hysterectomy. The reasons for these treatment failures are still not clear and deserve further study. For example, it is possible that those with HMB-O might be less likely to find satisfaction with EA than those women with HMB-E. Alternatively, given the apparent prevalence of otherwise occult von Willebrand disease, it is possible that some if not many of the "failures" may be related to undiscovered cases of coagulopathy.

In each comparative trial, there seem to be fewer serious or potentially serious complications such as uterine perforation or fluid overload when NREA techniques are used as compared to resectoscopic techniques, even though these procedures were done by experts. Nevertheless, NREA techniques are not exempt from serious complications as uterine perforation and bowel injury has been reported in association with each of the approved devices.

There are other limitations to current NREA technology. To a greater or lesser extent, each NREA system has limitations related to one or a combination of the size and configuration of the endometrial cavity that prevents general application of any device to the HMB population. Ultimate judgment of the value of EA awaits the results of more of carefully crafted long-term longitudinal studies that compare the economic, social, and medical benefits of hysterectomy to EA for the treatment of AUB.

References

1. Fritsch H. Uterusvapokauterisation, tod durch septische peritonitis nach spontaner sekundarer perforation. *Centralblatt fur Gynakologie*. 1898;**52**:1409–18.

2. Bardenheuer F. Elektrokoagulation der Uterusschleimhaut zur Behandlungklimakterischer Blutungen. *Zentralblatt fur Gynakologie*. 1937;**4**:209–11.

3. Cahan WG, Brockunier A, Jr. Cryosurgery of the uterine cavity. *Am J Obstet Gynecol*. 1967;**99**(1):138–53.

4. Droegemueller W, Greer BE, Makowski EL. Preliminary observations of cryocoagulation of the endometrium. *Am J Obstet Gynecol*. 1970;**107**(6):958–61.

5. Droegemueller W, Greer BE, Makowski EL. Cryosurgery in patients with dysfunctional uterine bleeding. *Obstet Gynecol*. 1971; **38**(2):256–8.

6. Goldrath MH, Fuller TA, Segal S. Laser photovaporization of endometrium for the treatment of menorrhagia. *Am J Obstet Gynecol*. 1981;**140**(1):14–19.

7. DeCherney AH, Diamond MP, Lavy G, Polan ML. Endometrial ablation for intractable uterine bleeding: hysteroscopic resection. *Obstet Gynecol*. 1987;**70**(4):668–70.

8. Vancaillie TG. Electrocoagulation of the endometrium with the ball-end resectoscope. *Obstet Gynecol*. 1989; **74**(3 Pt 1):425–7.

9. Vercellini P, Oldani S, Yaylayan L, Zaina B, De Giorgi O, Crosignani PG. Randomized comparison of vaporizing electrode and cutting loop for endometrial ablation. *Obstet Gynecol*. 1999;**94**(4):521–7.

10. Glasser MH. Endometrial ablation and hysteroscopic myomectomy by electrosurgical vaporization. *J Am Assoc Gynecol Laparosc*. 1997;**4**(3):369–74.

11. Overton C, Hargreaves J, Maresh M. A national survey of the complications of endometrial destruction for menstrual disorders: the MISTLETOE study. Minimally invasive surgical techniques – laser, endothermal or endorescetion. *Br J Obstet Gynaecol*. 1997;**104**(12):1351–9.

12. Istre O, Skajaa K, Schjoensby AP, Forman A. Changes in serum electrolytes after transcervical resection of endometrium and submucous fibroids with use of glycine 1.5% for uterine irrigation. *Obstet Gynecol*. 1992;**80**(2):218–22.

13. Kim AH, Keltz MD, Arici A, Rosenberg M, Olive DL. Dilutional hyponatremia during hysteroscopic myomectomy with sorbitol-mannitol distention medium. *J Am Assoc Gynecol Laparosc*. 1995; **2**(2):237–42.

14. Taskin O, Buhur A, Birincioglu M, Burak F, Atmaca R, Yilmaz I, et al. Endometrial Na+, K+-ATPase pump function and vasopressin levels during hysteroscopic surgery in patients pretreated with GnRH agonist. *J Am Assoc Gynecol Laparosc*. 1998; **5**(2):119–24.

15. Isaacson K, Nardella P. Development and use of a bipolar resectoscope in endometrial

electrosurgery. *J Am Assoc Gynecol Laparosc.* 1997;**4**(3):385–91.

16. Vilos GA. Intrauterine surgery using a new coaxial bipolar electrode in normal saline solution (Versapoint): a pilot study. *Fertil Steril.* 1999;**72**(4):740–3.

17. Donnez J, Vilos G, Gannon MJ, Stampe-Sorensen S, Klinte I, Miller RM. Goserelin acetate (Zoladex) plus endometrial ablation for dysfunctional uterine bleeding: a large randomized, double-blind study. *Fertil Steril.* 1997; **68**(1):29–36.

18. Goldenberg M, Zolti M, Bider D, Etchin A, Sela BA, Seidman DS. The effect of intracervical vasopressin on the systemic absorption of glycine during hysteroscopic endometrial ablation. *Obstet Gynecol.* 1996;**87**(6):1025–9.

19. Townsend DE, McCausland V, McCausland A, Fields G, Kauffman K. Post-ablation-tubal sterilization syndrome. *Obstet Gynecol.* 1993; **82**(3):422–4.

20. Valle RF, Baggish MS. Endometrial carcinoma after endometrial ablation: high-risk factors predicting its occurrence. *Am J Obstet Gynecol.* 1998;**179**(3 Pt 1):569–72.

21. Neuwirth RS, Loffer FD, Trenhaile T, Levin B. The incidence of endometrial cancer after endometrial ablation in a low-risk population. *J Am Assoc Gynecol Laparosc.* 2004;**11**(4):492–4.

22. Pooley AS, Ewen SP, Sutton CJ. Does transcervical resection of the endometrium for menorrhagia really avoid hysterectomy? Life table analysis of a large series. *J Am Assoc Gynecol Laparosc.* 1998;**5**(3):229–35.

23. Seidman DS, Bitman G, Mashiach S, Hart S, Goldenberg M. The effect of increasing age on the outcome of hysteroscopic endometrial resection for management of dysfunctional uterine bleeding. *J Am Assoc Gynecol Laparosc.* 2000;**7**(1):115–19.

24. McCausland V, McCausland A. The response of adenomyosis to endometrial ablation/resection. *Hum Reprod Update.* 1998;**4**(4):350–9.

25. Bae IH, Pagedas AC, Barr CA, Alexander C, Bae DS. Retrospective analysis of 305 consecutive cases of endometrial ablation and partial endomyometrial resection. *J Am Assoc Gynecol Laparosc.* 1996;**3**(4):549–54.

26. Browne DS. Endometrial resection – a comparison of techniques. *Aust N Z J Obstet Gynaecol.* 1996;**36**(4):448–52.

27. Eskandar MA, Vilos GA, Aletebi FA, Tummon IS. Hysteroscopic endometrial ablation is an effective alternative to hysterectomy in women with menorrhagia and large uteri. *J Am Assoc Gynecol Laparosc.* 2000;**7**(3):339–45.

28. El-Toukhy T, Chandakas S, Grigoriadis T, Hill N, Erian J. Outcome of the first 220 cases of endometrial balloon ablation using Cavaterm plus. *J Obstet Gynaecol.* 2004; **24**(6):680–3.

29. Mettler L. Long-term results in the treatment of menorrhagia and hypermenorrhea with a thermal balloon endometrial ablation technique. *JSLS.* 2002;**6**(4):305–9.

30. Singer A, Almanza R, Gutierrez A, Haber G, Bolduc LR, Neuwirth R. Preliminary clinical experience with a thermal balloon endometrial ablation method to treat menorrhagia. *Obstet Gynecol.* 1994; **83**(5 Pt 1):732–4.

31. Neuwirth RS, Duran AA, Singer A, MacDonald R, Bolduc L. The endometrial ablator: a new instrument. *Obstet Gynecol,* 1994;**83**(5 Pt 1):792–6.

32. McAllister KF, Bigrigg A. Uterine balloon therapy for menorrhagia: a feasibility study of its use in the community setting. *J Fam Plann Reprod Health Care.* 2002; **28**(3):133–4.

33. Marsh F, Thewlis J, Duffy S. Thermachoice endometrial ablation in the outpatient setting, without local anesthesia or intravenous sedation: a prospective cohort study. *Fertil Steril.* 2005;**83**(3):715–20.

34. Mangeshikar PS, Kapur A, Yackel DB. Endometrial ablation with a new thermal balloon system. *J Am Assoc Gynecol Laparosc.* 2003;**10**(1):27–32.

35. Ulmsten U, Carstensen H, Falconer C, Holm L, Lannér L, Nilsson S, et al. The safety and efficacy of MenoTreat, a new balloon device for thermal endometrial ablation. *Acta Obstet Gynecol Scand.* 2001;**80**(1):52–7.

36. Vihko KK, Raitala R, Taina E. Endometrial thermoablation for treatment of

menorrhagia: comparison of two methods in outpatient setting. *Acta Obstet Gynecol Scand.* 2003;**82**(3):269–74.

37. Glasser MH, Zimmerman JD. The Hydro ThermAblator system for management of menorrhagia in women with submucous myomas: 12- to 20-month follow-up. *J Am Assoc Gynecol Laparosc.* 2003;**10**(4):521–7.

38. Rosenbaum SP, Fried M, Munro MG. Endometrial hydrothermablation: a comparison of short-term clinical effectiveness in patients with normal endometrial cavities and those with intracavitary pathology. *J Minim Invasive Gynecol.* 2005;**12**(2):144–9.

39. Jack SA, Cooper KG, Seymour J, Graham W, Fitzmaurice A, Perez J. A randomised controlled trial of microwave endometrial ablation without endometrial preparation in the outpatient setting: patient acceptability, treatment outcome and costs. *BJOG.* 2005;**112**(8):1109–16.

40. Laberge PY, Sabbah R, Fortin C, Gallinat A. Assessment and comparison of intraoperative and postoperative pain associated with NovaSure and ThermaChoice endometrial ablation systems. *J Am Assoc Gynecol Laparosc.* 2003;**10**(2):223–32.

41. Gallinat A, Nugent W. NovaSure impedance-controlled system for endometrial ablation. *J Am Assoc Gynecol Laparosc.* 2002;**9**(3):283–9.

42. Cooper J, Gimpelson R, Laberge P, Galen D, Garza-Leal JG, Scott J, et al. A randomized, multicenter trial of safety and efficacy of the NovaSure system in the treatment of menorrhagia. *J Am Assoc Gynecol Laparosc.* 2002;**9**(4):418–28.

43. Donnez J, Polet R, Rabinovitz R, Ak M, Squifflet J, Nisolle M. Endometrial laser intrauterine thermotherapy: the first series of 100 patients observed for 1 year. *Fertil Steril.* 2000;**74**(4):791–6.

44. Van Vugt DA, Krzemien A, Roy BN, Fletcher WA, Foster W, Lundahl S, et al. Photodynamic endometrial ablation in the nonhuman primate. *J Soc Gynecol Investig.* 2000;**7**(2):125–30.

45. Mhawech P, Renaud A, Sene C, Lüdicke F, Herrmann F, Szalay-Quinodoz I, et al. High efficacy of photodynamic therapy on rat endometrium after systemic administration of benzoporphyrin derivative monoacid ring A. *Hum Reprod.* 2003;**18**(8):1707–11.

46. Degen AF, Gabrecht T, Mosimann L, Fehr MK, Hornung R, Schwarz VA, et al. Photodynamic endometrial ablation for the treatment of dysfunctional uterine bleeding: a preliminary report. *Lasers Surg Med.* 2004;**34**(1):1–4.

47. Kucuk M, Okman TK. Intrauterine instillation of trichloroacetic acid is effective for the treatment of dysfunctional uterine bleeding. *Fertil Steril.* 2005;**83**(1):189–94.

48. Kucukozkan T, Kadioglu BG, Uygur D, Moroy P, Mollamahmutoglu L, Besli M. Chemical ablation of endometrium with trichloroacetic acid. *Int J Gynaecol Obstet.* 2004;**84**(1):41–6.

49. Gurtcheff SE, Sharp HT. Complications associated with global endometrial ablation: the utility of the MAUDE database. *Obstet Gynecol.* 2003;**102**(6):1278–82.

50. Sowter MC, Lethaby A, Singla AA. Pre-operative endometrial thinning agents before endometrial destruction for heavy menstrual bleeding. *Cochrane Database Syst Rev.* 2002;**3**:CD001124.

51. Seymour J, Wallage S, Graham W, Parkin D, Cooper K. The cost of microwave endometrial ablation under different anaesthetic and clinical settings. *BJOG.* 2003;**110**(10):922–6.

52. Farrugia M, Hussain SY. Hysteroscopic endometrial ablation using the Hydro ThermAblator in an outpatient hysteroscopy clinic: feasibility and acceptability. *J Minim Invasive Gynecol.* 2006;**13**(3):178–82.

53. Hassan L, Gannon MJ. Anaesthesia and analgesia for ambulatory hysteroscopic surgery. *Best Pract Res Clin Obstet Gynaecol.* 2005;**19**(5):681–91.

Chapter 6

Endometrial sampling

Chapter summary

- Endometrial sampling includes the traditional dilation and curettage (D&C) and catheter-based techniques that collectively are termed "endometrial biopsy" (EB).
- Endometrial biopsy is more comfortable for the patient if local anesthesia is used.
- Endometrial biopsy has been shown to be approximately as accurate as D&C for the detection of endometrial neoplasia in women with postmenopausal bleeding.

Introduction

Histological evaluation of the endometrium (short of hysterectomy) requires that a representative sample be obtained, either with blind or image-guided techniques. Blind techniques include brush biopsy, endometrial aspiration biopsy using a hollow catheter, and acquisition of tissue with sharp curettes. When dilation of the cervix is necessary to allow access of the curette to the endometrial cavity, the process is termed "dilation and curettage" or "D&C." Hysteroscopy is the most commonly used image-guided technique; requiring that an endoscope with an instrument channel be placed in the endometrial cavity to allow targeted sampling with a biopsy forceps. Such an approach offsets the major deficiency of blind systems, namely, the inability to sample focal lesions.

Background

Usually a sample of endometrial tissue will be representative of the entire endometrium and will allow for an accurate histopathological analysis. Traditionally, such samples were obtained using cervical D&C using endometrial curettes, usually with regional or general anesthesia, in the setting of an operating room. More recently, endometrial biopsy (EB) with office-based techniques using a narrow, flexible, hollow suction catheter has been shown to be nearly equivalent to the "formal" D&C [1–5] (Class II-2).

Whereas catheter-based, blind endometrial sampling is equivalent to D&C in postmenopausal women, it is important to note that there some evidence that it is slightly less sensitive for the detection of endometrial neoplasia in premenopausal women [6, 7]. For purely postmenopausal bleeding, the sensitivity of the Pipelle® device (Prodimed, Neuilly en Thelle, France) to the detection of endometrial carcinoma is 99.6%; this falls to 91% in studies reporting on a mixture of pre- and postmenopausal subjects [1]. The sensitivity of the Pipelle device for atypical hyperplasia is about 82.3% in studies with mixed pre- and postmenopausal subjects; there are too few studies available evaluating purely postmenopausal subjects to make any comment. The Pipelle device seems to offer superior sensitivity to other catheter-based techniques such as the Vabra aspirator [7] (Class I-1).

Endometrial biopsy

Preparing the patient

The patient should undergo the process of informed consent whereby she is counseled to understand the rationale for the procedure, the amount of discomfort anticipated, and the types of problems or complications that could occur, including failure to gain access to the endometrial cavity, or to obtain an adequate specimen. Indications for EB as well as devices, equipment, and techniques for catheter biopsy are reviewed in Figure 16.1, Tables 16.1–16.5, and Video 16.1.

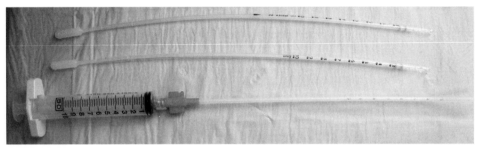

Figure 16.1 Flexible endometrial biopsy catheters. Top: Pipelle® in 4- and 3-mm outside diameters; bottom: Endorette®. Each has a system for applying suction to the catheter lumen either with an integrated suction piston or using an attachable syringe.

Table 16.1 Indications and contraindications for endometrial biopsy.

Indications:

1. Postmenopausal bleeding:

   • Primary assessment

   • When EEC by TVS is > 5 mm

2. Persistent AUB in the late reproductive years:

   • High risk of endometrial cancer

   • More than 12 months of AUB

3. Abnormal bleeding at any age (esp. > 35) if high risk

4. Very high risk asymptomatic women:

   • Morbid obesity

   • Unopposed estrogen

5. Chronic anovulation

6. AUB refractory to medical therapy

7. Evaluation of endometrium for trophoblast in nonviable gestations suspicious for ectopic pregnancy

Contraindications:

1. Viable pregnancy

2. Acute pelvic inflammatory disease

3. Acute cervicitis

AUB, abnormal uterine bleeding; EEC, endometrial echo complex; TVS, transvaginal ultrasound.

Table 16.2 Endometrial biopsy devices and manufacturer details.

Endometrial biopsy devices:
• Tao brush™
• EndoCurette® endometrial suction curette
• Pipet Curet®
• Wallach Endocell disposable endometrial cell sampler
• Tis-U-Trap endometrial cannula-curette with built-in specimen container (note large and small sizes; large size can also be used to empty contents of uterine cavity in addition to function of small size for obtaining endometrial tissue for histology)
• Novak metal curette (reusable)
• Ipas™ manual vacuum aspirator (MVA)
• Vabra aspirator

Manufacturer details:
• Tao brush™: Cook Medical Inc, Bloomington, IN, USA
• EndoCurette®: Utah Medical Products Inc, Midvale, UT, USA
• Pipet Curet®: Milex Products Inc, Chicago, IL, USA
• Wallach Endocell: Wallach Surgical Devices Inc, Orange, CT, USA
• Tis-U-Trap: Milex Products Inc, Chicago, IL, USA
• Novak: CooperSurgical, Inc, Trumbull, CT, USA
• Ipas™ manual vacuum aspiration: Ipas, Chapel Hill, NC, USA
• Vabra aspirator: Berkeley Medevices, Inc, Richmond, CA, USA

Sources of discomfort or pain with EB include that experienced with grasping of the cervix with a tenaculum, dilation of the cervical canal, and acquisition of the biopsy from the endometrial surface with the specimen acquisition device. If cervical stenosis is anticipated, there is high quality evidence that administration of either 200 μg of vaginal, or 400 μg oral misoprostol approximately 12 hours before the procedure will reduce the force required to dilate the cervix. [8, 9] (Class I-2). If such an approach is chosen, the patient must be provided with a prescription for the agent by at least the day before and counseled to anticipate mild lower abdominal cramping, possibly some slight diarrhea, and slight bleeding in the hours following this administration. *Post*procedure discomfort and pain may be reduced with the use of orally administered mefenamic acid 500 mg, or other NSAIDS like sodium naproxen or ibuprofen, approximately 1 hour prior to the procedure [10] (Class I-2).

Procedure

The patient is positioned on a gynecological examination table with her feet placed in comfortable stirrups with the buttocks advanced to the table's edge. Video 16.1 Bimanual examination of the uterus is performed to determine both version and flexion (Figure 2.4) in addition to size and shape. A uterus very enlarged and/or distorted with leiomyomas may influence both the technique and the ability to obtain an adequate specimen. A warm speculum of appropriate length, width, and contour is carefully inserted into the vagina to

Table 16.3 Equipment and supplies for endometrial biopsy with suction catheter.

General equipment:

- Absorbent pad to place beneath patient
- Povidone-iodine or disinfectant solution of choice to cleanse cervix
- Anesthetic agents and supplies. A combination of topical anesthetic jelly or spray (e.g., lidocaine or benzocaine), and injectable 0.5–2.0% lidocaine; spinal needle (20–22 gauge) and 10–20 mL syringe (Chapter 23)
- Completed labels and container(s) with required preservative for endometrial sample (depends on sampling device and laboratory requirements; may be formalin or CytoRich® Red solution)
- Personal protective equipment
- 2 × 2-inch pieces of lens or filter paper

Sterile equipment:

- Gloves (may not need to be sterile with 'no-touch' technique)
- Vaginal speculum
- Endocervical curette (if used)
- Gauze pads
- Scissors (if needed to cut catheter tip to place sample in container for laboratory)
- Ring forceps
- Tenaculum (should be on sterile tray so it is immediately available if needed)
- Biopsy catheter

Optional equipment:

- Cervical dilators and/or "os finders" should be available but sterile packaging does not need to be open until it is determined that one (or more) is needed

Table 16.4 Pipelle® technique: a summary.

1. Position the patient in the modified lithotomy position
2. Determine uterine size, version, and flexion
3. Insert speculum
4. Apply topical anesthetic as necessary
5. Wait the appropriate time for anesthetic effect (at least 5 minutes)
6. Apply topical antiseptic solution (povidone-iodine)
7. Apply tenaculum to 12 o'clock at anterior cervical lip (usually)
8. Use cough technique if no anesthesia injected or applied
9. Insert suction catheter via cervical os to fundus; note uterine length (sound)
10. Withdraw internal piston
11. Move catheter tip in and out encompassing the entire length of the cavity (without exiting), while twisting to cover 360° – repeat to create 3–4 such cycles
12. Withdraw catheter when filled with tissue
13. Expel sample into formalin using the internal piston. If tissue volume is perceived to be inadequate, consider a second aspiration

Table 16.5 Other suction catheters.

Novak's curette:
- Metal curette requiring the attachment of a 10 mL syringe to apply suction and hold tissue
- More useful than Pipelle® when endometrial tissue is needed in patients that are actively bleeding
- Difficult to use in patient with a stenotic cervix because curette is large in diameter and rigid
- Serrated teeth may "catch the myometrium", cause more pain, and may require more analgesia/local block

Vabra aspirator:
- Stainless steel or *rigid* plastic with outside diameter of 3 mm – difficult to use with stenotic os
- Suction is initiated via a device that generates vacuum of 600 mm Hg
- Produces a sample that is comparable to that of dilation and curettage
- May require intravenous analgesia

expose the cervix and the external os. Should there be apparent substantial stenosis of the external os; the clinician should consider available options for dealing with inability to access the endocervical canal (see "Troubleshooting" below).

The cervix is generally cleansed with an antiseptic solution such as poviodone-iodine solution, using a rectal swab or gauze/small sponge held by ring or long tissue forceps. Prior to any other manipulations, local anesthetic agents may be applied to the exocervix, the endocervical canal, the cervical stroma, paracervical tissue, and/or the endometrial cavity (Chapter 14, Video 14.1). Evidence supporting the use of local anesthetic agents for the performance of catheter-based EB has been inconsistent. While it is possible that some women have minimal discomfort or pain associated with EB, the clinician should carefully evaluate the patient's history and anatomy if routine anesthesia is not used. If the patient, for example, is nulliparous and has an anatomically narrow cervical os, anesthesia may be more likely to be of value.

The cervix is grasped with a single tooth tenaculum, usually at 12 o'clock, but in cases of severe retroversion, on the posterior aspect or lip. Gentle traction should be applied to the tenaculum both to reduce the flexion at the isthmus and to stabilize the cervix, thereby providing countertraction that facilitates passage of the biopsy acquisition device through the cervical canal into the endometrial cavity.

Flexible catheters

Catheter-based biopsy systems come in a variety of designs with outside diameters of typically ranging from 3 to 4 mm. This description will apply to flexible, disposable, catheters like the Pipelle and summarized in Figure 16.2. After placing the cervix on gentle traction, the semiflexible catheter is passed through the exocervical os, the cervical canal, and into the endometrial cavity until it is perceived that the tip has reached the uterine fundus. After noting this sounded length of the uterus, the internal rod or piston is withdrawn providing suction (Figure 16.2) (Video 16.1). Then the catheter is systematically partially withdrawn and rotated in a fashion that allows coverage of a maximal amount of the endometrial surface [11]. Typically, but not always, the clinician will observe a mixture of fluid and tissue being withdrawn into the transparent catheter. The process should be extended and/or repeated until there is confidence that an optimal specimen has been obtained. Still applying suction, the catheter is removed, and then held over the

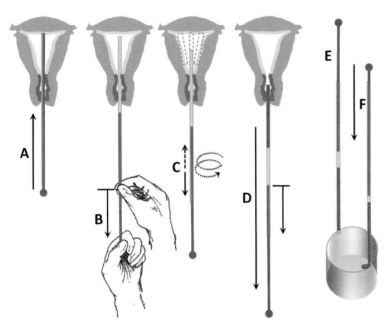

Figure 16.2 Technique for suction catheter endometrial biopsy, in this case with the Pipelle® system. (A) The unit is passed through the cervical canal into the endometrial cavity to the uterine fundus. In some instances it will be necessary to attach a tenaculum to the anterior lip of the cervix (after the administration of appropriate anesthesia), and uncommonly, dilation will be required. (B) While holding the external catheter with one hand, the other applies suction by withdrawing the piston or inner rod. (C) Then, maintaining this suction with one hand the other hand systematically withdraws and advances the system while rotating the catheter to optimize the surface area sampled. (D) Maintaining suction, the system is removed and then (E) held over a formalin-containing specimen container. (F) The piston is pushed forward expelling the tissue into the container. If the impression is that an inadequate amount of tissue was obtained, the process can be repeated.

formalin-containing specimen bottle. The internal rod/piston is now used to eject the tissue out the end of the catheter into the container. This specimen should be observed and, if tissue is not observed and it is suspected that there is inadequate tissue, a second aspiration should be considered. It is important not to reinsert a catheter into the endometrial cavity that has been dipped in the formalin solution.

Rigid catheters

The Novak curette (Figure 16.3) is a rigid, hollow catheter with a toothed side fenestration near the tip of the device that allows aspiration of the tissue specimen. Suction is created with a standard (usually 10 mL) syringe, attached to the proximal Luer adaptor. The most common OD of this device is 4 mm, but there exist a variety of ODs starting with 1 mm. Many perceive that this device is superior when a biopsy is performed in the context of active uterine bleeding and that pain associated with scraping the endometrium is more common. Otherwise the technique is similar to that used for flexible catheters with suction applied by withdrawing the piston of the syringe.

Tao brush™

Another method of obtaining cells for histopathological evaluation is the *Tao brush*™ (Figure 16.4; Cook Medical Inc., Bloomington, IN). There is evidence that this technique

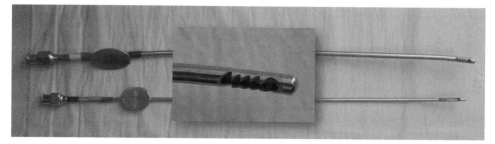

Figure 16.3 The Novak curette. This is a rigid, reusable endometrial biopsy device designed to work with an aspirating syringe attached with a Luer adaptor. The inset shows the toothed nature of the aperture that may facilitate acquisition of endometrial tissue in some instances.

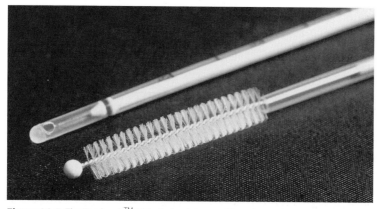

Figure 16.4 The Tao brush™. This device is inserted into the endometrial cavity in a similar-sized catheter and in a fashion similar to that for endometrial biopsy (catheter pictured behind). Once within the endometrial cavity, the brush is deployed, rotated, and then withdrawn into the catheter, which is removed with the specimen transferred into a special cytology-preserving solution. There is evidence that this technique is associated with a reduced frequency of inadequate specimens when compared to the catheter-based endometrial biopsy techniques.

results in fewer inadequate specimens when compared to the Pipelle device, thereby reducing the requirement for repeat assessment [12] (Class 1). However, it is important for the clinician to know that, despite the fact that in about 80% of cases a histological specimen is obtained, the cornerstone assessment of Tao brush specimens is by cytology, a technique for which there must be special specimen containers, and specific training for the pathologist and laboratory team. The patient is prepared and set up similar to any EB technique. The brush is retracted into the external catheter and the assembly is passed through the cervix, using a tenaculum if necessary for stability. When the clinician perceives that the system has accessed the fundus, the outer catheter is withdrawn thereby exposing the brush to the endometrial surface. First the brush is rotated 360° clockwise and then 360° counterclockwise whereupon it is retracted into the catheter once again. The system is withdrawn and then inserted into a special bottle containing a cytofixative.

Troubleshooting

Stenotic external os

In some instances, the external os is extremely narrow or even seemingly obliterated or closed. Obliteration appears to be more commonly encountered in postmenopausal women, particularly with increasing years, and especially in those who have undergone cervical excisional procedures (e.g., loop excision or cone) and who have not previously had a vaginal delivery. If the external os is difficult to find, evaluation with a colposcope may aid in identification of the dimple that represents the external os.

There are a number of approaches to dealing with this anatomic aberration [13] but, regardless of the technique, a tenaculum and local injectable anesthetic agents are necessary to provide stability and pain prevention respectively (Chapter 14). Then, a narrow-caliber reusable dilator, a lachrymal probe, or, preferably, a small semiflexible device called an "os finder" can be useful in identifying and expanding the external os sufficient to allow the passage of the EB catheter. If only a small, blind, dimple identifies the obliterated external os even the passage of one of the above-named dilating devices will be impeded. When this configuration is encountered, a number 11 scalpel blade may be used to create two small cruciate incisions centered at the dimple.

Stenotic internal os

The catheter may be advanced through the external os, but encounter a higher obstruction, usually at the level of the internal os. In most instances this obstruction can be overcome with the use of a semirigid or rigid dilator (Figure 16.5) and modest pressure while holding the cervix in traction with a tenaculum, as previously described. In other instances, the obstruction is created by previous trauma from, for example, prior dilation, or may occur related to a previous cesarean section, or the presence of a lesion such as a leiomyoma. If such a situation is thought to exist it is useful to perform a transvaginal ultrasound (TVS) to try to identify the cervical canal, the endometrial echo complex (EEC), and the presence or absence of readily identifiable lesions.

If the canal and the EEC are identifiable, suitable anesthesia should be introduced (if not already established) and there can be a repeat attempt at dilation with mild to modest force directed in the direction of the identified canal. Alternatively, or if there is failure with such

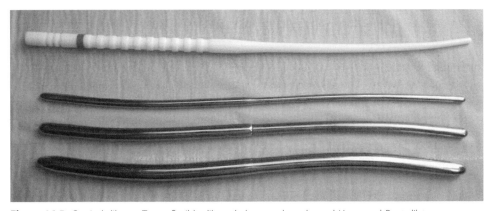

Figure 16.5 Cervical dilators. Top: a flexible dilator; below: graduated metal Hagar and Pratt dilators.

an approach, there are a number of options. Transrectal ultrasound, or, with a full bladder, transabdominal ultrasound, may be employed to direct the dilator along the canal, with modest force. While this approach is sometimes useful, it may be difficult to identify the canal and the EEC, particularly in postmenopausal women, and also difficult to align the image with the dilator.

We have found hysteroscopy to be the best technique for overcoming the apparently stenotic cervix (Video 21.2). A narrow caliber hysteroscope, preferably with the OD of the external sheath no more than 5 mm, an operating channel of 5-Fr, and with a telescope with foreoblique lens of 12–30°, is introduced through the external os to the level of the obstruction. Frequently the orientation of the internal os can be identified in this fashion. Then, in many instances, and with traction applied to the cervix with the attached tenaculum, the hysteroscope can be directed in a way that allows navigation to the endometrial cavity. When this is not possible, a 5 French (Fr) grasping or biopsy forceps can be passed into the observed and stenotic canal and then opened in a fashion that allows for dilation of the internal os. Then, the hysteroscope is directed past the obstructed area into the endometrial cavity.

If all of these approaches fail, it may be best to reconsider everything. In some instances, the use of misoprostol as described above and in the context of another session may make the difference between success and failure. If it is difficult for the patient to tolerate the above approaches, or if it is the considered opinion that the repeat procedure is better done in the context of a standard operating room with different anesthesia, suitable arrangements should be made.

Perforation known or suspected

Perforation of the uterus is rare with flexible catheters – the incidence is really unknown. More common causes of perforation are related to "sounding" with metal sounds, forceful attempts at dilation, or performing uterine manipulative procedures when the uterus is softened, such as is the case within 6–8 weeks following pregnancy. Even if perforation occurs, sounds, dilators, and flexible catheters are highly unlikely to perforate vessels or surrounding structures, unless, for example, bowel is attached to the perforation site by adhesions. Consequently, if the patient is stable and not hemorrhaging, expectant management is entirely appropriate and almost always successful. However, should the patient's condition evolve with increasing pain, tenderness, fever or other symptoms and/or signs of vascular or visceral perforation, it may be necessary to proceed to the operating room for exploratory laparoscopy or laparotomy, the approach determined by the clinical situation.

Inadequate specimen

In some instances the pathologist will report that there is inadequate endometrial tissue with which to make a diagnosis. This may occur because the clinician did not actually access the endometrial cavity because of a cervical stenosis or because of very atrophic endometrium.

In such a circumstance, TVS demonstrating an EEC of 5 mm or less is reassuring. Alternatively, a repeat attempt at sampling with another system may be an appropriate step, and, if a Tao brush technique was not attempted, this may be the time to do so. The preferential approach if a lesion is found, particularly if the EEC is thickened or in the face of persistent bleeding, is to perform a hysteroscopic evaluation with targeted biopsy.

Dilation and curettage

The term "D&C" is generally used to describe the process whereby the cervical canal is dilated adequate to pass "standard" endometrial curettes into the endometrial cavity to obtain a sample of the endometrium. Evidence has demonstrated that such a blind technique is not superior to catheter-based EB for postmenopausal bleeding, although, when the EEC is greater than 7 mm there is some evidence that catheter-based sampling is slightly inferior [6]. Regardless, the inferiority of both, and the implicit performance of D&C in a more standard operating room setting (even though it is probably not necessary with adequate anesthesia), suggest that D&C as a diagnostic procedure for AUB should preferably be performed only with hysteroscopy.

Prior to the procedure, the patient can be provided oral or vaginal misoprostol as described earlier in this section, or, a few hours prior to surgery, have a laminaria device inserted. These devices absorb surrounding fluid and dilate the cervix. Care must be exerted when using these devices, for, if they are inserted more than a few hours before the procedure, asymmetrical (dumbbell) dilation may fix the device in the cervical canal.

The patient is brought to the office procedure or operating room and positioned in the modified dorsal lithotomy position, in comfortable and secure stirrups (Video 16.3). Sufficient general, regional, or local anesthesia is instituted as appropriate (Chapter 14, Video 14.1). A careful manual examination is performed to determine or confirm uterine version, flexion, size, and consistency, important variables, particularly if blind instrumentation is to be performed. An appropriate speculum is positioned in the vagina, adequate to expose the cervix which is cleansed with an appropriate iodine-based solution. The cervix is then stabilized with a tenaculum, usually attached to the anterior exocervix and the cervical canal serially dilated, including internal os, being careful to consider the axis and relative relationships of both the cervix and the corpus. I do not use the malleable sound, preferring to use either a large diameter dilator, or, if hysteroscopy is performed, the hysteroscope to accurately sound the uterine length. The narrow sound is associated with perforation and, as evidence that we have produced in our institution shows, blind measurements are frequently inaccurate.

If hysteroscopy is to be performed, it is done when dilation has achieved a caliber sufficient to allow the external sheath to be inserted with relative ease. If hysteroscopy is not performed, or following the completion of hysteroscopy, the cervix is further dilated adequate to allow the passage of a uterine curette.

References

1. Machado F, Moreno J, Carazo M, León J, Fiol G, Serna R. Accuracy of endometrial biopsy with the Cornier Pipelle for diagnosis of endometrial cancer and atypical hyperplasia. *Eur J Gynaecol Oncol.* 2003;**24** (3–4):279–81.

2. Stovall TG, Ling FW, Morgan PL. A prospective, randomized comparison of the Pipelle endometrial sampling device with the Novak curette. *Am J Obstet Gynecol.* 1991;**165**(5 Pt 1): 1287–90.

3. Stovall TG, Photopulos GJ, Poston WM, Ling FW, Sandles LG. Pipelle endometrial sampling in patients with known endometrial carcinoma. *Obstet Gynecol.* 1991;**77**(6): 954–6.

4. Zorlu CG, Cobanoglu O, Işik AZ, Kutluay L, Kuşçu E. Accuracy of Pipelle endometrial sampling in endometrial carcinoma. *Gynecol Obstet Invest.* 1994;**38** (4):272–5.

5. Huang GS, Gebb JS, Einstein MH, Shahabi S, Novetsky AP, Goldberg GL. Accuracy of

preoperative endometrial sampling for the detection of high-grade endometrial tumors. *Am J Obstet Gynecol*. 2007; **196**(3):243,e1–5.

6. Epstein E, Skoog L, Valentin L. Comparison of Endorette and dilatation and curettage for sampling of the endometrium in women with postmenopausal bleeding. *Acta Obstet Gynecol Scand*. 2001; **80**(10):959–64.

7. Dijkhuizen FP, Mol BW, Brölmann HA, Heintz AP. The accuracy of endometrial sampling in the diagnosis of patients with endometrial carcinoma and hyperplasia: a meta-analysis. *Cancer*. 2000; **89**(8):1765–72.

8. Preutthipan S, Herabutya Y. Vaginal misoprostol for cervical priming before operative hysteroscopy: a randomized controlled trial. *Obstet Gynecol*. 2000; **96**(6):890–4.

9. Thomas JA, Leyland N, Durand N, Windrim RC. The use of oral misoprostol as a cervical ripening agent in operative hysteroscopy: a double-blind, placebo-controlled trial. *Am J Obstet Gynecol*. 2002;**186**(5):876–9.

10. Nagele F, Lockwood G, Magos AL. Randomised placebo controlled trial of mefenamic acid for premedication at outpatient hysteroscopy: a pilot study. *Br J Obstet Gynaecol*. 1997; **104**(7):842–4.

11. Sierecki AR, Gudipudi DK, Montemarano N, Del Priore G. Comparison of endometrial aspiration biopsy techniques: specimen adequacy. *J Reprod Med*. 2008; **53**(10):760–4.

12. Critchley HO, Warner P, Lee AJ, Brechin S, Guise J, Graham B. Evaluation of abnormal uterine bleeding: comparison of three outpatient procedures within cohorts defined by age and menopausal status. *Healthy Technol Assess* 2004;**8**(34):1–139.

13. Christianson MS, Barker MA, Lindheim SR. Overcoming the challenging cervix: techniques to access the uterine cavity. *J Low Genit Tract Dis*. 2008;**12**(1):24–31.

17 Hysterectomy

Chapter summary

- Total hysterectomy is surgical removal of the entire uterus.
- Supracervical hysterectomy is removal of the uterine corpus with retention of the cervix.
- Laparoscopic hysterectomy includes any procedure where the entire uterus is removed, partially or wholly, under laparoscopic direction.
- The type of hysterectomy associated with the least morbidity and cost is vaginal hysterectomy, while the greatest morbidity seems to be related to total abdominal hysterectomy.
- Available evidence suggests that supracervical hysterectomy is not associated with improved outcomes related to sexual or urinary tract function when compared to total hysterectomy.

Introduction

Hysterectomy is a procedure that results in removal of all or part of the uterus. Despite the advent of a plethora of medical and surgical alternatives for the treatment of AUB, hysterectomy remains a very commonly performed surgical procedure. While it is beyond the scope of this book to provide instruction on the performance of hysterectomy, it is prudent for any clinician caring for women with AUB to have a sound understanding of the various types of hysterectomy, and their relative advantages and disadvantages.

Hysterectomy types

The types of hysterectomy are summarized in Table 17.1. In short, hysterectomy may be perceived as either total or subtotal, the latter often called *supracervical* hysterectomy (SCH), reflecting the notion that the procedure results in removal of only the uterine corpus with retention of the uterine cervix. *Total hysterectomy* requires that a vaginal incision be made at the cervical-vaginal junction; with SCH, no such incision is necessary as the uterus is transected at the isthmus or junction of the cervix and corpus.

Abdominal hysterectomy implies that a laparotomy is made to perform the procedure; thus the procedures should probably be called *laparotomic* total or supracervical (or subtotal) hysterectomy to distinguish them from the laparoscopic hysterectomy variants. However, in practice, the term total abdominal hysterectomy (TAH) implies that the entire uterus is removed via the creation of a laparotomy; abdominal SCH, or subtotal abdominal hysterectomy similarly imply a laparotomic approach.

Vaginal hysterectomy (VH) almost always describes removal of the entire uterus through a vaginal incision without any of the components of the procedure being performed from "above." There is a vaginal supracervical technique that allows vaginally-directed removal of the corpus through an incision made between the bladder and the uterus, while retaining

Table 17.1 Hysterectomy types. Shown, from left to right, are the portion of uterus removed (total or corpus only), the different names for the same procedure, acronyms, the types and locations of incisions relating to the procedure, and then typical lengths of stay (LOS) in days and anticipated return to normal activity (RNA) in weeks. Length of stay varies dramatically between health care systems.

Portion of uterus removed	Procedure name(s)	Acronym(s)	Abdominal incisions		Vaginal incision	Typical LOS[b] (Days)	Typical RNA[c] (Weeks)
			Laparotomic[a]	Laparoscopic			
Total	Total abdominal hysterectomy, Laparotomic abdominal hysterectomy	TAH	Yes	No	Yes	3–7	6–8
	Vaginal hysterectomy	VH	No	No	Yes	< 1–4	3–6
	Laparoscopic hysterectomy, Laparoscopic assisted vaginal hysterectomy	LH, LAVH	No	Yes	Yes	< 1–2	3–6
Subtotal (corpus only)	Supracervical abdominal hysterectomy, Abdominal supracervical hysterectomy, Subtotal abdominal hysterectomy	ASH, STH	Yes	No	No	1–4	3–6
	Laparoscopic supracervical hysterectomy, Laparoscopic subtotal hysterectomy	LSH	No	Yes	No	< 1–2	1–3
	Vaginal supracervical hysterectomy, Vaginal subtotal hysterectomy, Döderlein hysterectomy	–	No	No	Yes	< 1–2	1–3

[a] Laparotomic: the creation of a relatively large abdominal incision; a laparotomy.
[b] LOS, length of stay.
[c] RNA, return to normal activities.

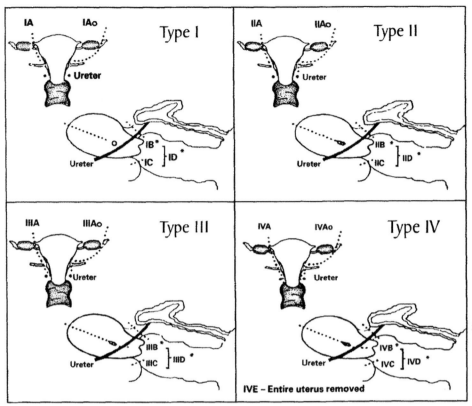

Figure 17.1 Classification of laparoscopic hysterectomy. Laparoscopic hysterectomy is a spectrum of techniques wherein part or all of the hysterectomy is performed under laparoscopic guidance. Type I procedures require that the ovarian vessels are taken laparoscopically; type II reflect laparoscopic occlusion and division of the uterine arteries; type III procedures require that some of the cardinal/uterosacral complex is dissected laparoscopically; while for type IV procedures the entire procedure is performed laparoscopically. The balance of the procedure in types I–III is performed vaginally. There may also be variations in the dissection of the bladder and cul-de-sac, which are reflected in the system by creating subgroups (B = bladder; C = culdotomy, D = both bladder dissection and culdotomy).

the cervix. This procedure, called the Döderlein hysterectomy after its inventor, is rarely performed [1].

Laparoscopic total hysterectomy describes a procedure that results in removal of the entire uterus, either partially or totally under laparoscopic direction. Originally, the laparoscope was used solely to direct a variable portion of the dissection, with the rest of the procedure completed vaginally; thus the term *laparoscopically assisted vaginal hysterectomy* (LAVH) [2]. However, with the evolution of equipment, technique, and experience, many surgeons now perform the entire procedure under laparoscopic guidance, including suturing for support and closure of the vaginal apex and incision (often called the vaginal cuff). The result of this technical development has been the evolution of a spectrum of confusing nomenclature for description of the procedural variants. Indeed, there may be a number of important differences in required equipment, technique, skill, and patient surgical risk depending upon which of these variants are performed for a given individual.

In the 1990s we attempted to create some order out of the confusion by publishing a classification system (Figure 17.1), adopted by the American Association of Gynecologic Laparoscopists, which can be used to help distinguish among the variants of hysterectomy performed partially or totally under the direction of a laparoscope, all of which we place under the umbrella term *laparoscopic hysterectomy*, or LH [3, 4]. The minimum dissection (type 0) is the division of adhesions under laparoscopic direction followed by VH; while other anatomical targets describe the extent of laparoscopic direction, with the remainder of the procedure performed vaginally. Consequently, laparoscopically-directed occlusion of the ovarian vessels define type I LH; the uterine vessels type II, part of the cardinal-uterosacral ligament type III, and dissection of the entire cardinal-uterosacral ligament(s) type IV. In recognition that there is variable dissection of structures located anteriorly and posteriorly on the cervix, there are three subtypes that describe the urinary bladder and anterior culdotomy incision (B), the creation of a posterior culdotomy (C), and (D) when both the anterior and posterior dissections are performed under laparoscopic direction.

Laparoscopic supracervical hysterectomy (LSH) replicates performance of subtotal hysterectomy following the creation of a laparotomy. The obvious challenge was the removal of the uterine corpus without the laparotomy incision. What is required is *morcellation* of the uterine corpus, a technique that can be performed with a standard knife and/or scissors through the umbilical laparoscopic incision, or using an electromechanical morcellator.

All of these procedures have their advantages and disadvantages, and their often passionate advocates and detractors, but clearly there is a place for all for appropriately selected women with AUB. The issue remains the selection of women appropriate for hysterectomy and then matching them with the technique that is considering best the uterine anatomy, coexistent pathology, and the clinical condition in the context of their own personal values and desires.

Assessment of hysterectomy by type

The relative value of the different types of hysterectomy is a process still under evaluation. There are many factors that impact the type and frequency of complications, and the direct and indirect costs of performing the procedure.

Direct costs include those directly associated with the operation including the time, personnel, and equipment and supplies used in the operating room, the duration and type of institutional care required after the procedure, and the cost of treating complications. Procedures that require expensive instruments, long periods of time in the operating room, prolonged hospital stay, and those associated with a higher incidence of complications will add to the direct costs of the operation. A cursory review of the literature by health care provider system demonstrates a relatively stunning variation in standard lengths of postoperative stay, even for the same operation. In some institutions, a hysterectomy that is performed as a day procedure with a postoperative stay measured in several hours is associated with a length of stay of several days in others.

Indirect costs include items such as the income lost by the patient during her period of disability related to the procedure, bills encountered for items such as additional child care, and the cost that her employer might have replacing a disabled employee. Understandably, indirect costs can be more difficult to measure, are less likely involved in clinical trials, and vary greatly depending upon the income of the individual; those women who are unemployed incur different indirect costs than do those with established employment.

Total abdominal hysterectomy requires a large incision and a variable but requisite number of days in hospital and, consequently, is generally associated with greater direct costs and morbidity than is VH [5] (Class II-2). Nationally reported data indicate that, in the United States, 64% of hysterectomies are performed abdominally [6, 7]. The postoperative complication rate has been estimated to be about 24.5% for VH and 42.8% for abdominal hysterectomy (AH). The morbidity and direct and presumed indirect costs of AH were factors that led to the development of LH.

Laparoscopic hysterectomy (Video 17.1) can clearly reduce the length of stay (over AH) and related costs, but it is a procedure that brings with it increased costs of its own, secondary to the need for more expensive equipment and supplies for performing the procedure. The value of LH varies in large part upon the training and ability of the surgeon and the type of equipment used to perform the procedure. Clearly, if VH can be performed and is appropriate for the patient, LH is unnecessary and more expensive [8]. Those with significant skill in VH find the laparoscopic technique to be of value only in a limited number of patients [5]; those with less training and skill in VH appropriately utilize LH more often to reduce the need for a laparotomy and its inherent morbidity and risk. Evaluation of the cost of LH is confounded by the cost of relatively expensive single use supplies such as laparoscopic trocar-cannula systems and hand instruments that are exemplified by energy-based blood vessel sealing and transection systems. Some health care systems and surgeons make extensive use of these instruments, while others use them sparingly, a circumstance that dramatically impacts the measured costs of the procedure. In the United States in particular, there is a profit motive driving the use of these disposable instruments for both the manufacturer and the hospital provider system, which can, essentially, make a profit reselling these instruments to the patient.

Supracervical hysterectomy, the subject of a modest renaissance, is potentially applicable to women with chronic AUB-E and -O but is controversial because of the perceived value of removing or retaining the cervix [9–12]. High quality evidence from three RCTs suggests that at least in the relatively short term (one to two years), both sexual and bladder function are similar following TAH and SCH [13–15] (Class I-2). However, these trials do not have individually or collectively, adequate sample size to evaluate potential differences in the occurrence of serious complications related to removal of the uterine cervix such as bowel, ureter, and bladder injury.

Laparoscopic supracervical hysterectomy (LSH) (Video 17.2) appears to have value in a number of circumstances, but controversy remains regarding its place compared with total hysterectomy. As an alternative to REA, LSH was associated with a significantly reduced incidence of subsequent surgery and an increased level of patient satisfaction in an Italian RCT studying women with AUB [16] (Class I-2). This outcome was achieved with both hospitalization times and return to normal preprocedural activities that were similar in the two groups. When AUB exists in women with uterine leiomyomas and/or other pathology that precludes VH, LSH is a viable way of treating the patient without the need for a laparotomic incision.

Appropriate selection of patients for SCH excludes those without existing preinvasive or invasive cervical neoplasia, and those in whom endometrial carcinoma is known or suspected as it is when atypical endometrial hyperplasia is diagnosed. Patients should be counseled that, in some instances, some degree of intermittent bleeding might persist following the procedure with an incidence that ranges from 2 to 25% [17]. At least some of this bleeding may relate to inadequate removal of the lower uterine segment, a component of the procedure that may vary with technique, and which may be the reason for the large variation in post-procedure bleeding rates. Well-designed studies comparing LSH and total or supracervical vaginal or abdominal hysterectomy are presently lacking.

Summary

There are a number of techniques by which hysterectomy can be performed, each with its own limitations and advantages and advocates and detractors. Variations in the training of individual surgeons, the pathological entities treated with the hysterectomy, and in the design of the related health care system all confound our ability to assess the relative value of the various procedure types in a satisfactory fashion. There is much to be said for the surgeon who performs hysterectomy in a fashion consistent with their training, experience, and comfort; but there is also much to be said for gynecologic surgeons to be adequately trained in all types of the procedure, so that the impact on the woman is more related to the characteristics of her case, and her personal desires regarding retention of the cervix, and not variations in the abilities of the surgeon. My personal perspective of cervical retention reflects my approach to health care interventions in general – it is incumbent on the individual advocating an intervention to provide evidentiary support for that intervention, not the other way around. Consequently, SCH has a place in the health care of women, and none should be made to feel pressured into removal of the entire uterus principally because of an advocacy position. Clearly there is need for more and better clinical trials and studies to provide more useful information for provider and patient alike.

References

1. Döderlein A, Kronig S. *Die techniquder vaginalen bauchholenoperationen.* Leipzig: Verlag von S Hirzel; 1906.
2. Reich H, de Caprio J, McGlynn F. Laparoscopic hysterectomy. *J Gynecol Surg.* 1989;5:213–15.
3. Munro MG, Parker WH. A classification system for laparoscopic hysterectomy. *Obstet Gynecol.* 1993;**82**(4 Pt 1):624–9.
4. Olive DL, Parker WH, Cooper JM, Levine RL. The AAGL classification system for laparoscopic hysterectomy. Classification Committee of the American Association of Gynecologic Laparoscopists. *J Am Assoc Gynecol Laparosc.* 2000;7(1):9–15.
5. Kovac SR. Hysterectomy outcomes in patients with similar indications. *Obstet Gynecol.* 2000;**95**(6 Pt 1):787–93.
6. Mushinski M. Average charges for three types of hysterectomy procedures: United States, 1998. *Stat Bull Metrop Insur Co.* 2000;**81**(2):27–36.
7. Farquhar CM, Steiner CA. Hysterectomy rates in the United States 1990–1997. *Obstet Gynecol.* 2002;**99**(2):229–34.
8. Summitt RL, Jr., Stovall TG, Lipscomb GH, Ling FW. Randomized comparison of laparoscopy-assisted vaginal hysterectomy with standard vaginal hysterectomy in an outpatient setting. *Obstet Gynecol.* 1992;**80**(6):895–901.
9. Lyons TL. Laparoscopic supracervical hysterectomy. A comparison of morbidity and mortality results with laparoscopically assisted vaginal hysterectomy. *J Reprod Med.* 1993;**38**(10):763–7.
10. Munro MG. Supracervical hysterectomy … a time for reappraisal. *Obstet Gynecol.* 1997;**89**(1):133–9.
11. Jones DE, Shackelford DP, Brame RG. Supracervical hysterectomy: back to the future? *Am J Obstet Gynecol.* 1999; **180**(3 Pt 1):513–15.
12. Scott JR, Sharp HT, Dodson MK, Norton PA, Warner HR. Subtotal hysterectomy in modern gynecology: a decision analysis. *Am J Obstet Gynecol.* 1997;**176**(6):1186–91; discussion 1191–2.
13. Learman LA, Summitt RL, Jr., Varner RE, McNeeley SG, Goodman-Gruen D, Richter HE, et al. A randomized comparison of total or supracervical hysterectomy: surgical

complications and clinical outcomes. *Obstet Gynecol.* 2003;**102**(3):453–62.

14. Thakar R, Ayers S, Clarkson P, Stanton S, Manyonda I. Outcomes after total versus subtotal abdominal hysterectomy. *N Engl J Med.* 2002;**347**(17):1318–25.

15. Gimbel H, Zobbe V, Andersen BM, Filtenborg T, Gluud C, Tabor A. Randomised controlled trial of total compared with subtotal hysterectomy with one-year follow up results. *BJOG.* 2003; **110**(12):1088–98.

16. Zupi E, Zullo F, Marconi D, Sbracia M, Pellicano M, Solima E, et al. Hysteroscopic endometrial resection versus laparoscopic supracervical hysterectomy for menorrhagia: a prospective randomized trial. *Am J Obstet Gynecol.* 2003;**188**(1): 7–12.

17. Johnson N, Barlow D, Lethaby A, Tavender E, Curr E, Garry R. Surgical approach to hysterectomy for benign gynaecological disease. *Cochrane Database Syst Rev.* 2005;**1**:CD003677.

Intrauterine progestin-releasing systems

Chapter summary

- The LNG-IUS releases norgestrel at a rate of 20 μg/day decreasing to 11 μg/day by the 5th post-insertion year.
- Insertion can be performed at any time in the cycle.
- In women with normal endometrial cavities there is an immediate reduction in menstrual flow by about 80% at 3 months and by as much as 96% at 12 months.
- Intermenstrual spotting and light bleeding will be experienced by the majority for up to 6 months; following that the rate of such spotting decreases to about 15–20%, with amenorrhea being experienced by 20% or more by the end of the 2nd year, increasing with subsequent years to reach about 50% by year 5.

Introduction

Intrauterine progestin-releasing systems were first developed in the 1970s for contraception, but their efficacy at reducing menstrual blood loss has led to these devices becoming a cornerstone in the management of HMB. The concept of an intrauterine drug delivery system provides high local concentration of the active agent, with minimal systemic absorption, thereby increasing the chance of a therapeutic effect while reducing the incidence and severity of systemic side effects. This approach will likely be a platform for the development of other agents for the treatment of local uterine conditions.

The device

The Mirena® intrauterine system (Bayer Schering Pharma AG, Berlin, Germany) has a shape and insertion technique similar to that of a copper-wrapped intrauterine device called the Nova-T, which is available in most countries throughout the world (Figure 18.1). The frame, which measures 32 mm in length, is made radiopaque by the barium-impregnated plastic construction. The stem of the device contains 52 mg of levonorgestrel (LNG) mixed with polydimethylsiloxane (PDMS) contained within a PDMS capsule that permits slow release of the progestin within the endometrial cavity at a rate of 20 μg/day, that decreases to 11 μg/day by the 5th post-insertion year. A nylon-like thread is attached to the lower tip of the device by a knot that functionally creates a double thread to facilitate removal. The device comes with an insertion system that includes an insertion catheter that is 4.5 mm in outside diameter.

Pharmacokinetics

Levonorgestrel, a 19-nortestosterone derivative, is a progestin with a high degree of endometrial activity, even at low doses. The systemic levels of levonorgestrel are extremely

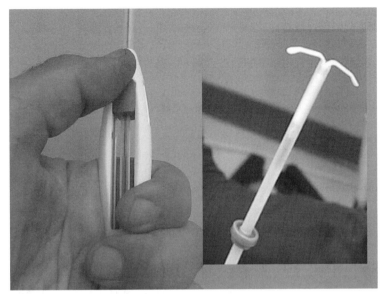

Figure 18.1 Levonorgestrel-releasing intrauterine system (LNG-IUS). The device is pictured in the inset, prior to retraction into the insertion catheter. The handle contains a slider that is manipulated by the thumb to facilitate loading and deployment.

low, even in the first year, ranging from 0.4 to 0.6 nmol/L, far lower than progestin-only contraceptive pills or levonorgestrel implants. On the other hand, the concentrations of levonorgestrel in the endometrium itself are 10^3 times greater than those associated with, for example, oral levonorgestrel therapy [1]. These high levels of local progestin have profound effects on the endometrium that appear to contribute to the mechanism of breakthrough bleeding, but which evolve over the weeks and months after initial insertion to reach a point where they stabilize by about six months. Details of the presumed mechanisms are described in Chapter 11.

As described previously, serum levels of levonorgestrel diminish over the five post-insertion years, a circumstance that does not appear to alter the contraceptive effect but may impact other functions. For example, ovulation may be suppressed initially, but only rarely following the first year.

Insertion

Preprocedure

First of all, the clinician inserting the LNG-IUS should have adequate training from individuals with expertise and experience in LNG-IUS use – reading a book, or watching a video, or supplement, does not supplant this need.

Patient selection

The evidence regarding the LNG-IUS in women with AUB has been discussed in detail in Chapter 8. In summary, women with HMB-E can expect an immediate reduction in menstrual flow by about 80% at 3 months and by as much as 96% at 12 months. The details of side effects are currently derived from the contraception studies, and may not exactly reflect the experience of women with HMB-E who are treated with the LNG-IUS. Intermenstrual spotting and light bleeding will be experienced by the majority for up to 6 months; following that the rate of such spotting decreases to about 15–20%, with amenorrhea being experienced by 20% or more by the end of the 2nd year, increasing with subsequent years to reach about 50% by year 5. The impact of the LNG-IUS on women with AUB/HMB-O or submucosal leiomyomas has not been assessed. Consequently, the ideal subject has been adequately investigated to make a diagnosis of HMB-E, does not wish to conceive in the short to intermediate term, and is comfortable with the notion of short-term intermenstrual spotting, and long-term very light periods or amenorrhea. The endometrial cavity should be essentially normally configured, without uterine septae and, preferably, without submucosal leiomyomas. Consistent with the risks of pelvic inflammatory disease, women should be celibate, or, if heterosexual, in a mutually monogamous sexual relationship.

Patient preparation

For those who are not postpartum, the Mirena® LNG-IUS can be inserted at any time. However, there may be a greater risk of spontaneous expulsion if inserted in the heavy days of the cycle, especially for women with HMB-E who may be passing substantial amounts of blood. The manufacturer supports insertion immediately following spontaneous or surgical pregnancy termination, but recommends a six week interval between delivery and positioning of the device. Indeed, lactating women, even those more than six weeks postpartum, appear to be at greater risk for uterine perforation [2].

There is no requirement for screening of patients for organisms such as gonococcus and *Chlamydia trachomatis*, but the clinician should use judgment and, if indicated, perform such testing either before or at the time of the insertion procedure. At the time of insertion, the clinician should ensure that as much as possible is done to evaluate for pregnancy, including routine use of a sensitive urine assay for hCG. Use of preprocedure analgesia such as ibuprofen, as discussed in Chapter 14, may have value, but there is no current evidence supporting such an approach.

The insertion procedure

Patient positioning and examination

After suitable informed consent and discussion of the essentials of the procedure, the patient is positioned in the modified dorsal lithotomy position in comfortable stirrups. The uterus is examined, or reexamined, to determine length, width, version, flexion, and then a plastic or warmed metal speculum of appropriate size, and coated with 2% lidocaine gel, is positioned in the vagina. At this time, uterine anesthesia is instituted, as appropriate, and as described in Chapter 15.

Insertion techniques (Video 18.1) (Figure 18.2)

At this point, I have to explain that there are basically two approaches to insertion. The manufacturer suggests using a rigid or semiflexible sound to measure the length of the uterus from fundus to exocervix. However, I prefer to "sound" with the insertion system and contained device itself, an approach that I feel may provide less risk of perforation because (a) the uterus is sounded once, and (b) the inserter with the contained device is wider and probably less likely to perforate than a uterine sound. The countervailing argument is that if you open the package, and are unable to insert the device, you may "waste" a LNG-IUS in the process. Functionally the two techniques are very similar.

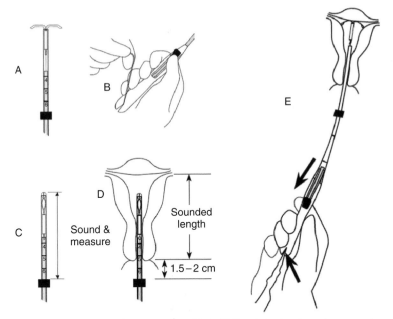

Figure 18.2 Insertion of the Mirena® LNG-IUS. (A) The device is oriented transversely so the numbers on the catheter face up. (B) One hand advances the slider toward the tip of the catheter and then holds it there as the strings are pulled withdrawing the device into the catheter. The strings are hooked into the slot at the proximal end of the handle. (C) The uterus can be sounded separately, although I typically use the device to do this to reduce instrumentation. (D) The stopper is set at the sounded length but the device is positioned so that the tip of the catheter is 1.5–2.0 cm from the fundus. (E) Holding the catheter in position, the slider is withdrawn to the first mark, a maneuver that releases the crossmembers of the T-shaped device. Then the catheter is advanced, positioning the device at the fundus, the slider withdrawn completely, and the entire apparatus removed. The strings are cut to about 3 cm from the external os.

Preparing the system for insertion

1. The system can be prepared without the need for sterile gloves.
2. The package is opened, placed on a firm table, the device removed, and the threads are released.
3. The insertion catheter is rotated so that the centimeter scale is visible (Figure 18.2 A).
4. The device should be held so that the arms of the system are horizontal; if not, the device can be held so that the arms of the T are against the sterile package bottom – rotation allows the T to assume the correct orientation.
5. The slider on the handle is advanced to its furthest (distal) position and held as the threads are pulled to withdraw the LNG-IUS into the insertion tube until the two arms are closed against each other (Figure 18.2 B).
6. When this has been accomplished, the flange is set:
   i. If the uterus has been sounded, the flange is oriented horizontally, planar with the arms of the T, and set so that the distal edge is located at the measured uterine length (Figure 18.2 C).
   ii. If the uterus has not been sounded, the clinician withdraws the flange to a point that is clearly longer than the anticipated length and rotates it so that its long axis is in the same plane as the arms of the T.

Positioning the device

1. If not already done, the cervix is grasped with a tenaculum and placed on slight traction.
2. The inserter is held with the thumb and forefinger holding the slider in the furthermost position and the assembly is moved carefully through the cervical canal.
   i. If the flange has been set based on uterine sounding, the advancement stops when the flange is about 1.5–2.0 cm from the external os (Figure 18.2 D).
   ii. If the uterus has not been previously sounded, the assembly is advanced until it is perceived to reach the fundus of the uterus. Then the flange can be advanced to be flush with the exocervix. The system is then withdrawn until its leading edge is 1.5–2.0 cm from the external os.
3. Now, while holding the insertion assembly steady, the LNG-IUS is opened by pulling the slider back until it reaches the dark mark located midway on the track.
4. With the arms now open, the inserter can be advanced the 1.5–2.0 cm needed to reach the fundus, or until the flange touches the exocervix.

Removing the insertion system

1. Holding the insertion tube in position, the slider is pulled all the way down, a motion that also releases the threads from the cleft in the handle (Figure 18.2 E).
2. Before the insertion tube is removed, check to be sure that the threads are running freely.
3. The threads are cut to leave at least 3 cm visible outside the cervix.

Troubleshooting

Cervical stenosis

The most common problem, assuming that anesthesia is used to minimize pain, is encountering a stenotic cervix. In such instances, the sound or device should be removed, appropriate anesthesia introduced (if not already done), and the cervix dilated, following the steps described in Chapter 16. Care must be taken not to exert too much force on the device.

Suspected perforation

Perforation has been reported to occur in 2.6 per 1000 insertions and it is likely that the vast majority, if not all, occur at the time of insertion [2]. If perforation is suspected, management depends upon the available resources. If an ultrasound unit with a transvaginal transducer is available, the clinician can perform a post-insertion scan to determine whether or not the IUD is in appropriate position. If such a resource is not available, the patient should be sent immediately to a radiology unit where ultrasound and, if necessary, plain X-rays can provide information on the location of the IUD. If indeed perforation has occurred, steps should be taken to remove the device. There is no emergency, and even the absolute need for removal of the device can be questioned, as it appears unlikely to elicit a clinically significant inflammatory response [3]. Generally, perforated IUDs can be found by laparoscopy, occasionally with the need for concomitant hysteroscopy.

Post-procedure management

Perforation may occur without symptoms and without any suspicion on the part of the clinician. Consequently, if a TVS is readily available, it is not unreasonable to perform a post-procedure exam to confirm appropriate placement. Certainly, the patient should be provided information about the strings and the potential for inducing transient deep dyspareunia for a male sexual partner, the possibility of expulsion (which is low), and to reiterate the expectations regarding the impact on bleeding iterated previously.

Removal

Removal of the LNG-IUS should take place if the patient wishes to become pregnant, at menopause, at five years post insertion, if the bleeding symptoms recur, or if other symptoms and findings dictate. There are no good data documenting the duration of the optimal effect of the LNG-IUS on HMB, but, from a contraceptive perspective, the limit is five years.

Removal is generally relatively easy. The procedure may be done at any time in the cycle, if there is one, and no special preparation is needed. The patient is placed in the modified lithotomy position, feet or legs in comfortable stirrups, and an appropriate-sized speculum positioned to expose the cervix. The strings of the device are grasped with a uterine packing or ring forceps and with mild to moderate traction the device is removed. If reinsertion of a new LNG-IUS is to be performed, it may be done at the same setting, remembering to administer appropriate anesthesia prior to removal of the original device.

If the strings are not visible, a cotton tipped applicator or a cytobrush (used for acquisition of endocervical cells for Pap smears) may be passed into the canal, rotated, and then removed. Frequently this maneuver retrieves the string(s). If this is not successful, a Novak curette (Chapter 16) can be passed into the endometrial cavity, rotated, and then removed. The serrated teeth of the Novak may capture the string, or, occasionally, the device thereby allowing removal. If these steps fail, it is reasonable to consider ultrasound to ensure that the device indeed is still in the endometrial cavity. If that is the case, then hysteroscopically-directed removal would be indicated.

References

1. Nilsson CG, Haukkamaa M, Vierola H, Luukkainen T. Tissue concentrations of levonorgestrel in women using a levonorgestrel-releasing IUD. *Clin Endocrinol (Oxf)*. 1982; **17**(6):529–36.
2. Van Houdenhoven K, van Kaam KJ, van Grootheest AC, Salemans TH, Dunselman GA. Uterine perforation in women using a levonorgestrel-releasing intrauterine system. *Contraception*. 2006; **73**(3):257–60.
3. Haimov-Kochman R, Doviner V, Amsalem H, Prus D, Adoni A, Lavy Y. Intraperitoneal levonorgestrel-releasing intrauterine device following uterine perforation: the role of progestins in adhesion formation. *Hum Reprod*. 2003; **18**(5):990–3.

Myoma ablation

Chapter summary
- Leiomyoma ablation is targeted destruction of a uterine leiomyoma using any of a number of techniques.
- Cryomyolysis may be performed under laparoscopic direction to target leiomyomas using freezing techniques.
- High-intensity focused ultrasound can be used to perform image guided myoma ablation using either ultrasound or MRI.
- Laser and radiofrequency techniques can also be used to target leiomyomas for hyperthermic ablation.
- In general, these techniques should not be used for women who desire future fertility.

Introduction
Techniques designed to destroy rather than remove leiomyomas have been termed *myolysis* or *myoma ablation*. Several such techniques are under development using liquid nitrogen for hypothermic ablation; laser or radiofrequency electricity and, more recently, focused ultrasound energy, directed and monitored by ultrasound or MRI for hyperthermic ablation. These approaches have shown some promise, but well-designed clinical trials are necessary not only to determine their efficacy but, even if efficacious, to compare them to other techniques for clinically relevant outcomes.

Hypothermic myoma ablation
The first publication of hypothermic treatment of leiomyomas was from the Yale group in New Haven, Connecticut in 1996 [1]. The technique, sometimes called *cryomyolysis*, uses probes cooled either by liquid nitrogen or by differential gas exchange, as described by Joule-Thompson. The probe is passed into a leiomyoma and then activated, resulting in a reduction of local temperature to less than –90°C, creating an ice ball, the size and shape reflecting features of the probe and the duration of application. Lethal tissue damage occurs at –20°C, but at the edge of the ice ball the tissue temperature is approximately 0°C and, consequently, is not destructive to the tissue [2]. A potential advantage of this technique over hyperthermic approaches is the ability to predict the limits of treated tissue by imaging the ice ball with ultrasound.

The extent of tissue necrosis may be secondary to the degree of vascular damage. When tissue cools, the damaged vascular endothelium detaches from the internal surface of vessel, a process that contributes to the development of edema and local activation of platelets. The resulting thrombosis then occludes the local circulation thereby enhancing

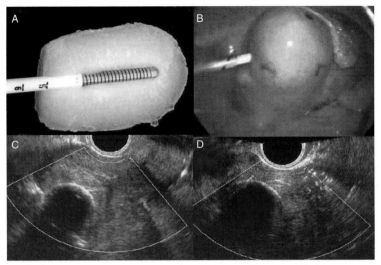

Figure 19.1 Hypothermic myoma ablation ("cryomyolysis"). (A) Cryoprobe with a typical surrounding iceball that reflects the typical lesion size. (B) The laparoscopic view of a uterus with a fundal myoma and the cryoprobe passed through a laparoscopic port into the substance of the fibroid. (C) and (D) demonstrate the progressive expansion of the iceball under ultrasound monitoring from [6] Zupi et al.

both local ischemia and tissue necrosis. The result is a graded response as histopathological examination shows complete necrosis in the central aspects of the target area and tissue sparing in the periphery of the previously frozen tissue. The relative uniformity of cell death in the zones that reach $-20°C$ or lower suggests that the principal clinical impact of cryomyolysis is one that is secondary to the vascular impact on tissue [2]. There is also evidence that leiomyomata may be more sensitive to freezing than normal myometrial tissue, whereas the effects of laser or electrosurgical energy are similar in myoma and adjacent healthy myometrium [3]. If this is accurate, hypothermic ablation techniques may have a degree of tissue specificity, and could aid the clinician in preserving neighboring myometrium.

In its present form, the technique is performed laparoscopically, usually under general anesthesia, with the telescope inserted through the umbilicus, or higher in the event of a large uterus (Figure 19.1). After exposure of the cervix with a speculum or retractors, a uterine manipulator is positioned and used to stabilize and manipulate the uterus, thereby optimally positioning the myomas for insertion of the probe ("cryoprobe"). The surgeon also positions additional ports as required for instrument access necessary to perform the procedure, the location and number determined at the time of the procedure based upon the size and location of the myomas to be treated. An incision in the uterus, over the leiomyoma, is made with a monopolar electrosurgical hook or blade to create a passageway that is 4–5 mm wide and a depth that is about 1 cm or less from the estimated inferior surface of the myoma. For myomas 4 cm or less in diameter, a single central incision is adequate, while for larger-diameter lesions, multiple incisions will be required The cryoprobe Her Option® (American Medical Systems Inc, Minnetonka, MN, USA) is then passed through the appropriate ancillary port and inserted into the myoma via the previously created tunnel. For larger myomas, it is thought useful to reduce the blood supply from both the serosa and from the endometrial vessels. Consequently, there exists a strategy of freezing the myoma superficially and then deeply using additional incisions, the number determined by the myoma volume [4–7].

There are a number of studies evaluating this technique. In most instances both myoma volume and related symptoms, including HMB, are reduced by approximately 50% at 6 months and even more at 12 months following therapy [4, 6–8] (Class II-3). These data are encouraging in that they suggest that hypothermic ablation is potentially a minimally invasive, safe, and feasible procedure in selected patients. There remain a number of questions including the impact of hypothermic ablation on fertility and future pregnancy, although a recent small series of nine patients demonstrated that such patients may remain fertile and have essentially normal pregnancy outcomes [9].

It is clear that these studies are insufficient to evaluate long-term outcomes and that further studies, with larger sample size and longer follow-up are needed to confirm the preliminary data. As a result, hypothermic ablation or cryomyolysis should still be considered an experimental procedure.

Hyperthermic myoma ablation

Laser and electrosurgical energy

In the early 1990s coagulation of leiomyomas was reported, under laparoscopic guidance, using either laser (Nd:YAG or infrared) energy [10–12] or a bipolar radiofrequency electrical probe [13, 14]. These different kinds of electromagnetic waveforms are converted first to mechanical energy, oscillating intracellular protein, and then to elevation of intracellular temperature that causes both coagulative necrosis and devascularization within the treated tissue. The volume of necrosis created is dependent on the amount of electromagnetic energy delivered to the tissue. There remain challenges related to predicting or monitoring the local distribution of this energy in tissue, although probes/electrodes with thermal couples that measure local temperature have some promise.

Hyperthermic myoma ablation is an investigational procedure that has been described via laparoscopy, hysteroscopy, and under ultrasound direction. When the procedure is performed laparoscopically, the laser fiber or bipolar electrodes are passed through the instrument channel of an operating laparoscope or ancillary cannula and are then used to pierce the myoma and advance into its core. An attempt is made to coagulate the entire myoma by repeated insertions at multiple concentric sites. A few investigators have described the use of hysteroscopically-directed application of laser energy to ablate myomas, or the portions of type 1 or 2 myomas that remain in the myometrium. The Nd:YAG fiber is guided through the instrument channel of an operating hysteroscope and positioned in the intramural myoma [12]. Unfortunately, positioning such a fiber without being able to view the uterine serosal surface is a concern. As a result, there is also some work underway evaluating the potential role of ultrasound-directed positioning of radiofrequency electrodes for the purpose of electrosurgical leiomyoma ablation, but no data are yet available [15].

There are some outcome data available for laparoscopic hyperthermic myoma ablation. Typically there is a decrease in myoma volume within 6 months of up to 50% of the original size [11–14] (Class II-3). There is also evidence of reduction in the volume of HMB but, in the study with the largest sample size, it is unclear how much of this reduction is related to concomitant hysteroscopically-directed treatment [14]. Post-ablation pregnancy is a lingering concern as a number of authors have reported adverse outcomes such as rupture of the uterus [16, 17].

Focused ultrasound energy

The potential for treatment of uterine leiomyomas using high-intensity focused ultrasound (HIFU) was first described in a multicenter feasibility study in 2003 [18]. Focusing ultrasound energy, essentially with a parabolic mirror, for the ablation of tissue is a noninvasive technique, first described in 1927 and then again in 1942 [19]. The technique was slow to develop because of limitations in the control of the process of coagulative necrosis. With improvements in real time imaging, including ultrasound and MRI, has come the potential for use of HIFU as a viable therapeutic instrument. Magnetic resonance guided focused ultrasound surgery (MRgFUS) has now been evaluated in a number of tissues including breast [20], brain [21], and prostate gland [22]. Under development is the use of diagnostic ultrasound for image-guided the direction of focused ultrasound energy [15, 23].

Technique

For the treatment of uterine leiomyomas, the procedure is performed in a specially-designed suite with the patient positioned on a procedure table overlying the ultrasound generator (Figure 19.2). This system functions to create an array of pulsed high-intensity ultrasound beams that are focused on the target tissue, directed by MRI or, possibly, ultrasound imaging. One such array generates a volume of tissue ablation that is in the range of 6 mm by 25 mm using 2-D measurements. The device is then refocused to an adjacent target and the process repeated until the desired volume of tissue ablation is reached. Tumor necrosis is also dependent upon the time of exposure. With MRI, the degree of tumor necrosis can, to a degree, be estimated allowing the ability to thermally

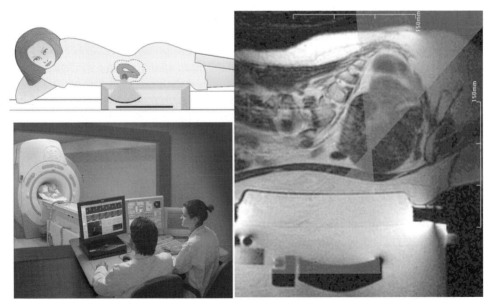

Figure 19.2 Magnetic resonance guided focused ultrasound (MRgFUS). *Upper left*: Diagram demonstrating the positioning of the patient over the ultrasound system which focuses the sonic energy on the leiomyoma within the uterus. *Upper right*: An MRI image demonstrating the aiming mechanism with the energy targeted on the MRI-imaged leiomyomas in the uterus. *Lower left*: The MRI suite with the patient lying within the magnetic coil and on top of the focused ultrasound unit.

"map" the region of the target tissue to a prespecified temperature as measured by the proton resonance frequency shift [24, 25]. However, preliminary studies comparing MRI-based treatment volume with the volume of nonperfused or necrotic tissue based on post-procedure hysterectomy and histological examination, reveal that the volume of myoma or myometrial necrosis is threefold higher that that predicted by MRI [26].

For uterine leiomyomas, the currently available data are almost totally derived from MRgFUS techniques. The patient is treated in an MRI suite where she is placed in the prone position with the abdomen resting over the treatment device. Conscious sedation is generally administered with a variable combination of narcotics and anxiolytics. The FUS comprises a spherically-curved radiator contained within a sealed water bath. Then MRI is performed to ensure that bladder and bowel are not in the path of the ultrasound beams and, if so, manipulation or repositioning of the patient used in an attempt to remedy the situation. Treatment, called "sonication," is performed in a systematic fashion with typical treatment times to date being about two hours and time in the suite about three hours. Patients are discharged home about one hour following the end of the procedure.

Results

The first published clinical study was a seven-center multi-national multi-institutional trial that described a series of 109 patients, treated with the ExAblate® 2000 system (InSightec, Haifa, Israel) [27] (Class III). The mean *fibroid* volume of these patients, depending on the number of myomas, was 294–346 cm^3 while the mean *treatment* volume was only 32–36 cm^3, or about 10–11% of the total. There were relatively few treatment-related serious outcomes, but only 79.3% of the patients were available for followup at 6 months. The mean fibroid volume reduction was 13.5% ± 32 and, using the multidimensional Uterine Fibroid Symptoms and Quality of Life Questionnaire (UFS-QOL), there was a mean 27.3 point reduction in the score compared with baseline.

In a subsequent study, and one that resulted in US FDA approval of the ExAblate 2000 device for use in the United States, 109 of 176 women enrolled were treated in 7 sites in the United States, Europe, and Israel [28]. In this trial the mean uterine volume was 595.0 ± 362.5 cm^3, the mean myoma volume was 284.7 ± 225.4 cm^3, and the mean treated myoma volume as estimated by MRI was 25.6 ± 18.4 cm^3. Several mild skin burns resulted and one patient had a sciatic nerve injury that had resolved by the 12-month evaluation. The mean reduction in UFS-QOL was 23.8 and, at 12 months, with only 82 of the original cohort available for evaluation, 51.2% of the women reached the targeted reduction of at least 10 points.

More recently, and in a well-designed comparative trial, the preprocedural use of GnRHa has been shown to potentiate the effect of focused ultrasound energy as measured by intraprocedural MRI [29]. In a subsequent reported clinical series evaluating 49 women, and followed for 12 months, UFS-QOL reductions of 45% were seen at 12 months and 83% achieved at least a 10-point reduction in the scale [30]. The reduction in targeted myoma volume was 37% at 12 months in the patients available for evaluation.

The clinical results associated with MFgFUS are promising, but both myoma reduction and the measured relief of symptoms seem disproportionate to the amount of myoma treated. The feasibility study, previously discussed, demonstrated that the volume of tumor necrosis exceeded the treated volume by a factor of three. More recently, a retrospective comparison was published, comparing predicted volume of treated tissue, treatment volume based on MRI-determined temperature elevation, and MRI-determined volume of post-treatment nonperfused tissue [31]. In this comparison, and only in larger areas of sonication, the volume of nonperfused tissue was double that of the "treated" volume based on MRI-measured tissue temperature. The authors suggest that this larger area of necrotic tissue may have been caused by vascular occlusion and "downstream" ischemia, but the possibility exists that MR is not as accurate as thought for the determination of treated tissue in these lesions.

Summary

Despite the apparent promise of leiomyoma ablation, there are still no published trials comparing any of the three procedures with experimental or established approaches such as uterine artery embolization or occlusion, medical therapy, myomectomy or hysterectomy. Indeed, some patients, who have symptoms related to type II submucosal myomas, may be candidates for endometrial ablation by any of a number of techniques. Furthermore, while the impact of myoma ablation on fertility and pregnancy is unknown, the few adverse outcomes reported following hyperthermic ablation with MRgFUS must be reason for concern. It is also clear that a number of patient characteristics including myoma size, location, the presence of adhesions, or abdominal scarring, may, to a greater or lesser extent impact or even preclude some patients from undergoing myoma ablation.

The MR or ultrasound-guided FUS are the only techniques that have, to date, delivered energy to tissue without direct contact by the energy source with the treated tissue. Consequently, this approach offers the potential for "incisionless" surgery, at least for the selected patients who would qualify for therapy. However, the issue of prediction of the treatment volume must remain an area for concern given the structures that surround the uterus and the possibility for injury.

Despite all of the aforementioned reservations, these procedures seem to be promising techniques to reduce the invasiveness of traditional surgery and should be subjected to appropriately designed clinical trials that can better define their role in the management of the myriad clinical circumstances associated with uterine leiomyomas.

For the present, the techniques must still be considered experimental and should be performed in a structured environment by well-experienced groups with patients carefully selected and counseled considering all available options. Careful observation and reporting of all results, both positive and negative, will help to define the role that myoma ablation has in the management of symptoms, including AUB, related to uterine leiomyomas.

References

1. Olive DL, Rutherford T, Zreik T, Palter S. Cryomyolysis in the conservative treatment of uterine fibroids. *J Am Assoc Gynecol Laparosc.* 1996;3(4 Suppl):S36.

2. Devireddy RV, Coad JE, Bischof JC. Microscopic and calorimetric assessment of freezing processes in uterine fibroid tumor tissue. *Cryobiology.* 2001;42(4):225–43.

3. Rupp CC, Nagel TC, Swanlund DJ, Bischof JC, Coad JE. Cryothermic and hyperthermic treatments of human leiomyomata and adjacent myometrium and their implications for laparoscopic surgery. *J Am Assoc Gynecol Laparosc.* 2003;10(1):90–8.

4. Zreik TG, Rutherford TJ, Palter SF, Troiano RN, Williams E, Brown JM, et al. Cryomyolysis, a new procedure for the conservative treatment of uterine fibroids. *J Am Assoc Gynecol Laparosc.* 1998;5(1):33–8.

5. Odnusi KO, Rutherford TJ, Olive DL, Bia F, Parkash V, Brown J, et al. Cryomyolysis in the management of uterine fibroids: technique and complications. *Surg Technol Int.* 2000;8:173–8.

6. Zupi E, Piredda A, Marconi D, Townsend D, Exacoustos C, Arduini D, et al. Directed laparoscopic cryomyolysis: a possible alternative to myomectomy and/or

hysterectomy for symptomatic leiomyomas. *Am J Obstet Gynecol.* 2004;**190**(3):639–43.

7. Ciavattini A, Tsiroglou D, Piccioni M, Lugnani F, Litta P, Feliciotti F, et al. Laparoscopic cryomyolysis: an alternative to myomectomy in women with symptomatic fibroids. *Surg Endosc.* 2004; **18**(12):1785–8.

8. Zupi E, Marconi D, Sbracia M, Exacoustos C, Piredda A, Sorrenti G, et al. Directed laparoscopic cryomyolysis for symptomatic leiomyomata: one-year follow up. *J Minim Invasive Gynecol.* 2005;**12**(4):343–6.

9. Ciavattini A, Tsiroglou D, Litta P, Vichi M, Tranquilli AL. Pregnancy outcome after laparoscopic cryomyolysis of uterine myomas: report of nine cases. *J Minim Invasive Gynecol.* 2006; **13**(2):141–4.

10. Nisolle M, Smets M, Malvaux V, Anaf V, Donnez J. Laparoscopic myolysis with the Nd:YAG laser. *J Gynecol Surg.* 1993;**9** (2):95–9.

11. Zaporozhan VN. Intratissue laser thermotherapy in treatment of uterine myomata. *J Am Assoc Gynecol Laparosc.* 1996;**3**(4 Suppl):S56.

12. Jourdain O, Roux D, Cambon D, Dallay D. A new method for the treatment of fibromas: interstitial laser hyperthermia using the Nd:YAG laser. Preliminary study. *Eur J Obstet Gynecol Reprod Biol.* 1996; **64**(1):73–8.

13. Goldfarb HA. Comparison of bipolar electrocoagulation and Nd:YAG laser coagulation for symptomatic reduction of uterine myomas. *J Am Assoc Gynecol Laparosc.* 1994;**1**(4 Pt 2):S13.

14. Phillips DR, Milim SJ, Nathanson HG, Haselkorn JS. Experience with laparoscopic leiomyoma coagulation and concomitant operative hysteroscopy. *J Am Assoc Gynecol Laparosc.* 1997;**4**(4):425–33.

15. Hurst BS, Elliot M, Matthews ML, Marshburn PB. Ultrasound-directed transvaginal myolysis: preclinical studies. *J Minim Invasive Gynecol.* 2007; **14**(4):502–5.

16. Arcangeli S, Pasquarette MM. Gravid uterine rupture after myolysis. *Obstet Gynecol.* 1997;**89**(5 Pt 2):857.

17. Vilos GA, Daly LJ, Tse BM. Pregnancy outcome after laparoscopic electromyolysis. *J Am Assoc Gynecol Laparosc.* 1998;**5** (3):289–92.

18. Tempany CM, Stewart EA, McDannold N, Quade BJ, Jolesz FA, Hynynen K. MR imaging-guided focused ultrasound surgery of uterine leiomyomas: a feasibility study. *Radiology.* 2003; **226**(3):897–905.

19. Lynn JG, Zwerner, R.L., Chick, A.J., Miller, A.E. A new method for the generation and use of focused ultrasound in experimental biology. *J Gen Physiol.* 1942;**26**:179–203.

20. Hynynen K, Pomeroy O, Smith DN, Huber PE, McDannold NJ, Kettenbach J, et al. MR imaging-guided focused ultrasound surgery of fibroadenomas in the breast: a feasibility study. *Radiology.* 2001;**219**(1):176–85.

21. McDannold N, Moss M, Killiany R, Rosene DL, King RL, Jolesz FA, et al. MRI-guided focused ultrasound surgery in the brain: tests in a primate model. *Magn Reson Med.* 2003;**49**(6):1188–91.

22. Smith NB, Buchanan MT, Hynynen K. Transrectal ultrasound applicator for prostate heating monitored using MRI thermometry. *Int J Radiat Oncol Biol Phys.* 1999;**43**(1):217–25.

23. Zhou XD, Ren XL, Zhang J, He GB, Zheng MJ, Tian X, et al. Therapeutic response assessment of high intensity focused ultrasound therapy for uterine fibroid: utility of contrast-enhanced ultrasonography. *Eur J Radiol.* 2007;**62** (2):289–94.

24. Hynynen K, Freund WR, Cline HE, Chung AH, Watkins RD, Vetro JP, et al. A clinical, noninvasive, MR imaging-monitored ultrasound surgery method. *Radiographics.* 1996;**16**(1):185–95.

25. Chung AH, Jolesz FA, Hynynen K. Thermal dosimetry of a focused ultrasound beam in vivo by magnetic resonance imaging. *Med Phys.* 1999; **26**(9):2017–26.

26. Stewart EA, Gedroyc WM, Tempany CM, Quade BJ, Inbar Y, Ehrenstein T, et al. Focused ultrasound treatment of uterine fibroid tumors: safety and feasibility of a noninvasive thermoablative technique. *Am J Obstet Gynecol.* 2003; **189**(1):48–54.

27. Hindley J, Gedroyc WM, Regan L, Stewart E, Tempany C, Hynyen K, et al. MRI guidance of focused ultrasound therapy of uterine fibroids: early results. *AJR Am J Roentgenol.* 2004; **183**(6):1713–19.

28. Stewart EA, Rabinovici J, Tempany CM, Inbar Y, Regan L, Gostout B, et al. Clinical outcomes of focused ultrasound surgery for the treatment of uterine fibroids. *Fertil Steril.* 2006; **85**(1):22–9.

29. Smart OC, Hindley JT, Regan L, Gedroyc WG. Gonadotrophin-releasing hormone and magnetic-resonance-guided ultrasound surgery for uterine leiomyomata. *Obstet Gynecol.* 2006;**108**(1):49–54.

30. Smart OC, Hindley JT, Regan L, Gedroyc WM. Magnetic resonance guided focused ultrasound surgery of uterine fibroids – the tissue effects of GnRH agonist pre-treatment. *Eur J Radiol.* 2006; **59**(2):163–7.

31. McDannold N, Tempany CM, Fennessy FM, So MJ, Rybicki FJ, Stewart EA, et al. Uterine leiomyomas: MR imaging-based thermometry and thermal dosimetry during focused ultrasound thermal ablation. *Radiology.* 2006;**240**(1):263–72.

Chapter summary

- Myomectomy is targeted removal of uterine leiomyomas.
- Myomectomy may be performed from within the endometrial cavity using a resectoscope, or abdominally either via laparoscopic or laparotomic direction.
- Resectoscopic myomectomy requires that the leiomyoma be either type 0, type 1, or type 2 with an adequate margin of myometrium between the myoma and the uterine serosa.
- Laparoscopic myomectomy may be restricted by the number, size, and location of the myomas and the ability of the surgeon.

Introduction

Myomectomy refers to a collection of procedures that are designed to remove leiomyomas from the uterus. For most women, the overall goal is to treat symptoms of bleeding or pressure while preserving or enhancing fertility. Others simply wish to retain the integrity of their reproductive tract.

General issues

Removal of leiomyomas via laparotomy (abdominal myomectomy) was first reported by Atlee in 1845 [1]. Despite, and perhaps because of its early introduction into gynecologic practice, abdominal myomectomy has not been subjected to rigorous clinical evaluation comparing it with expectant, medical, and other surgical approaches to the various manifestations of uterine leiomyomata. Consequently, there remains controversy regarding its value, particularly for the treatment of infertility.

The advent of operative endoscopy added new surgical options for the woman with symptomatic leiomyomas. A number of potential candidates for the abdominal approach were removed with the introduction of hysteroscopically-directed management of submucosal myomas by Neuwirth in 1978 [2]. Although Semm and Mettler first described laparoscopic myomectomy [3], Dubuisson et al. published the first series of laparoscopically-directed myomectomies as a potentially less morbid alternative to a laparotomy-based approach [4].

Indications for myomectomy by any approach are currently being re-evaluated, as cost containment incentives, medical therapy, consumer pressure, and academic introspection combine to reinforce the long known fact that most myomas are asymptomatic and do not require treatment. The incidence of leiomyosarcoma is so rare, even in rapidly growing leiomyomata, that in the vast majority of instances, malignancy is not a relevant consideration [5]. Even in the face of symptoms, it is prudent not to assume that patient complaints are caused by the myoma felt on examination or imaged on ultrasound.

Patient selection for myomectomy

The etiology of AUB-L is presumed to be secondary to alterations in the endometrial vasculature and the local synthesis of agents necessary for hemostasis by submucosal lesions (Chapter 5). Consequently, the clinician should seek to evaluate the endometrial cavity for leiomyomas using SIS or hysteroscopy, and/or attempt medical therapy with tranexamic acid, COX inhibitors or oral contraceptives before concluding that myomectomy is an appropriate therapeutic option for AUB.

Leiomyosarcoma is extremely rare, particularly in premenopausal women [5, 6), and, contrary to some perceptions, likely represents a de novo neoplasm, not a result of malignant transformation of a benign tumor (Chapter 9). Understanding that a myoma is almost certainly benign should give confidence to both the patient and her physician that expectant or medical approaches, if effective, are appropriate alternatives to surgery. Growth of apparent myomas in postmenopausal women is likely a contraindication to conservative surgical procedures like myomectomy.

Preoperative preparation and evaluation

Counseling and evaluation

Preparation for myomectomy is undertaken in view of the need of the patient to under-stand the procedure, considering the expectant, medical, and other surgical options. The patient should have a clear understanding of potential complications as well as the expected and the possible degree of postoperative disability. The potential for unanticipated hys-terectomy should be reviewed. All of this information should be documented in the clinical notes and the informed consent document.

Most would find it prudent to preoperatively confirm tubal patency (if the procedure is designed to preserve or improve fertility) and to obtain as much information as pos-sible regarding the location and extent of the myomas using one or a combination of hysterosalpingogram, SIS, and hysteroscopy. Such information may help in the selection of incision sites and, perhaps, in determining the route of access. If there is clinical suspicion that the masses in the uterus represent adenomyosis, MRI scanning may be appropriate as, in such instances, conservative surgery is unlikely to improve reproductive performance. Ancillary investigations should be performed as appropriate; however, a hemoglobin or hematocrit is essential. In addition, because of the potential for blood loss, the patient should be provided the opportunity for collection and storage of autologous blood, provided her hemoglobin levels and the time available before surgery permit.

Gonadotropin releasing hormone analogs

Preoperative administration of gonadotropin releasing hormone analogs (GnRHa) may provide value for the woman with anemia, as creation of amenorrhea can be expected to facilitate the restoration of hemoglobin levels, provided sufficient amounts of iron are administered over an adequate amount of time [7] (Class I-2). In such instances, autologous blood may more safely be obtained. Consequently, the duration of administration of the analog is related to the pre-existing degree of anemia and the response of the patient to iron or other appropriate therapy.

There is controversy regarding the impact of prelaparotomic myomectomy GnRHa use on the ability of the surgeon to detect small myomas intraoperatively and on the subsequent risk of "recurrence." One RCT suggested that surgeons were more likely to miss myomas when the patient was treated with GnRHa while another showed no such relationship [8, 9] (Class I-2). A Cochrane Systematic Review of RCTs concluded that, in addition to improving both pre- and postoperative hemoglobin levels, preoperative GnRHa also reduced operating time and the rate of vertical skin incisions [10] (Class I-1).

Resectoscopic myomectomy poses problems associated with systemic fluid absorption and with the mechanical aspects of removing masses from within the endometrial cavity. There is evidence that systemic absorption of fluid is greater during resectoscopic myomectomy, particularly when deep type I and type II submucosal myomas require dissection into the myometrium [11]. There is also evidence that preoperative GnRHa reduces operative time, perhaps related in part to a reduction the volume of leiomyomas in general, a feature that would be expected to facilitate the performance of resectoscopic myomectomy [11]. As a result of the above, it would seem preferable to use preoperative GnRHa in patients undergoing resectoscopic myomectomy, but specific prospective studies are needed to further investigate this issue.

In summary, GnRHa are clearly useful in allowing otherwise anemic women to enter surgery with normal hemoglobin and stored autologous blood. Their value in changing the clinical outcomes associated with myomectomy is less clear. There seems little doubt that the size of at least intramural lesions may reduce following the use of preoperative agonist therapy, and that the maximum effect is usually realized in three months. If, in the judgment of the surgeon, such a change would facilitate the procedure then selective use can be justified. Clearly, larger multicenter trials are necessary to more adequately assess the impact of preoperative GnRHa on clinically relevant parameters such as operative time, transfusion rates, and subsequent fertility.

Procedures

The principles of contemporary abdominal myomectomy were established by Bonney with his publications of 20 years of experience and amplified by his 1946 report of 806 cases [12]. The low morbidity and mortality were rather remarkable with only 2 deaths in the last 400 cases (overall mortality of 1.1%). The limitations (and advantages) of laparoscopy have given rise to reconsideration of these classical approaches. In addition, the advent of GnRHa and adhesion prevention techniques have given rise to new controversies in the technique of myomectomy. Finally, hysteroscopic myomectomy appears to represent an important and less morbid alternative to abdominal and laparoscopic approaches in selected women with submucosal leiomyomas.

Resectoscopic (hysteroscopic) myomectomy

Resection (Video 20.2) and vaporization (Video 20.1) are resectoscopic techniques used to remove leiomyomata, with limitations related to the size, number, and location of the tumors, especially in the cornual region and to the proportion of the tumor that is in the myometrium. In addition, the goals of the patient with respect to fertility are important as, for optimal retention or enhancement of fertility, complete excision of the myoma with maximum preservation of endometrial and myometrial integrity may be required. Resectoscopic myomectomy is more likely to result in improved bleeding symptoms (> 90%) than successful treatment of infertility (53–70%) [13–15] (Class II-2).

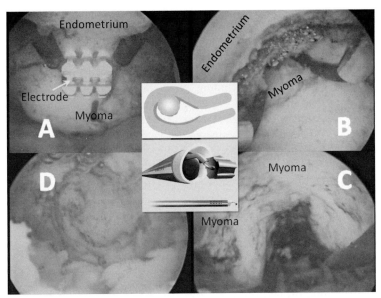

Figure 20.1 Resectoscopic myomectomy. The technique described combines resectoscopic dissection, partial vaporization, and mechanical excision of the anterior type 1 submucosal myoma shown in (A) and depicted in the top central inset. A loop electrode was used to make an endometrial incision at the myoma base (B), which allowed blunt dissection of the myoma from the myometrium using the spiked bulk vaporizing electrode (lower inset; also seen in (A)). Once the majority of the lesion is dissected away, the bulk vaporizing electrode is activated and the myoma is cytoreduced using electrosurgical vaporization until it is small enough to remove with Corson forceps (Figure 21.4) leaving a depression in the myometrium where the myoma once was located (D). The myometrium will generally expand to a near normal thickness, but there will be a variable amount of scarring where the endometrium was removed with the myoma.

Preoperative imaging is important, not only to select appropriate patients for resectoscopic surgery, but also to plan the technical approach itself. Lesions that are totally within the endometrial cavity (type 0, and superficial type 1) and that are appropriately sized (generally ≤ 5 cm diameter) can generally be vaporized and excised with relative ease. However, for those lesions that penetrate into the myometrium to a substantial degree (deep type I and type II tumors), careful planning and substantial skill with the resectoscope are important requisites (Video 20.3). The margin between the uterine serosa and the deepest extent of the myoma(s) should be measured [16] and if it is less than 5–8 mm I suggest that intraoperative ultrasound and/or laparoscopy may be necessary to prevent injury to extrauterine structures such as bowel.

In most instances resectoscopic myomectomy is performed in a standard operating room under appropriate anesthesia. The patient is positioned in the dorsal lithotomy position, the cervix dilated, and the resectoscope inserted with a suitable electrode and attached to an electrosurgical generator. I typically use a combination of dissection, vaporization (Figure 20.1), and removal of the residual myoma with a "Corson" forceps (Figure 21.4) (Video 21.4). Resection of deep submucosal myomas is more often associated with systemic absorption of substantial amounts of distending fluid, a feature that should be made clear to patients for, in such instances, the procedure may have to be aborted and completed at a later time [14, 17] (Class II-3).

Laparotomic myomectomy

Laparotomic myomectomy may be performed if there are many leiomyomas, if they are very large (Figure 20.2), or if they may involve adjacent structures in a way not suitable for the safe conduct of laparoscopic technique. At laparotomy, there exist a number of approaches that may reduce blood loss, including preoperative GnRHa, mechanical vascular tourniquets, myometrial injection of vasoactive substances, and careful dissection technique. Vascular tourniquets are applied after creating windows in the broad ligaments that allow straps (usually urethral catheters or Penrose drains) to be placed around the uterine isthmus occluding the blood supply from the uterine arteries. The vessels in the infundibulopelvic ligaments can be occluded bilaterally with vascular clamps, thereby obstructing the blood supply from the ovarian arteries, but in practice I rarely take this step [18, 19]. The vasoactive substance of choice is dilute vasopressin, 20 units in 60–100 mL of normal saline, injected around the myomas taking care to avoid intravascular infusion [20].

Minimizing the number of posterior incisions is important as they have been associated with a greater incidence of postoperative adhesions [21] (Class II-2) and it is prudent to apply microsurgical techniques including meticulous hemostasis, careful tissue handling, and the use of fine caliber suture on peritoneal surfaces. There is some information supporting the use of adhesion barriers over myomectomy incisions [22, 23] (Class II-3). Unfortunately, no data exists comparing the impact of adhesion barriers on fertility.

Morbidity at laparotomic myomectomy was recently reviewed in 128 patients operated upon by 46 surgeons with varying amounts of training; a likely measure of procedure *effectiveness* or the results in the hands of a spectrum of surgeons [24] (Class II-3). The average uterine size was consistent with 14 weeks gestation and the average estimated blood loss was 342 mL. Five had blood loss in excess of 1 L, the transfusion rate was 20%, and one patient required intraoperative hysterectomy. Postoperative complications included wound infection [1], deep venous thrombosis [1], and postoperative fever [15].

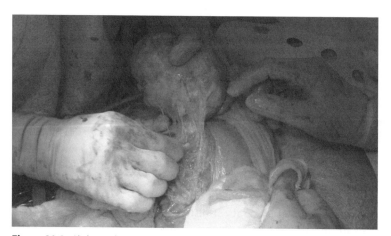

Figure 20.2 Abdominal myomectomy. Here a laparotomy has been performed and the surgeon is dissecting a large, fist-sized leiomyoma from the myometrium.

Laparoscopic myomectomy

Laparoscopically-directed myomectomy is just what it seems – removal of uterine leio-myomas under laparoscopic direction (Figure 20.3) (Video 20.4). The procedure is in some ways controversial, but it has been demonstrated to be effective in a number of observa-tional studies [25–29], and, at least with selected patients and expert surgeons, shorter hospitalization, faster recovery, fewer adhesions, and reduced blood loss [30]. However, the spectrum of myoma size and location, the difficulty with morcellation and removal, and the technical requirements for manipulation of needles and suture with which to close the uterine incisions make the procedure difficult to perform. Nevertheless, retrospective comparative studies [31] (Class II-2) and available RCTs [32] (Class I-2) suggest that, in selected patients, fertility outcome is about 50–60% with both the laparoscopic and laparotomic approaches. Another outcome important to women undergoing myomectomy is pregnancy outcome. Currently available evidence suggests that patients selected for laparoscopic myomectomy and operated upon by skilled surgeons will have similar preg-nancy outcomes compared to those who have laparotomic myomectomy [33].

It is thought useful to review some of the advantages, limitations, and concerns regarding laparoscopic myomectomy. The principle potential advantage, compared to the laparotomic approach, is the reduction of both direct and indirect costs. The small abdominal incisions generally reduce the need for analgesia, allow earlier mobilization and alimentation, and facilitate earlier hospital discharge, frequently on the same day of surgery [34] (Class I-2). In addition, the lack of a significant abdominal incision allows a faster return to economic productivity thereby reducing the indirect cost of care.

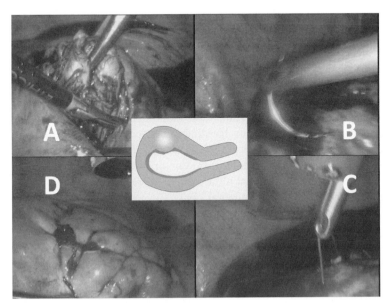

Figure 20.3 Laparoscopic myomectomy. The myoma is a type 2 lesion that is largely intramural with only about 5% of the diameter distorting the endometrial cavity (inset). (A) An incision has been made, the myoma grasped with a tenaculum, and an ultrasonic dissecting system is being used to dissect the myoma from the myometrium. (B) Laparoscopic needle drivers are used to position suture, and laparoscopic knot manipulators are used to transfer knots tied externally and secure them tightly. (D) The completed closure.

197

Theoretically at least, the reduced need for packs and manual retraction would minimize tissue trauma and subsequent adhesions. On the other hand, multiple myomas cannot usually be removed through the same incision and the surgeon loses the ability to palpate uterine tissue, detecting smaller myomas. It is also more difficult to apply laparoscopic technique to myomas in problem areas such as the region of the uterine arteries or the cornua thereby preserving tubal patency. As is the case with any laparoscopic procedure, there are geometrical limitations posed by the location of the instrument ports. In some instances at least, it may be more difficult to reapproximate myometrial and serosal tissue, a feature that may enhance the development of adhesions and which may increase the risk of uterine rupture should pregnancy occur. Morcellation of the tissue is now less difficult because of the development of efficient endomechanical morcellators [35] (Class II-3). All of these factors conspire to increase operating time, frequently offsetting the reduction in postoperative direct costs intrinsically associated with laparoscopic surgery.

Minilaparotomy (± laparoscopic assistance)

Frequently, laparoscopically-directed technique is not feasible for a component of the case, such as dissection near the cornua near the oviduct [36]. In such instances, a relatively small suprapubic incision can be enlarged sufficient to complete that portion of the dissection or other component of the procedure, often with externalization of the myoma and/or uterus. This approach can also be used primarily without laparoscopic assistance.

It seems that from a short-term perspective, myomectomy by "minilaparotomy" or laparoscopic myomectomy with minilaparotomy have similar short-term outcomes, including time to discharge, postoperative pain, and return to normal activity, when each are compared to the standard laparotomic approach [37]. Consequently, for clinicians who are not experienced or skilled with laparoscopic myomectomy, minilaparotomy-based approaches may provide patients with many of the benefits of minimal access surgery.

Vaginal myomectomy

There are a number of instances where removal of a leiomyoma can be performed vaginally. The most obvious situation is when a submucosal myoma prolapses through the cervical canal so that it can be removed simply by transecting or avulsing the stalk. This is typically accomplished by grasping the lesion with a tenaculum or ring forceps and twisting it until the lesion separates. Clinically significant bleeding rarely occurs. In many instances the procedure can be performed in the office or procedure room with no or local anesthesia, or, in some instances, systemically administered anxiolysis or anesthesia. There may be value to performing postprocedure transvaginal ultrasound or hysteroscopy to evaluate for the presence of additional lesions in the endometrial cavity.

For submucosal leiomyomas that have not prolapsed through the cervical canal, vaginal myomectomy has also been described following dilation of the cervix with laminaria, which are natural (elm) or synthetic rods that osmotically absorb existing fluid and slowly dilate the canal [38]. The myomas can be removed intact, while morcellation can be used to remove larger lesions.

Another approach is *vaginal hysterotomy*, a technique that I use, where incisions are made in the cervix to facilitate removal [39]. This approach is used for leiomyomas that are present in the lower uterine segment and extending to the cervical canal, a location that is extremely challenging to accomplish resectoscopically. To facilitate the procedure, the urinary bladder is dissected from the cervix in a fashion similar to that used for vaginal hysterectomy. Then, anterior and/or posterior longitudinal incisions are made in the cervix and extended as high as necessary to allow access to the myoma and dissection from the uterus. The incisions are closed with full thickness, continuous, delayed absorbable suture. I usually perform a second-look hysteroscopic procedure three to four weeks later to dissect free adhesions that may occlude the canal. Although successful for bleeding, the impact of this approach on fertility has not been evaluated so patients must be cautioned in this regard.

References

1. Atlee WL. Case of successful extirpation of a fibrous tumor of the peritoneal surface of the uterus by the large peritoneal section. *Am J Med Sci*. 1845;**9**:309–35.

2. Neuwirth RS. A new technique for and additional experience with hysteroscopic resection of submucous fibroids. *Am J Obstet Gynecol*. 1978;**131**(1):91–4.

3. Semm K, Mettler L. Technical progress in pelvic surgery via operative laparoscopy. *Am J Obstet Gynecol*. 1980;**138**(2):121–7.

4. Dubuisson JB, Lecuru F, Foulot H, Mandelbrot L, Aubriot FX, Mouly M. Myomectomy by laparoscopy: a preliminary report of 43 cases. *Fertil Steril*. 1991; **56**(5):827–30.

5. Parker WH, Fu YS, Berek JS. Uterine sarcoma in patients operated on for presumed leiomyoma and rapidly growing leiomyoma. *Obstet Gynecol*. 1994;**83**(3):414–18.

6. Leibsohn S, d'Ablaing G, Mishell DR, Jr., Schlaerth JB. Leiomyosarcoma in a series of hysterectomies performed for presumed uterine leiomyomas. *Am J Obstet Gynecol*. 1990;**162**(4):968–74; discussion 74–6.

7. Stovall TG, Muneyyirci-Delale O, Summitt RL, Jr., Scialli AR. GnRH agonist and iron versus placebo and iron in the anemic patient before surgery for leiomyomas: a randomized controlled trial. Leuprolide Acetate Study Group. *Obstet Gynecol*. 1995;**86**(1):65–71.

8. Fedele L, Vercellini P, Bianchi S, Brioschi D, Dorta M. Treatment with GnRH agonists before myomectomy and the risk of short-term myoma recurrence. *Br J Obstet Gynaecol*. 1990;**97**(5):393–6.

9. Friedman AJ, Daly M, Juneau-Norcross M, Fine C, Rein MS. Recurrence of myomas after myomectomy in women pretreated with leuprolide acetate depot or placebo. *Fertil Steril*. 1992;**58**(1):205–8.

10. Kongnyuy EJ, van den Broek N, Wiysonge CS. A systematic review of randomized controlled trials to reduce hemorrhage during myomectomy for uterine fibroids. *Int J Gynaecol Obstet*. 2008;**100**(1):4–9.

11. Parazzini F, Vercellini P, De Giorgi O, Pesole A, Ricci E, Crosignani PG. Efficacy of preoperative medical treatment in facilitating hysteroscopic endometrial resection, myomectomy and metroplasty: literature review. *Hum Reprod*. 1998; **13**(9):2592–7.

12. Bonney V. *The Technical Minutia of Extended Myomectomy and Ovarian Cystectomy*. London: Cassel; 1946.

13. Emanuel MH, Wamsteker K, Hart AA, Metz G, Lammes FB. Long-term results of hysteroscopic myomectomy for abnormal uterine bleeding. *Obstet Gynecol*. 1999;**93**(5 Pt 1):743–8.

14. Vercellini P, Zaina B, Yaylayan L, Pisacreta A, De Giorgi O, Crosignani PG. Hysteroscopic myomectomy: long-term effects on menstrual pattern and fertility. *Obstet Gynecol*. 1999;**94**(3):341–7.

15. Fernandez H, Sefrioui O, Virelizier C, Gervaise A, Gomel V, Frydman R. Hysteroscopic resection of submucosal myomas in patients with infertility. *Hum Reprod*. 2001;**16**(7):1489–92.

16. Leone FP, Lanzani C, Ferrazzi E. Use of strict sonohysterographic methods for preoperative assessment of submucous myomas. *Fertil Steril*. 2003;**79**(4):998–1002.

17. Propst AM, Liberman RF, Harlow BL, Ginsburg ES. Complications of hysteroscopic surgery: predicting patients at risk. *Obstet Gynecol*. 2000;**96**(4):517–20.

18. Ginsburg ES, Benson CB, Garfield JM, Gleason RE, Friedman AJ. The effect of

operative technique and uterine size on blood loss during myomectomy: a prospective randomized study. *Fertil Steril.* 1993;**60**(6):956–62.

19. DeLancey JO. A modified technique for hemostasis during myomectomy. *Surg Gynecol Obstet.* 1992;**174**(2):153–4.

20. Fletcher H, Frederick J, Hardie M, Simeon D. A randomized comparison of vasopressin and tourniquet as hemostatic agents during myomectomy. *Obstet Gynecol.* 1996;**87**(6):1014–18.

21. Tulandi T, Murray C, Guralnick M. Adhesion formation and reproductive outcome after myomectomy and second-look laparoscopy. *Obstet Gynecol.* 1993;**82**(2):213–15.

22. March CM, Boyers S, Franklin R, Haney AF, Hurst B, Lotze E, et al. Prevention of adhesion formation/reformation with the Gore-Tex Surgical Membrane. *Prog Clin Biol Res.* 1993;**381**:253–9.

23. Mais V, Ajossa S, Piras B, Guerriero S, Marongiu D, Melis GB. Prevention of de-novo adhesion formation after laparoscopic myomectomy: a randomized trial to evaluate the effectiveness of an oxidized regenerated cellulose absorbable barrier. *Hum Reprod.* 1995;**10**(12):3133–5.

24. LaMorte AI, Lalwani S, Diamond MP. Morbidity associated with abdominal myomectomy. *Obstet Gynecol.* 1993;**82**(6):897–900.

25. Nezhat FR, Roemisch M, Nezhat CH. Long-term follow-up of laparoscopic myomectomy. *J Am Assoc Gynecol Laparosc.* 1996;**3**(4 Suppl):S35.

26. Dubuisson JB, Chapron C, Verspyck E, Foulot H, Aubriot FX. [Laparoscopic myomectomy: 102 cases.] *Contracept Fertil Sex.* 1993;**21**(12):920–2.

27. Daniell JF, Kurtz BR, Taylor SN. Laparoscopic myomectomy using the argon beam coagulator. *J Gynecol Surg.* 1993;**9**(4):207–12.

28. Parker WH, Rodi IA. Patient selection for laparoscopic myomectomy. *J Am Assoc Gynecol Laparosc.* 1994;**2**(1):23–6.

29. Hasson HM, Rotman C, Rana N, Sistos F, Dmowski WP. Laparoscopic myomectomy. *Obstet Gynecol.* 1992;**80**(5):884–8.

30. Myers ER, Barber MD, Gustilo-Ashby T, Couchman G, Matchar DB, McCrory DC. Management of uterine leiomyomata: what do we really know? *Obstet Gynecol.* 2002;**100**(1):8–17.

31. Taylor A, Sharma M, Tsirkas P, Di Spiezio Sardo A, Setchell M, Magos A. Reducing blood loss at open myomectomy using triple tourniquets: a randomised controlled trial. *BJOG.* 2005;**112**(3):340–5.

32. Zullo F, Palomba S, Corea D, Pellicano M, Russo T, Falbo A, et al. Bupivacaine plus epinephrine for laparoscopic myomectomy: a randomized placebo-controlled trial. *Obstet Gynecol.* 2004;**104**(2):243–9.

33. Dubuisson JB, Fauconnier A, Deffarges JV, Norgaard C, Kreiker G, Chapron C. Pregnancy outcome and deliveries following laparoscopic myomectomy. *Hum Reprod.* 2000;**15**(4):869–73.

34. Mais V, Ajossa S, Guerriero S, Mascia M, Solla E, Melis GB. Laparoscopic versus abdominal myomectomy: a prospective, randomized trial to evaluate benefits in early outcome. *Am J Obstet Gynecol.* 1996;**174**(2):654–8.

35. Carter JE, McCarus S. Time savings using the Steiner Morcellator in laparoscopic myomectomy. *J Am Assoc Gynecol Laparosc.* 1996;**3**(4 Suppl):S6.

36. Nezhat C, Nezhat F, Bess O, Nezhat CH, Mashiach R. Laparoscopically assisted myomectomy: a report of a new technique in 57 cases. *Int J Fertil Menopausal Stud.* 1994;**39**(1):39–44.

37. Cagnacci A, Pirillo D, Malmusi S, Arangino S, Alessandrini C, Volpe A. Early outcome of myomectomy by laparotomy, minilaparotomy and laparoscopically assisted minilaparotomy. A randomized prospective study. *Hum Reprod.* 2003;**18**(12):2590–4.

38. Goldrath MH. Vaginal removal of the pedunculated submucous myoma: the use of laminaria. *Obstet Gynecol.* 1987;**70**(4):670–2.

39. Goldrath MH. Vaginal removal of the pedunculated submucous myoma. Historical observations and development of a new procedure. *J Reprod Med.* 1990;**35**(10):921–4.

Polypectomy

Chapter summary

- Polypectomy may be performed blindly or under hysteroscopic direction.
- There is evidence that hysteroscopically-directed polypectomy is associated with reduced recurrence.

Introduction

As described in Chapter 5, uterine polyps are localized proliferations of endothelial tissue usually emanating from either the endometrium or the columnar epithelium of the cervix. It is likely that most polyps are asymptomatic, but when they present, symptoms include bleeding (AUB-P), typically IMB, infertility, and, uncommonly, pain. Although there is some controversy regarding the need for removal of asymptomatic endometrial polyps, the rate of malignancy in symptomatic polyps ranges from 0.5 to 4.7% justifying routine excision when AUB is a presenting symptom [1, 2].

Techniques

Removal of exocervical polyps can be achieved using forceps that either excise or twist off the lesion, usually with relative ease. However endometrial and endocervical polyps are best removed under direct visualization using mechanical and/or electrosurgical technique. While blind removal or avulsion techniques can be performed, there is evidence that the recurrence/ persistence rate is up to 15 times higher [3] (Class II-3). A nonrandomized comparative trial demonstrated that it preferable to remove the lesions under direct hysteroscopic visualization with one or a combination of hysteroscopic scissors, biopsy forceps, or an electrosurgical cutting loop. In a case control study, grasping forceps were associated with a 15% incidence of recurrence compared to the other techniques at 0–4% [4] (Class II-2).

Instrumentation

There are a number of techniques for hysteroscopically-directed endometrial or endo-cervical polypectomy. For office procedure rooms, it is generally best to use a system that comprises a hysteroscope and a continuous flow sheath system that includes at least a 5 Fr (1.7 mm diameter) operating channel, in addition to discrete inflow and outflow channels. In an operating room environment, a continuous-flow resectoscope may be used, fitted either with a bridge to allow passage of a 5–7 Fr (2.3 mm) operating instrument, or with the electrosurgical element and loop electrode. The continuous flow system is important to maintain distention and to evacuate blood that may be present in the endometrial cavity.

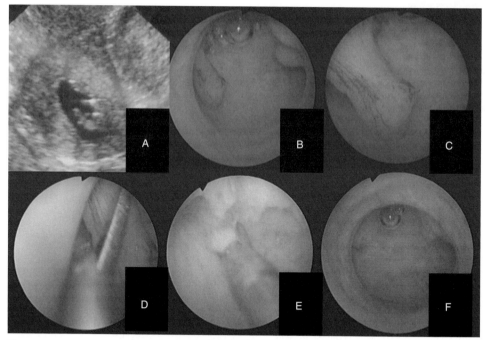

Figure 21.1 Hysteroscopic polypectomy with scissors. The polyp is shown both in a transverse image from a preprocedure saline infusion sonography (A), and hysteroscopically (B); the largest polyp is seen on the right side of the endometrial cavity together with a smaller polyp on the left side. (C) The largest polyp is seen close up as the scissors are brought in via the operating channel (D). Image (E) shows the end of the dissection on the right side while (F) shows the postpolypectomy appearance. The glistening bubble at 12 o'clock is an air bubble in the fluid media. This procedure was performed in the office setting under local anesthesia.

Currently, such operating systems are 5.0–5.5 mm in maximum diameter while resectoscopes are about 7–9 mm in outside diameter.

The endoscope-light source system should be one that provides enough illumination to allow precise identification of the lesion in its entirety. My preference is for a 12–15° foreoblique lens, a selection that affords the best combination of near and far vision. In some instances, such as cornual polyps, a 25–30° lens may have value. Fluid-distending media should be used preferentially to gas media; risks of gas emboli are greater when transecting lesions from within the endometrial cavity [5]. The type of media used is dictated by the use of radiofrequency (RF) electricity and the type of electrosurgical instrumentation used. Bipolar RF instruments will require that isotonic media like normal saline be used, while unipolar RF instruments will mandate a nonelectrolyte-containing solution such as dextrose in water, 1.5% sorbital, 3% glycine, or mannitol.

There are a number of instruments that can be used to transect and remove the polyp. Simple mechanical scissors are generally very effective; hooked or flat at the discretion of the surgeon (Figure 21.1). Unipolar or bipolar RF electrodes can be used to transect the base as well, although there is some evidence that these are no more effective or efficient than scissors (Figure 21.2). We have found that electrosurgical polyp snares are particularly useful for long polyps, especially those attached at the fundus where it is sometimes difficult to direct scissors or an electrode (Figure 21.3).

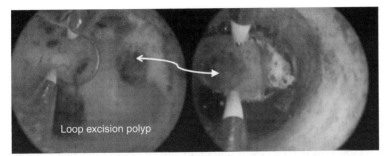

Figure 21.2 Resectoscopic loop electrosurgical polypectomy. The photograph on the left shows the polyp on the left side of the endometrial cavity as well as the loop electrode extended. The photograph on the right shows the polyp after removal with the loop electrode. This procedure was performed in a standard operating room.

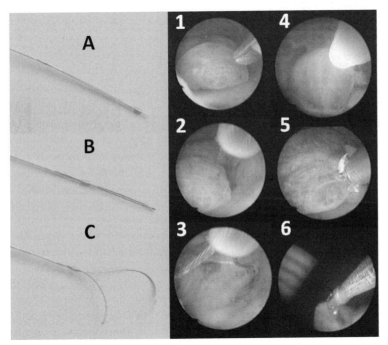

Figure 21.3 Endometrial polypectomy with an electrosurgical snare. The left panel displays the 5 Fr diameter snare: (A) the 5-Fr catheter with the undeployed snare; (B) the loop extruded but not opened; (C) the fully deployed snare. The electrode is connected to a radiofrequency electrosurgical generator. The photographic series in the right panel demonstrates the snare polypectomy. (1) The polyp is demonstrated. (2) The snare catheter is brought in the vicinity of the polyp and deployment is started with the configuration similar to that in (B). (3) The snare, now deployed as in (C), is being positioned around the base of the polyp, and in (4) the electrosurgical generator is being activated to transect the polyp at the base. (5) A cup biopsy forceps is used to grasp the polyp allowing it to be withdrawn from the endometrial cavity (6). This procedure was performed under local anesthetic in the office setting.

Patient preparation

No endometrial preparation is mandatory, but in premenopausal women, a thin endometrium will allow for more precise identification of the polyps, especially small ones, and, there will be less blood and debris to obscure the operative field. Of course, this is not generally an issue with postmenopausal women, or those who have been on GnRHa therapy for at least four weeks. Consequently, in premenopausal women, it is preferable to institute a course of progestin-based therapy for at least four weeks using a continuous combination oral or transvaginal contraceptive, or an oral progestin such as MPA 20 mg twice daily. If prepolypectomy medical preparation is not practicable, then the polyp resection should be performed early in the follicular phase, just after menses, when the endometrium is still thin.

Cervical preparation may be useful for vaginally nulliparous women or for those who are suspected or known to have cervical stenosis. A number of regimens employing oral or vaginal misoprostol have been reported in the context of high quality clinical trials [6, 7] (Class I-2). Mechanical preparation with laminaria is also an option, but this does not usually deal with the problem of cervical stenosis, and is perhaps more useful if one anticipates the use of a large-diameter instrument. In our experience, laminaria provide only occasional value.

Anesthesia

Anesthesia for hysteroscopy is discussed in (Chapter 14).

Procedure

Positioning of a hysteroscope or resectoscope in the endocervical canal or endometrial cavity is described in Chapter 23 (Video 23.4). It is important to evaluate the entire cavity and endometrial canal. Occasionally, flat polyps can be compressed against the endometrium in a cornual area or at the fundus making it important to evaluate these areas closely.

If scissors are used, they should be navigated to the base of the lesion and used to transect the polyp as closely as possible to the endometrial surface. Cutting obliquely increases the work, and possibly increases the amount of bleeding encountered. Once the polyp is transected, the scissors can be replaced with grasping or biopsy forceps of similar diameter and the lesion grasped and removed under direct vision, simultaneously removing the hysteroscope and sheath.

The technique used with RF electrodes depends in part on the electrode design, and, in part, on the characteristics of the polyps. Should a loop electrode be employed, in conjunction with a resectoscope, the loop can be used to "scoop" out the base of the polyp (Video 21.3). The polyp snare, described above, that is useful for long polyps, is opened once it is positioned in the endometrial cavity, allowing capture of the polyp (Video 21.xx). Then the introducer is navigated so that the base of the loop is as close as possible to the base of the polyp. This instrument is best attached to an RF electrosurgical generator which is activated as the loop is tightened, thereby transecting the polyp at the base. A needle or other linear cutting electrode is simply directed to the base of the polyp where it is activated to transect the lesion.

For any of the techniques described above, and following removal of the lesion, it is advisable to reposition the endoscope in the endometrial cavity and to use scissors or an electrode to remove any visible base of the lesion. For some large polyps it may be necessary to morcellate the lesion or to take it off in sequential steps. Furthermore, the lesion may be too large to remove through the cervix because of inadequate dilation. In such instances, the hysteroscope should be removed, and the cervical canal dilated to the degree necessary to retrieve the polyp. Such overdilation may make it necessary to use additional clamps or

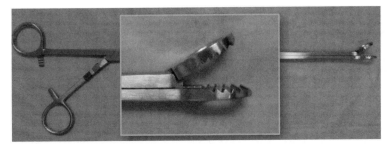

Figure 21.4 Corson biopsy forceps. Useful instruments for grasping and removing large polyps and myomas from the endometrial cavity. Unlike standard polyp forceps, these forceps are distally articulated and the tooth design (inset) facilitates tenacious grasping of the lesion.

tenaculi on the cervix to allow the creation of an adequate seal to allow cavity distention. Another useful technique is to use a polyp forceps, or, preferably a Corson myomectomy forceps to grasp and remove the polyp blindly (Figure 21.4). The distal articulation of the Corson forceps makes it particularly useful in this situation.

With multiple polyps, visualization may be compromised as blood and debris from the dissection cloud the field, particularly in the office situation. In such instances, it may be necessary to complete the procedure in a separate session.

References

1. Anastasiadis PG, Koutlaki NG, Skaphida PG, Galazios GC, Tsikouras PN, Liberis VA. Endometrial polyps: prevalence, detection, and malignant potential in women with abnormal uterine bleeding. *Eur J Gynaecol Oncol.* 2000;**21**(2):180–3.

2. Shushan A, Revel A, Rojansky N. How often are endometrial polyps malignant? *Gynecol Obstet Invest.* 2004;**58**(4):212–15.

3. Liberis V, Dafopoulos K, Tsikouras P, Galazios G, Koutlaki N, Anastasiadis P, Maroulis G. Removal of endometrial polyps by use of grasping forceps and curettage after diagnostic hysteroscopy. *Clin Exp Obstet Gynecol.* 2003;**30**(1):29–31.

4. Preutthipan S, Herabutya Y. Hysteroscopic polypectomy in 240 premenopausal and postmenopausal women. *Fertil Steril.* 2005;**83**(3):705–9.

5. Groenman FA, Peters LW, Rademaker BM, Bakkum EA. Embolism of air and gas in hysteroscopic procedures: pathophysiology and implication for daily practice. *J Minim Invasive Gynecol.* 2008;**15**(2):241–7.

6. Preutthipan S, Herabutya Y. Vaginal misoprostol for cervical priming before operative hysteroscopy: a randomized controlled trial. *Obstet Gynecol.* 2000; **96**(6):890–4.

7. Thomas JA, Leyland N, Durand N, Windrim RC. The use of oral misoprostol as a cervical ripening agent in operative hysteroscopy: a double-blind, placebo-controlled trial. *Am J Obstet Gynecol.* 2002;**186**(5):876–9.

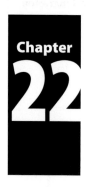

Chapter 22

Uterine artery embolization or occlusion

Chapter summary

- Uterine artery embolization is radiographically-directed occlusion of the uterine arteries using particles such as microspheres.
- Uterine artery occlusion refers to occlusion of the uterine arteries extraluminally under laparoscopic or laparotomic direction, or intraluminal occlusion performed by radiographic catheter-based techniques.
- Both techniques been demonstrated effective in the treatment of bulk symptoms and bleeding associated with uterine leiomyomas.

Introduction

In the mid 1990s Ravina et al., from France, described the use of an interventional radiology technique to perform bilateral uterine artery embolization with polyvinyl alcohol (PVA) microspheres positioned by a catheter passed through the right femoral artery [1]. Initially used as a method for reducing blood loss at myomectomy, it soon became apparent that the procedure resulted in substantial reduction in the volume of AUB-L, pressure symptoms, and the size of the leiomyomas.

Uterine artery embolization

Uterine artery embolization (UAE) is performed under conscious sedation in an interventional radiology suite with fluoroscopic guidance (Figure 22.1) (Video 22.1). The embolic agent is generally either PVA microspheres or gelatin-coated trisacryl spheres, which are supplied in diameters that typically range from 300 to 500 μm, but can range from 150 to 700 μm depending upon the technique of the radiologist.

The right femoral artery is usually selected, catheterized, and a narrow caliber catheter with guidewire passed retrograde up the right external iliac and common iliac arteries, then over the bifurcation and down the left common and internal iliac arteries to the uterine vessel. There, the embolic agent is injected until there is no uterine artery blood flow. Then, the catheter is withdrawn back into the right common iliac artery where it is directed to the right internal iliac artery and then positioned in the right uterine artery, where the same particles are injected until there is cessation in right uterine artery flow. The total treatment time typically ranges from 30 to 60 minutes.

Immediate post-procedure pain is generally substantial, requiring institutional admission at least overnight, typically with a requirement for narcotic analgesia. In about 20–35% of patients, a delayed response may occur in 1–5 days characterized by fever, nausea, vomiting, and general malaise, a constellation of symptoms that has been termed

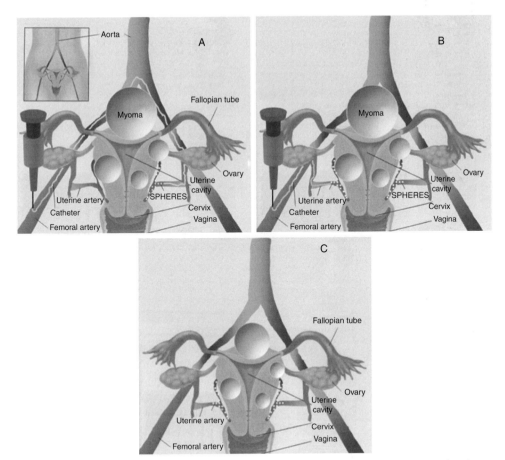

Figure 22.1 Stylized depiction of uterine artery embolization. (A) The right femoral artery is accessed and a catheter is advanced under fluoroscopic control to the left uterine artery where the microspheres or other embolic agents are deposited until there is no uterine artery flow. (B) Then the catheter is withdrawn to the right side where the right uterine artery is cannulated and microspheres injected until the cessation of uterine artery flow. The catheter is removed, the femoral artery compressed and bandaged, and the patient sent to the recovery area. (C) Abnormal uterine bleeding/heavy menstrual bleeding seems to stop immediately, but it takes several months to achieve the typical 50% volume reduction of the uterus and myomas.

post-embolization syndrome. Complications are relatively infrequent but include, in addition to the post-embolization syndrome, misembolization of tissues that include the ovary, ureter, and other structures, and infection which has been associated with severe sepsis and, rarely, death. In about 10% of cases, collateral circulation, most often from the ovarian arteries, may provide substantial supply to the uterine fundus, a feature that may be a reason for ultimate failure of the procedure [2].

The indications for the procedure are discussed in Chapter 9, but there are a number of situations where it may be advisable to delay therapy or choose another approach. First of all, the procedure should not be performed with a current pregnancy or in the face of active or recent pelvic infection. Pedunculated submucosal leiomyomas should generally be removed using resectoscopic technique, but, if UAE is performed when such lesions are present, patients should be counseled that there may be a delayed and painful process of

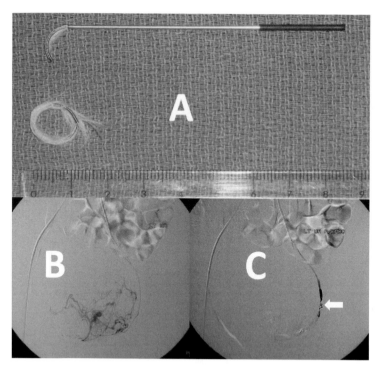

Figure 22.2 Intravascular "micro" coils. (A) These elongated coils are permanent (steel and platinum) but result in localized occlusion of a vessel rather than embolic occlusion distant to the site of deposition. (B) A perfused uterus before occlusion. (C) The post-occluded appearance.

"delivery" of the myoma at a time remote from the embolic procedure [3, 4]. In some instances this process may require surgical dilation of the cervix to facilitate expulsion. Patients should be also counseled that myomas larger than 8–9 cm are associated with a higher risk of UAE failure [3, 4].

Uterine artery occlusion

Localized uterine artery occlusion (UAO) using laparoscopically-directed techniques has also been described. The uterine vessels are occluded with electrodessication or clips without the need for embolization (Figure 22.2). A number of series have been published with results similar to those available for UAE [5] (Class II-2) [6] (Class III). A prospective comparative trial has demonstrated that clinical results may be similar and that patients undergoing UAO seem to experience much less pain than the patients who are treated with embolization [7] (Class II-1).

Another way to perform local occlusion of the uterine arteries is using a transcatheter technique with "coils" instead of microspheres (Figure 22.3). A pilot RCT, done in our center, compared transcatheter UAE to UAO and demonstrated that there was much less pain associated with focal occlusion of the vessels with the coils [8]. However, comparative studies comparing long-term clinical results with the two techniques are not yet available.

References

1. Ravina JH, Merland JJ, Ciraru-Vigneron N, Bouret JM, Herbreteau D, Houdart E, et al. [Arterial embolization: a new treatment of menorrhagia in uterine fibroma.] *Presse Med.* 1995;**24**(37):1754.

2. Razavi MK, Wolanske KA, Hwang GL, Sze DY, Kee ST, Dake MD. Angiographic classification of ovarian artery-to-uterine artery anastomoses: initial observations in uterine fibroid embolization. *Radiology.* 2002;**224**(3):707–12.

3. Mehta H, Sandhu C, Matson M, Belli AM. Review of readmissions due to complications from uterine fibroid embolization. *Clin Radiol.* 2002;**57**(12):1122–4.

4. Spies JB, Roth AR, Jha RC, Gomez-Jorge J, Levy EB, Chang TC, et al. Leiomyomata treated with uterine artery embolization: factors associated with successful symptom and imaging outcome. *Radiology.* 2002;**222**(1):45–52.

5. Liu WM, Ng HT, Wu YC, Yen YK, Yuan CC. Laparoscopic bipolar coagulation of uterine vessels: a new method for treating symptomatic fibroids. *Fertil Steril.* 2001;**75**(2):417–22.

6. Lichtinger M, Hallson L, Calvo P, Adeboyejo G. Laparoscopic uterine artery occlusion for symptomatic leiomyomas. *J Am Assoc Gynecol Laparosc.* 2002;**9**(2):191–8.

7. Hald K, Langebrekke A, Klow NE, Noreng HJ, Berge AB, Istre O. Laparoscopic occlusion of uterine vessels for the treatment of symptomatic fibroids: Initial experience and comparison to uterine artery embolization. *Am J Obstet Gynecol.* 2004;**190**(1):37–43.

8. Cunningham E, Barreda L, Ngo M, Terasaki K, Munro MG. Uterine artery embolization versus occlusion for uterine leiomyomas: a pilot randomized clinical trial. *J Minim Invasive Gynecol.* 2008;**15**(3):301–7.

23 Uterine imaging

Chapter review

- Uterine imaging refers to visualization of the uterus using ultrasound, radiologic, magnetic resonance imaging (MRI), or endoscopic (hysteroscopic) techniques.
- Transvaginal ultrasound (TVS) is effective at identification of women with post-menopausal bleeding at low risk for hyperplasia or malignancy.
- Saline infusion sonography (SIS) is as effective as hysteroscopy at detecting intrauterine lesions such as polyps and leiomyomas, but is less effective at identifying lesions in the endocervical canal.
- Hysteroscopy can be used to evaluate the endometrial cavity and can be used to direct simultaneous removal of targeted lesions such as polyps.
- Magnetic resonance imaging may be especially useful in women or children who are virginal, and in the differentiation of leiomyomas from adenomyomas.
- Ultrasound may be almost effective as MRI at diagnosing diffuse adenomyosis.

Introduction

Accurate structural evaluation of the endometrial cavity and the myometrium requires imaging by one or a combination of ultrasonography, MRI, and direct inspection with hysteroscopy.

Transvaginal ultrasound

Transvaginal sonography (TVS) is generally performed using a transducer with a frequency of 5.0–7.5 megahertz (MHz) passed into the vagina to the level of the cervix (Figure 23.1). The proximity of the transducer to the target organs and tissue allows for the acquisition of images with much greater resolution than those generally seen with abdominal ultrasound. Transvaginal ultrasound can be performed without anesthesia very comfortably in the clinician's office or in a sonology or radiology suite [1].

Ultrasound for imaging

The term "ultrasound" refers to all acoustic energy that has a frequency above 20 KHz, the upper limit perceived by the human ear. The ultrasound "probe" is actually a handheld instrument containing an array of piezoelectric transducers that convert electrical pulses from the base unit into ultrasonic waves at the desired frequency. These waves travel through the underlying structures and then, to a variable degree, are reflected back to the transducer. At this point, the piezoelectric transducer functions in reverse – the reflected ultrasonic wave is converted into a mechanical vibration that, in turn, is transformed into

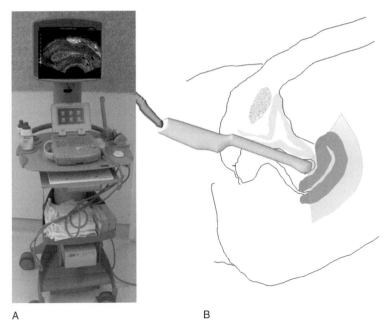

A   B

Figure 23.1 (A) Portable ultrasound unit. (B) With the bladder emptied, the vaginal transducer is positioned in the anterior fornix of the vagina oriented in the sagittal plane imaging almost the entire length of the uterus. The field of view is shaded and the image obtained displayed on the ultrasound unit's monitor. Note that with this anterverted and anteflexed uterus, the anterior wall is oriented closest to the transducer.

an electrical pulse that travels to the base unit where it contributes to the formation of an image.

The image is created considering the strength of the echo (if one is received) and the amount of time taken from transmission to receipt. This first calculation allows for determination of the location of the pixel on the screen as a function of the distance from the transducer head. The second calculation measures the strength of the echo that determines the proportion of the original wave reflected back to the transducer. Calcified areas reflect nearly all of the transmitted waves allowing the machine to light a bright white pixel in accordance with their "hyperechoic" or "echodense" composition. Dark areas depict an absence or near absence of received waves, and are therefore called "hypoechoic" or "sono-lucent," and are typical for clear, fluid-filled structures. Tissues with intermediate echodensity manifest in a spectrum of image intensity that ranges from dark to white and are called "grayscale" images, depicting the ability of contemporary ultrasound to display a range of image densities depending upon the reflectance of the target tissue.

The depth and resolving ability of diagnostic ultrasound is in large part a function of the frequency of the transducer. Typical diagnostic ultrasound operates in a frequency range of 2–18 MHz; lower frequencies are capable of imaging deeper structures, but they do so at the expense of reduced resolution.

Doppler sonography employs the Doppler effect or, more commonly, pulsed waves to determine if blood is moving towards or away from the transducers, and can estimate the velocity of the blood flow. Such information is displayed on the screen using a spectrum of colors that depict the intensity and velocity of blood flow in the targeted area. This functionality can allow determination of the presence or absence of blood flow, for example, in a tumor, and is especially useful in uterine imaging for the identification of arteriovenous malformations.

Multiple, parallel, or simultaneous two dimensional (2-D) ultrasound images can be captured in a structured format and reassembled into a three-dimensional (3-D) image [2]. The "structured format" may involve manual capture or, more accurately, an automated process. The image can be displayed 3-D in a fashion that is very similar to MRI. In addition, saline infusion can be performed to provide contrast for evaluation of the endometrial cavity. Three-dimensional imaging has a number of potentially useful advantages over 2-D techniques, particularly the ability to create a coronal plane, not possible with standard transvaginal sonography. Currently, the utility of 3-D ultrasound is undergoing evaluation.

Performing TVS and SIS

Transvaginal ultrasound

The evaluation is best performed with an empty bladder, unlike the situation for abdominal scanning where the full bladder is necessary to provide an ultrasound "window" (Video 23.1). A full bladder may push the anteverted and anteflexed uterus posteriorly, compromising optimal evaluation. The vaginal transducer is covered by a condom-like sheath that contains, at its distal tip, the water-based gel used for coupling with the vaginal epithelium. Following insertion of the transducer into the vagina, and identification of the uterus, images are generally obtained in the sagittal and transverse planes and other orientations as feasible and appropriate to evaluate the cervix, the myometrium, and the entire endometrium.

Saline infusion sonography

Saline infusion sonography is the sonographic (usually transvaginal) evaluation of the endometrial cavity following the transcervical instillation of saline [3], an approach with a diagnostic accuracy for the endometrial cavity that is comparable to hysteroscopy [4, 5] (Figure 23.2) (Video 23.2, 23.3). Saline infusion sonography should not be performed during menses, for blood, clot, and debris confounds evaluation, and, while it can be performed at any other time in the cycle, it is best done in the early follicular phase, following the cessation of bleeding. Saline infusion sonography is best interpreted by the examiner evaluating the "real-time" dynamic images.

The patient is asked to empty her bladder for the same reasons elucidated above for TVS. She is placed in the modified dorsal lithotomy position, and an open-sided vaginal speculum is used to expose the cervix, which is cleansed with an antiseptic solution. Then a narrow-caliber insemination, infant feeding tube, or specialized SIS catheter is attached to a syringe containing 20–30 mL of contrast fluid, usually normal saline, and flushed to extrude air.[1] The catheter is then introduced into the cervical canal and passed into the endometrial cavity. In some instances, difficulty will be encountered entering the endometrial cavity, a situation that can usually be overcome by injecting a small amount of anesthetic, placing a tenaculum on the anterior cervix and applying gentle traction. If this is not effective, the use of a narrow flexible or rigid dilator may be necessary.

---

[1]   Any sterile low viscosity fluid may be used, including 5% dextrose in water, Ringer's lactate, 3% sorbitol, 1.5% glycine, or 5% mannitol.

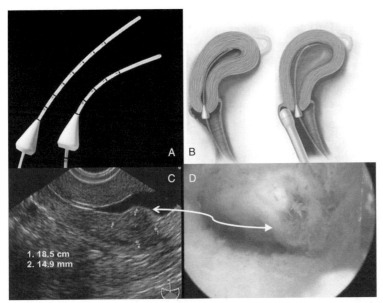

Figure 23.2 Saline infusion sonography, also known as sonohysterography. (A) Goldstein catheters. The adjustable conical stopper minimizes egress of fluid with a patulous cervix. (B) Catheter after being positioned with the tip in the endometrial cavity, left, with the ultrasound transducer placed in the appropriate vaginal fornix. (C) and (D) Saline infusion sonography demonstrating a type 2 leiomyoma (C) and the appearance under hysteroscopic imaging (D).

Once the catheter is positioned, the speculum, and, if it has been used, the tenaculum, are removed and the vaginal transducer placed in the vagina to identify the endometrial echo complex as for TVS (see above). Once a sagittal view has been obtained, fluid is gently injected at a rate sufficient to distend the endometrial cavity and allow a contrast-enhanced evaluation.

A systematic approach to evaluation is essential. The transducer is moved horizontally, keeping the uterus in a sagittal plane, scanning from cornua to cornua evaluating the entire endometrial cavity in the sagittal plane. Then, with rotation of the transducer by 90°, transverse "cuts" can be obtained from the internal cervical os to the fundus, thereby completing the assessment in a way that allows the examiner to mentally assemble a 3-D image.

Generally the process is relatively painless and the imaging can be performed quickly and accurately. In some instances, patients experience pain, a circumstance that may be overcome by instilling a 1% or 2% lidocaine solution first and leaving sufficient time for the anesthetic effect to take hold [6].

In vaginally parous patients, insemination catheters or feeding tubes may be insufficient to provide a seal against the surrounding cervical epithelium, and there is enough vaginal spill of saline to prevent separation of the endometrial surfaces adequate to allow satisfactory examination. In such instances a specialized catheter that has an integrated stopper or balloon may be used successfully to occlude the cervical canal.

Normal appearance of the endometrium

The endometrial echo complex (EEC) is, by definition, the sonographic representation of the two juxtaposed layers of the endometrium. Ideally, three echogenic lines are seen; one at the endomyometrial junction on each side, and another representing the interface between the two endometrial layers. Thickness of the EEC is determined by measuring the length of a line drawn in a perpendicular fashion between the myometrial-endometrial junction on one side to that on the opposite side (Figure 23.3). When fluid is present in the endometrial cavity, the EEC is determined by summing the thickness of the two endometrial echoes, ignoring the contribution of the fluid (Figure 23.4).

The normal appearance (echogenicity and thickness) of the EEC varies with exposure to gonadal steroids, being relatively *hypo*echoic in the follicular phase when under the influence of unopposed estradiol, changing to a relatively *hyper*echoic pattern when progesterone is added in the luteal phase following ovulation. The double layer thickness

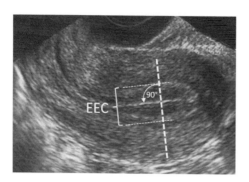

Figure 23.3 Endometrial echo complex (EEC). In this image of a late follicular phase endometrium, measurement of the EEC is demonstrated as the combined thickness of the two adjacent endometrial linings as measured by the distance between the echodense white lines of the opposing endomyometrial junctions.

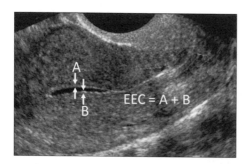

Figure 23.4 Transvaginal ultrasound showing the endometrial echo complex in a patient with endometrial fluid. In this instance, the thickness is calculated as the sum of the two endometrial echos, not the distance between the two opposing endomyometrial junctions.

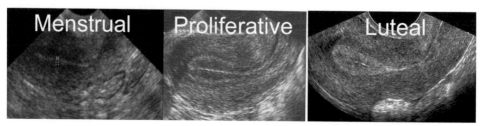

Figure 23.5 Cycle-related changes in the endometrial echo complex (EEC) appearance. On the left is the relatively thin echodense EEC of the menstrual phase; in the center, the thicker sonolucent endometrium of the estradiol-dominated late follicular phase; while on the right is the still thick but relatively echodense EEC that reflects progesterone exposure in the mid to late luteal phase.

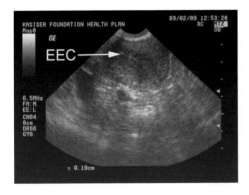

Figure 23.6 Normal postmenopausal endometrium. In this case the endometrial echo complex (EEC) measures 1.9 mm. To be normal, the EEC should be homogeneous and less than or equal to 5 mm thick.

of the EEC of ovulatory women ranges from a few millimeters in the early follicular phase to as much as 12 mm in the luteal phase (Figure 23.5). When there is little or no estrogen exposure, such as for postmenopausal women not on gonadal steroid replacement therapy, the normal endometrium appears as a thin hyperechoic line 5 mm or less in thickness (Figure 23.6). For women using HRT, the EEC appearance and thickness will depend on a number of factors including estrogen dose, the type, dose, and scheduling of progestins, and, in the case of cyclic progestins, the time in the replacement cycle. In all instances, the thickness of the EEC should be consistent throughout the endometrium, a feature that demands careful scanning in both the sagittal and transverse planes.

Using TVS and/or SIS to evaluate the endometrium and endometrial cavity

In the nonpregnant, reproductive-aged woman with AUB, a normal EEC in combination with an absence of leiomyomas near to the endometrial "stripe" is usually associated with a negative hysteroscopic examination [7]. Normal includes all of the following: an echodense line in the middle of the uterus with a homogeneous endometrium and a distinct endometrial myometrial interface. Any of the following: deformation of the lining, the absence of the central echodense line, variable echodensity, and the presence of any structure with or without well-defined margins exclude the diagnosis of "normal." Using these criteria, a normal TVS should predict a normal hysteroscopic examination in about 97% of cases [7].

Endometrial polyps

Endometrial polyps have a variable appearance on TVS, but can elude TVS detection as they can be present with a normal EEC thickness of 5 mm [8, 9]. When visible on TVS, they typically manifest as either hyper- or hypoechoic areas located in the middle of the EEC (Figure 23.7). They are best seen early in the follicular phase when the normal endometrium is the thinnest. Large, long polyps may be difficult to distinguish from a thickened endometrium.

Saline infusion sonography generally can easily distinguish between thickened endometrium and the presence of a polyp (Figure 23.2). The technique also allows the examiner to distinguish polyps that are attached to the endometrium by a narrow stalk or pedicle from sessile lesions that attach to the endometrium over a larger area.

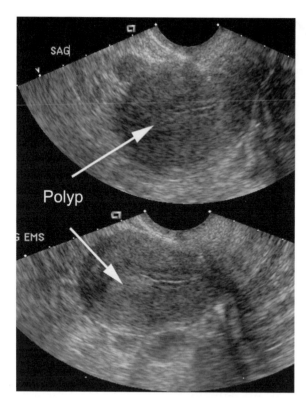

Figure 23.7 Endometrial polyp. This endometrial polyp can be seen on simple transvaginal ultrasound in the mid follicular phase. Note that in the top image the otherwise normal proliferative endometrium is interrupted adjacent to the fundus while on the bottom image the hyperechoic lesion can be seen. The polyp was attached to the fundus on the right side and measured about 2 cm in length.

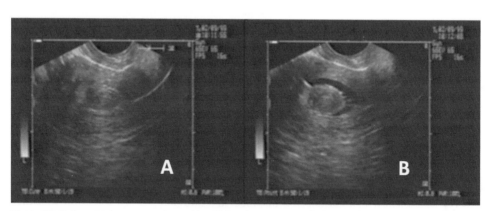

Figure 23.8 Type 1 leiomyoma as imaged by (A) baseline transvaginal ultrasound and (B) saline infusion sonography.

Leiomyomas (myomas, fibroids)

Leiomyomas are usually detectable on TVS but vary in appearance, having calcified, hypoechoic, echogenic or isoechoic, and mixed echogenic patterns. Degenerating fibroids often appear cystic. The relationship of myomas to the endometrium is less readily determined because they often attenuate the sound beam and have ill-defined borders [10]. Saline infusion sonography provides an increased degree of accuracy for the identification of submucosal leiomyomas and should be performed liberally when it is necessary to confirm this relationship, particularly when TVS is equivocal [9] (Figure 23.8).

Saline infusion sonography generally allows myomas to be easily and accurately classified by location, size, and degree of intramural extension. Further, they can be evaluated for resectability in a way not feasible by hysteroscopy, because of the ability to determine the depth of myometrial involvement (Video 20.3). Only pedunculated submucosal fibroids can be fully assessed with hysteroscopy. However, SIS imaging may be compromised in the presence of a myometrial wall laden with leiomyomatous tissue, for the mass effect may inhibit the ability to distend the endometrial cavity sufficient to adequately classify the myomas. In such instances, subsequent evaluation with hysteroscopy or MRI imaging may be necessary.

Ultrasound for the myometrium

The myometrium is assessed to determine the presence of leiomyomas, the extent of submucous myoma involvement, to identify adenomyosis, or to distinguish between leiomyomas and adenomyomas [11]. Ultrasound has been demonstrated useful for the evaluation of myomas in the myometrium, although variations in echogenicity can, in some instances, reduce the sensitivity of the examination (Figures 23.9 and 23.10).

Transvaginal ultrasound is relatively effective in diagnosing adenomyosis if real-time imaging is used and if the uterus is small enough to be evaluable by the transvaginal technique. The findings are related to a combination of the amount and location of endometrial glands and stroma in the myometrium and the associated myometrial hypertrophy and hyperplasia (Figure 23.11). From an overall perspective, adenomyosis commonly manifests with diffuse thickening of the myometrium and/or localized thickening, most often in the posterior myometrial wall. More specific sonographic findings in adenomyosis include myometrial heterogeneity, increased echogenicity, decreased echogenicity, and anechoic lacunae or myometrial cysts. Adenomyotic tissue extending into the inner myometrium can give the appearance of echogenic linear striations and, when these striations are small or indistinct, there may be the appearance of

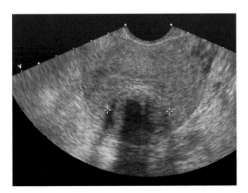

Figure 23.9 Types 3–5 leiomyoma. This relatively sonolucent 3.5 cm diameter leiomyoma can be well seen in the posterior myometrium of this patient. She presented with irregular and heavy menstrual bleeding unrelated to this leiomyoma.

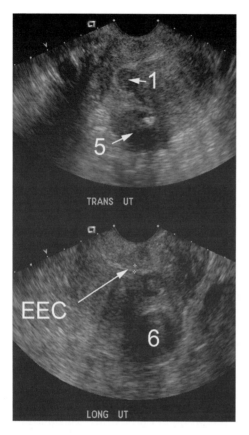

Figure 23.10 Transvaginal ultrasound in a patient with relatively sonolucent leiomyomas. In the transverse view (top) a type 1 leiomyoma is seen deflecting the endometrial echo complex and a type 5 myoma is seen subserosally. In the longitudinal image (bottom) a type 6 (subserosal) myoma can be seen emanating from the posterior myometrial wall. If the leiomyomas have an echodensity similar to that of the myometrium, they are much less readily seen.

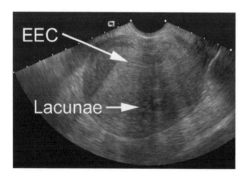

Figure 23.11 Adenomyosis. This transvaginal sonogram demonstrates heterogeneity and disproportionate thickening of the posterior myometrium. Some tiny anechoic lacunae can be seen posteriorly, and the striations are visible, appearing to radiate from the endometrium into the myometrium. There is a relatively indistinct endomyometrial junction. Compare this with the pathological images of Figure 5.2.

widening of the endomyometrial junction. Typically, but not always, three or more of these findings should be present to diagnose adenomyosis [12].

The presence of myometrial cysts within a poorly defined area with abnormal echotexture is highly specific for adenomyosis [13, 14]. Distinguishing focal adenomyosis from leiomyomas can be difficult using TVS, but one distinguishing feature is the blood vessels which course around the myoma but retain their normal vertical course with adenomyosis, a feature that is best be seen using Doppler imaging [15].

Diagnostic hysteroscopy

Hysteroscopy is the evaluation of the endometrial cavity and cervical canal using an endoscope. The ability of diagnostic hysteroscopy to provide information not predictably obtainable by blind endometrial sampling has been adequately documented [16]. For women with AUB, the goal of evaluation of the uterine cavity is either to obtain a sample of the endometrium, usually for the detection of hyperplasia or neoplasia, or to identify structural abnormalities such as polyps and myomas. In many instances, polyps can be removed at the same session with scissors or using one or a combination of a variety of transection techniques [17].

For most patients, diagnostic hysteroscopy can be performed in an office- or clinic-based procedure room with minimal discomfort and at a much lower cost than in an operating room. For some, concerns about patient comfort or a preexisting medical condition may preclude office hysteroscopy.

Prior to the procedure

Visualization of the endometrial cavity can be compromised with active bleeding, or even in the presence of thick proliferative or secretory endometrium. Consequently, the success, duration, and even comfort of the procedure are enhanced if hysteroscopy is performed in the early proliferative phase of the cycle, if it can be identified, or if endometrial suppressive or "thinning" agents are used for a sufficient time prior to the procedure (Table 23.1 [18]). I generally use medical suppression to increase the chance of procedural success and comfort and to facilitate scheduling – matching menstrual cycle time to bookable procedure-room hours is a difficult task.

If a stenotic cervix is anticipated, there is value in the use of preprocedure techniques to facilitate or initiate cervical dilation. One approach is the use of a laminaria tent, inserted in the cervix three to eight hours before the procedure. However, if laminaria are left in place too long (e.g., longer than 24 hours), the cervix may overdilate, which is particularly counterproductive for CO_2 insufflation. A second approach, and one that I prefer, is the use of oral or vaginal prostaglandin E_1 (misoprostol) to ripen the cervix 12–24 hours prior to the procedure (400 µg orally or 200 µg vaginally) [19, 20]. Some data suggest a benefit to the use of COX inhibitors, such as 800 mg of ibuprofen, at least an hour prior to the procedure, to reduce the severity of post-procedure pain [21] (Class I-2).

Part of the patient preparation and the process of informed consent for any procedure is discussion of the inherent risks. In the case of diagnostic hysteroscopy, the risks are relatively low but include those related to anesthesia, perforation, bleeding, and the distention media. The patient should also be informed about post-procedure expectations. She should anticipate slight vaginal bleeding and occasionally, lower abdominal cramps. If CO_2 is used as the distending media, severe cramps, dyspnea, and upper abdominal and right shoulder pain can develop if CO_2 passes into the peritoneal cavity. Regardless, the patient should be advised to have a friend or relative available to accompany her home.

Equipment and technique

The surgeon must be knowledgeable about the equipment, its mechanisms, and the technical specifications that collectively facilitate efficiency, optimal clinical outcome, and a decreased probability of complications. A typical hysteroscopy setup for diagnostic and minor operative procedures is shown in Figures 23.12 and 23.13 and in Video 23.4. Core competencies required for hysteroscopy are as follows:

Table 23.1 Visualization at both diagnostic and operative hysteroscopy is facilitated by suppressing the endometrium. Any of the below approaches will result in a thinned endometrium; those that are progestin-based are generally acceptable at 4 weeks but are not optimal until about 2 months.

Agent type	Drug	Dose	Duration
Androgen	Danazol[a]	200 mg orally three times daily	28–42 days
GnRHa	Leuprolide acetate	3.75 mg IM × 1	28–35 days
Progestin	MPA	10–20 mg orally twice daily	28+ days
Combination estrogen and progestin contraceptives	E.g., EE and NET	EE 35 µg and NET 1 mg orally once daily	28+ days
Antiprogestin, antiestrogen, and antiandrogen	Gestrinone[a]	2.5 mg orally twice weekly	28–35 days

[a] Triolo et al. [18] (Class 1–2)
EE, ethinyl estradiol; GnRHa, gonadotropin releasing hormone agonists; IM, intramuscularly; MPA, medroxyprogesterone acetate; NET, norethindrone.

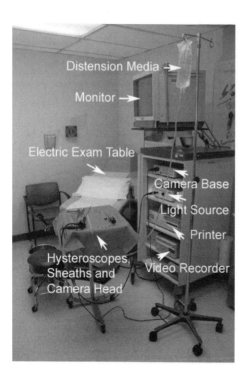

Figure 23.12 Office hysteroscopy setup. Basic components include an electrical examination table with "stirrups"; a "Tower" that includes light source, the camera base, a printer, and video recorder; and a tray comprising of hysteroscopic instrumentation and the camera head.

1. Patient positioning and cervical exposure
2. Anesthesia
3. Cervical dilation
4. Uterine distention
5. Imaging
6. Intrauterine manipulation.

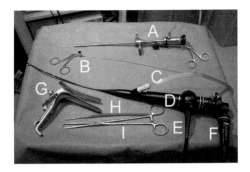

Figure 23.13 Office hysteroscopy tray. (A) Rigid hysteroscope in a continuous flow sheath with an operating channel. (B) Five-French semirigid biopsy forceps. (C) Inflow tubing attached to (D), a flexible and steerable fiberoptic hysteroscope with attached light cable (E) and digital camera (F). An open-sided speculum (G), flexible dilator (H), and a single toothed tenaculum (I) are demonstrated.

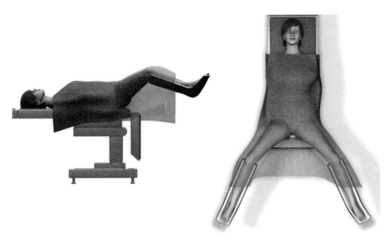

Figure 23.14 Patient positioning for office hysteroscopy. The patient is placed in a modified lithotomy position, preferably using supportive "stirrups" or leg supports with the buttocks at the edge of the examining table.

Patient positioning and exposure

Hysteroscopy is performed in a modified dorsal lithotomy position while the legs are positioned in stirrups (Figure 23.14). Stirrups that hold and support the knees, calves, and ankles permit prolonged procedures with greater comfort. The so-called "candy cane" stirrups should be avoided when hysteroscopic procedures are performed on conscious patients.

The cervix is exposed with the smallest caliber speculum required to provide adequate exposure of the cervix. A bivalve speculum hinged on only one side allows its removal without disturbing the position of the tenaculum and hysteroscope. The speculum should be warmed in its entirety to minimize the discomfort of cold metal on skin; for whatever value it provides, we lubricate the speculum with 2% lidocaine gel (Chapter 14). The use of weighted specula should be avoided in conscious patients because of the discomfort involved.

Anesthesia

The need for anesthesia for office hysteroscopy varies greatly, depending on a number of factors that include the patient's level of anxiety, the status of her cervical canal, the procedure, and the outside diameter of the hysteroscope or sheath. In some patients, diagnostic hysteroscopy is possible without anesthesia, especially if the patient is parous or if narrow-caliber (< 3 mm in outside diameter) hysteroscopes and sheaths are used. A detailed description of local anesthetic techniques is found in Chapter 14 Video 14.1.

Cervical dilation

Dilation of the cervix, although apparently simple, can be incorrectly performed in a way that compromises the whole procedure. If the objective lens of the hysteroscope cannot be placed in the endometrial cavity, the hysteroscopy cannot be done. The cervix should be dilated as atraumatically as possible. It is best to avoid using a uterine sound because it can traumatize the canal or the endometrium, causing unnecessary bleeding and uterine perforation. If cervical stenosis is encountered, and misoprostol or laminaria have not been used or were ineffective, there is evidence that intracervical injection of vasopressin (0.05 U/mL, 4 mL at 4 and 8 o'clock) also substantially reduces the force required for cervical dilation [22]. Care must be taken with the use of vasopressin, particularly in a nonmonitored environment, as systemic injection can result in a number of cardiorespiratory complications. Consequently, this step should probably be reserved for hysteroscopy in a setting where appropriate resuscitative measures can be taken.

Imaging

Endoscopes

Hysteroscopes can generally be classified as being flexible or rigid in design. Flexible hysteroscopes use optical fibers for transmission of both light and image, and, consequently, have lower resolution than rigid instruments of a similar diameter that use optical lenses for image acquisition. An advantage of flexible hysteroscopes is the capability to design a relatively durable narrow caliber instrument that can be steered within the endometrial cavity (Figure 23.13, D). Rigid hysteroscopes are more durable and usually provide a superior image (Figure 23.15). The most commonly used hysteroscopes are 3–4 mm in diameter, although those smaller than 2 mm in diameter are available.

The field of view of a rigid endoscope is dependent in large part on viewing angle of the lens. Zero-degree lenses have a panoramic or central field of view, but are deficient when it is necessary to visualize structures below or lateral to the endoscope. Those with an angled (*foreoblique*) lens allow better visualization of, and access to, structures like the cornua and are available in 12–15° and 25–30° models, suitable for hysteroscopic use (Figure 23.16).

Light sources and cables

Adequate illumination of the endometrial cavity is essential. Because it runs from a standard 110- or 220-volt wall outlet, the light source requires no special electrical connections. For most cameras and endoscopes, the element must have at least 150 watts of power for direct viewing and preferably 250 watts or more for video and operative procedures [23].

Video imaging

Diagnostic hysteroscopy may be performed with direct visualization. The value of a video camera and monitor is fourfold. First, video imaging allows the surgeon to sit and work in a more comfortable position. Second, the support staff have the ability to anticipate surgeon needs since they can see the procedural image, a circumstance not possible if the surgeon has the only view through the telescope. Third, video imaging provides the opportunity for

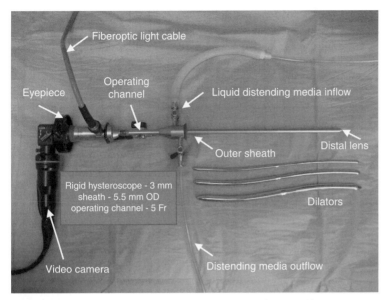

Figure 23.15 Diagnostic/operative hysteroscopic system. This is an Olympus 3 mm outside diameter (OD) hysteroscope in a 5.5 mm OD continuous flow sheath that includes a 5 Fr operating channel. As depicted, the system is attached to fluid media inflow and outflow channels, a fiberoptic light cable, and a CCD medical video camera. Dilators are used if necessary to facilitate positioning of the assembled system into the endometrial cavity.

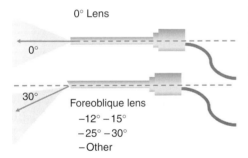

Figure 23.16 Zero-degree and thirty-degree foreoblique lenses. Typical foreoblique lenses used in gynecologic procedures include 0° for diagnostic purposes, 12–15° for general purposes and endometrial procedures, and 25–30° for procedures involving instrumentation of the fallopian tubes.

still or video documentation of the procedure. Finally, the conscious patient can generally appreciate the findings and have a better understanding about what was or was not found. The camera must be adequately sensitive to light because of the narrow diameter of the endoscope and the frequently dark background of the endometrial cavity, particularly when it is enlarged.

Sheaths

Flexible or fiberoptic hysteroscopes typically have integrated inflow and, in some instances, outflow channels. A rigid hysteroscope requires a system that interfaces with the media source, allowing inflow and, in *continuous flow* systems, outflow of the distending media from the endometrial cavity. These devices are called "sheaths" and have a design and diameter that reflects both the dimensions of the endoscope and the purpose of the instrument. Diagnostic

223

hysteroscopes have a sheath slightly wider than the telescope, allowing infusion, and, preferably, a separate channel for outflow of the distention media. Sheaths for operative hysteroscopes are typically from 5–8 mm in diameter and have yet another one or two channels that permit the insertion of semirigid instruments, either 5 or 7 Fr in diameter.

Uterine distention

Distention of the endometrial cavity is necessary to create a viewing space. The choices include CO_2 gas, high-viscosity 32% dextran 70, and a number of low-viscosity fluids, including solutions of glycine, sorbitol, mannitol, saline, and dextrose in water. A pressure of 45 mm Hg or higher is generally required for adequate distention of the uterine cavity. To minimize extravasation, this pressure should not exceed the mean arterial pressure. For each of the fluids, there are several methods used to create this pressure by infusion into the endometrial cavity.

Media

Carbon dioxide gas is an excellent media for diagnostic purposes, but it is unsuitable for operative hysteroscopy and for diagnostic procedures when the patient is bleeding because there is no effective way to remove blood and other debris from the endometrial cavity. The gas is transmitted to the sheath from an insufflator specially designed for the procedure, with rubberized tubing. To minimize the risk of CO_2 embolus the intrauterine pressure is kept below 100 mm Hg, and the flow rate is maintained at less than 100 mL/min.

Normal saline (NS) is a useful and safe medium for procedures that do not require radiofrequency (RF) electricity from standard monopolar instruments. Even if there is absorption of a substantial volume of solution, saline does not cause electrolyte imbalance and, consequently is a good choice for minor procedures performed in the office. The development of bipolar RF instrumentation for hysteroscopic surgery has allowed the application of saline as a distending medium in even more advanced and complex procedures.

Dextran 70 is useful for patients who are bleeding, because it does not mix with blood. This agent is generally drawn up in a 50 mL syringe, attached to standard caliber connector tubing, and attached to the inflow port of the sheath. The media is expensive and tends to "caramelize" on instruments, which must be disassembled and thoroughly cleaned in warm water immediately after each use. Dextran 70 should never be used with flexible endoscopes. Use of this agent is rarely associated with anaphylactic reactions and, despite the low volume of infused fluid, fluid overload and electrolyte disturbances can occur.

The so-called "low viscosity" media, which include 3% sorbitol, 1.5% glycine, 5% mannitol, and combined solutions of sorbitol and mannitol, are commonly used when RF electrosurgery is to be performed using monopolar instruments because they are nonionic, and, therefore, do not disperse current. This circumstance can be a liability with operative hysteroscopy when substantial amounts of the distending media are absorbed into the systemic circulation, a circumstance that can result in hyponatremia. In the office environment, for diagnostic and simple procedures, this is rarely a concern.

Media delivery systems — Large capacity syringes can be used for office diagnostic procedures, but are most practicable for infusing dextran 70 solution. The syringe can be operated by either the surgeon or an assistant and is either connected directly to the sheath or attached by connecting tubing.

Continuous hydrostatic pressure is effectively achieved by elevating the vehicle containing the distention media above the level of the patient's uterus using an IV pole or other suitable adjustable device. The achieved pressure is proportional to both the width of the connecting tubing and the elevation – for operative hysteroscopy with 10-mm tubing, intrauterine pressure ranges from 70 to 100 mm Hg when the bag is between 1.0 and 1.5 m above the uterine cavity. The tubing is connected to the endoscope inflow port using wide connector tubing that allows the creation of adequate pressure. A pressure cuff may be placed around the infusion bag to elevate the pressure in the system. Caution must be exercised, however, because this technique causes increasing extravasation if intrauterine pressure rises above the mean arterial pressure.

A variety of infusion pumps are available, ranging from simple devices to instruments that maintain a preset intrauterine pressure. Simple pump devices continue to press fluid into the uterine cavity regardless of resistance, whereas the pressure-sensitive pumps reduce the flow rate when the preset level is reached, thereby impeding the efflux of blood and debris and compromising the view. In my opinion, there is little value to using these systems in the office diagnostic setting.

Findings and documentation

With a good hysteroscopic view, the normal endometrial cavity can readily be determined (Video 23.5). Should abnormalities such as polyps (Videos 23.6, 23.7, 23.8) or submucosal myomas (Videos 23.8, 23.9, 23.10, 23.11) be found, it is important to document the presence, size, location, and, in the case of leiomyomas, the "type" of lesion based upon the proportion of the lesion in the endometrial cavity (Figure 4.1).

Magnetic resonance imaging

Evaluation of the endometrial cavity

Magnetic resonance imaging has been shown to be accurate in the evaluation of the endometrial cavity in women with AUB, although it can miss polyps otherwise detected by SIS and it does not seem to be superior to hysteroscopy [9] (Class I-2). Nevertheless, it may have value in selected patients in whom SIS or hysteroscopy are not feasible (e.g., virginal women).

Evaluation of the myometrium

The use of MRI in the evaluation of the myometrium for leiomyomas and adenomyosis has been demonstrated effective at distinguishing one from the other [24] (Class II-1) (Figure 23.17). Magnetic resonance imaging also appears superior to transvaginal sonography, SIS, and hysteroscopy for measuring the myometrial extent of submucosal leiomyomas [9] and, particularly when leiomyomas have an echodensity similar to that of the myometrium, MRI is superior to ultrasound for the detailed myoma localization that is important when laparoscopic or abdominal myomectomy is contemplated (Figure 22.18). These characteristics may be important when evaluating a patient for myomectomy. For example, hysteroscopic myomectomy is feasible if it is clear that there exists a margin of myometrium between the deepest edge of the myoma and the overlying serosa. In many instances, this determination cannot be determined completely and accurately using ultrasound alone, while MRI allows detailed examination of the entire edge of the myoma. Another important value of MRI is the distinction of leiomyomas from focal adenomyosis or adenomyomas (Figure 23.17), for attempted excision of adenomyotic lesions is associated with bleeding, incomplete excision, and a lack of evidence of efficacy. The cost of the MRI is far less than the impact of a hysterotomy that has no therapeutic value.

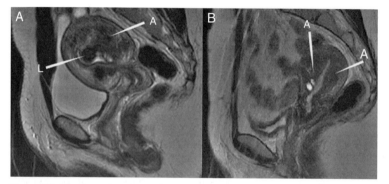

Figure 23.17 Magnetic resonance imaging of the uterus – adenomyosis versus leiomyomas. (A) The patient demonstrates a type 1 leiomyoma (L) from the posterior myometrium and adenomyosis (A) largely localized to the posterior myometrial wall. (B) The patient had what appeared to be a similar leiomyoma from the anterior myometrium, but on MRI has a junctional zone that is 13 mm thick, two thirds of the myometrial thickness; a finding consistent with adenomyosis (A) and two low intensity (bright) areas suggestive of an adenomyoma.

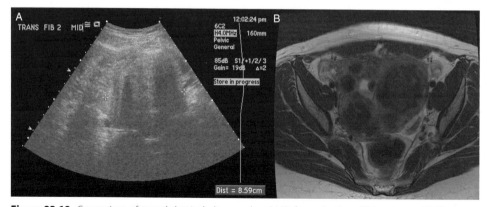

Figure 23.18 Comparison of transabdominal ultrasound and MRI for evaluation of leiomyomas. (A) The transabdominal, transversely-oriented ultrasound of a woman with a uterus enlarged to about 14-weeks size. Her leiomyomas are indistinct because the echodensity is similar to that of the myometrium. (B) The MRI of the same patient in approximately the same region, also in the transverse plane with the leiomyomas clearly seen, including their relationship to the endometrial cavity.

References

1. Loken K, Steine S, Laerum E. Patient satisfaction and quality of care at four diagnostic imaging procedures: mammography, double-contrast barium enema, abdominal ultrasonography and vaginal ultrasonography. *Eur Radiol.* 1999;**9** (7):1459–63.

2. Timor-Tritsch IE, Monteagudo A. Three and four-dimensional ultrasound in obstetrics and gynecology. *Curr Opin Obstet Gynecol.* 2007;**19**(2):157–75.

3. Bonilla-Musoles F, Simon C, Serra V, Sampaio M, Pellicer A. An assessment of hysterosalpingosonography (HSSG) as a diagnostic tool for uterine cavity defects and tubal patency. *J Clin Ultrasound.* 1992;**20** (3):175–81.

4. Widrich T, Bradley LD, Mitchinson AR, Collins RL. Comparison of saline infusion

sonography with office hysteroscopy for the evaluation of the endometrium. *Am J Obstet Gynecol.* 1996;**174**(4):1327–34.

5. Saidi MH, Sadler RK, Theis VD, Akright BD, Farhart SA, Villanueva GR. Comparison of sonography, sonohysterography, and hysteroscopy for evaluation of abnormal uterine bleeding. *J Ultrasound Med.* 1997;**16**(9):587–91.

6. Guney M, Oral B, Bayhan G, Mungan T. Intrauterine lidocaine infusion for pain relief during saline solution infusion sonohysterography: a randomized, controlled trial. *J Minim Invasive Gynecol.* 2007;**14**(3):304–10.

7. Emanuel MH, Verdel MJ, Wamsteker K, Lammes FB. A prospective comparison of transvaginal ultrasonography and diagnostic hysteroscopy in the evaluation of patients with abnormal uterine bleeding: clinical implications. *Am J Obstet Gynecol.* 1995;**172**(2 Pt 1):547–52.

8. Breitkopf DM, Frederickson RA, Snyder RR. Detection of benign endometrial masses by endometrial stripe measurement in premenopausal women. *Obstet Gynecol.* 2004;**104**(1):120–5.

9. Dueholm M, Lundorf E, Hansen ES, Ledertoug S, Olesen F. Evaluation of the uterine cavity with magnetic resonance imaging, transvaginal sonography, hysterosonographic examination, and diagnostic hysteroscopy. *Fertil Steril.* 2001;**76**(2):350–7.

10. Farquhar C, Ekeroma A, Furness S, Arroll B. A systematic review of transvaginal ultrasonography, sonohysterography and hysteroscopy for the investigation of abnormal uterine bleeding in premenopausal women. *Acta Obstet Gynecol Scand.* 2003;**82**(6):493–504.

11. Togashi K, Nishimura K, Itoh K, Fujisawa I, Noma S, Kanaoka M, et al. Adenomyosis: diagnosis with MR imaging. *Radiology.* 1988;**166**(1 Pt 1):111–14.

12. Dueholm M, Lundorf E, Hansen ES, Sorensen JS, Ledertoug S, Olesen F. Magnetic resonance imaging and transvaginal ultrasonography for the diagnosis of adenomyosis. *Fertil Steril.* 2001;**76**(3):588–94.

13. Reinhold C, Atri M, Mehio A, Zakarian R, Aldis AE, Bret PM. Diffuse uterine adenomyosis: morphologic criteria and diagnostic accuracy of endovaginal sonography. *Radiology.* 1995;**197**(3):609–14.

14. Bazot M, Darai E, Rouger J, Detchev R, Cortez A, Uzan S. Limitations of transvaginal sonography for the diagnosis of adenomyosis, with histopathological correlation. *Ultrasound Obstet Gynecol.* 2002;**20**(6):605–11.

15. Chiang CH, Chang MY, Hsu JJ, Chiu TH, Lee KF, Hsieh TT, et al. Tumor vascular pattern and blood flow impedance in the differential diagnosis of leiomyoma and adenomyosis by color Doppler sonography. *J Assist Reprod Genet.* 1999;**16**(5):268–75.

16. Goldrath MH, Sherman AI. Office hysteroscopy and suction curettage: can we eliminate the hospital diagnostic dilatation and curettage? *Am J Obstet Gynecol.* 1985;**152**(2):220–9.

17. Iossa A, Cianferoni L, Ciatto S, Cecchini S, Campatelli C, Lo Stumbo F. Hysteroscopy and endometrial cancer diagnosis: a review of 2007 consecutive examinations in self-referred patients. *Tumori.* 1991;**77**(6):479–83.

18. Triolo O, De Vivo A, Benedetto V, Falcone S, Antico F. Gestrinone versus danazol as preoperative treatment for hysteroscopic surgery: a prospective, randomized evaluation. *Fertil Steril.* 2006;**85**:1027–31.

19. Thomas JA, Leyland N, Durand N, Windrim RC. The use of oral misoprostol as a cervical ripening agent in operative hysteroscopy: a double-blind, placebo-controlled trial. *Am J Obstet Gynecol.* 2002;**186**(5):876–9.

20. Preutthipan S, Herabutya Y. Vaginal misoprostol for cervical priming before operative hysteroscopy: a randomized controlled trial. *Obstet Gynecol.* 2000;**96**(6):890–4.

21. Nagele F, Lockwood G, Magos AL. Randomised placebo controlled trial of mefenamic acid for premedication at outpatient hysteroscopy: a pilot study. *Br J Obstet Gynaecol.* 1997;**104**(7):842–4.

22. Phillips DR, Nathanson HG, Milim SJ, Haselkorn JS. The effect of dilute vasopressin solution on the force needed for cervical dilatation: a randomized controlled trial. *Obstet Gynecol.* 1997; **89**(4):507–11.

23. Brill AI. Energy systems for operative hysteroscopy. *Obstet Gynecol Clin North Am.* 2000;**27**(2): 317–26.

24. Mark AS, Hricak H, Heinrichs LW, Hendrickson MR, Winkler ML, Bachica JA, et al. Adenomyosis and leiomyoma: differential diagnosis with MR imaging. *Radiology.* 1987; **163**(2):527–9.

Glossary

Abdominal supracervical hysterectomy	See Supracervical abdominal hysterectomy
Abnormal uterine bleeding (AUB)	Is nonphysiologic bleeding, emanating from the uterus, and unrelated to pregnancy. Any uterine bleeding that exists prior to menarche or after menopause is abnormal. In the reproductive years bleeding between menstrual periods is abnormal as are disorders in frequency, volume, duration, or predictability of the onset of menstrual flow. Unscheduled bleeding associated with suppressive medical therapy is a type of AUB called "breakthrough bleeding"
Activin	A peptide from the transforming growth factor β family produced in the pituitary and in the granulosa cells, which has a role in the regulation of menstrual function that is essentially the opposite of inhibin. Activin enhances FSH synthesis and secretion and in the follicle increases FSH binding as well as FSH-induced aromatization of androgens to estrogens
Adenomyoma	A benign tumor composed of muscular and glandular elements; in the uterus implies localized adenomyosis; may be difficult to distinguish from a leiomyoma
Adenomyosis	When endometrial tissue exists in the myometrium beneath the basalis of the endometrium
Adnexa	The uterine adnexa include the ovaries and fallopian tubes
Adrenarche	An increase in the production of androgens by the adrenal cortex that usually occurs during the eighth or ninth year of life and typically results in the development of axillary and pubic hair
Alkaline hematin test	A research quantification of menstrual blood loss whereby the patient (or subject in a study) collects all menstrual tampons and pads and submits them to a laboratory that extracts the total amount of hemoglobin (as hematin) to determine an exact volumetric amount
Angiogenesis	The formation and differentiation of blood vessels
Anovulatory	Not involving or associated with ovulation, such as "anovulatory bleeding"

Anteversion	A condition of being anteverted – when used to describe the uterus means the long axis of the cervix is anterior to the long axis of the vagina
Aromatase	An enzyme or complex of enzymes that promotes the conversion of an androgen into an estrogen; e.g., testosterone to estradiol
Aromatase inhibitor	A pharmaceutical agent that inhibits the action of the aromatase enzyme
Arteriovenous malformation (AVM)	A rare localized proliferation of arterial and venous channels with fistula formation and an admixture of small capillary like channels that may cause abnormal uterine bleeding. In the uterus may be congenital or acquired and can occur in association with AVM at other sites
AUB	See Abnormal uterine bleeding
AVM	See Arteriovenous malformation
Basalis (of the endometrium)	The basal part of the endometrium that is not shed during menstruation
Breakthrough bleeding	Abnormal flow of blood from the uterus in women on contraceptive hormones, postmenopausal hormone replacement therapy, or other hormonal therapy otherwise designed to suppress endometrial function
Cardinal ligament	The condensation of the most inferior portion of the broad ligament that serves as a major support structure for the cervix, and, therefore, the rest of the uterus
Cervix	The narrow lower (caudal) or outer end of the uterus that attaches to the vagina
Climacteric	A period of life characterized by physiological and psychic change that marks the end of the reproductive capacity of women that includes menopause – see Perimenopause
COC	See Combination oral contraceptives
Combination oral contraceptives (COC)	Orally administered hormonal contraceptive agents for women that contain both an estrogen and a progestin
Corpus	The main part or body of the uterus that contains the endometrial cavity, and which is intimately attached to the cervix and the fallopian tubes – see Uterine corpus
COX	See Cyclooxygenase
COX-1	See Cyclooxygenase-1
COX-2	See Cyclooxygenase-2
COX inhibitors	Pharmaceutical agents that block or inhibit the activity of cyclooxygenase enzymes. The main COX inhibitors are nonsteroidal anti-inflammatory drugs (NSAIDS), but

	these can be categorized as nonselective or the selective COX-2 inhibitors that have been associated with an increased risk of thrombosis, heart attack and stroke through relative increases in thromboxane.
Cul-de sac (Cul-de-sac of Douglas)	A deep peritoneal recess between the uterus and the upper vaginal wall anteriorly and the rectum posteriorly – called also *Douglas's cul-de-sac, Douglas's pouch*
Cyclooxygenase (COX)	An enzyme that catalyzes the conversion of arachidonic acid to prostaglandins, that is inactivated by aspirin and other NSAIDs, and that has two isoforms, COX-1, and COX-2
Cyclooxygenase-1	Prostaglandins that are synthesized by the cyclooxygenase-1 enzyme, or COX-1, are responsible for maintenance and protection of the gastrointestinal tract
Cyclooxygenase-2	Prostaglandins that are synthesized by the cyclooxygenase-2 enzyme, or COX-2, are responsible for inflammation, pain, and are expressed in abundance in the late luteal and early menstrual phases of the cycle
Danazol	A synthetic androgenic derivative ($C_{22}H_{27}NO_2$) of ethisterone that suppresses gonadotropin secretion by the adenohypophysis and is used especially in the treatment of endometriosis
Depot medroxyprogesterone acetate (DMPA)	An injectable synthetic progestational steroid hormone ($C_{24}H_{34}O_4$) that is used for treatment of endometriosis and as a contraceptive
Depo-Provera®	See Depot medroxyprogesterone acetate
Dilate	Verb, to enlarge, stretch, or cause to expand – dilate the cervix. *Intransitive verb*: to become expanded – the cervix was *dilating*
Dilator	An instrument for expanding a tube, duct, or cavity – a device for dilating the uterine cervix
Disordered endometrium	The histopathological appearance of endometrium that has had excessive and prolonged estrogen stimulation, usually associated with anovulation
Dysfunctional uterine bleeding (DUB)	Abnormal uterine bleeding in the reproductive years that is not associated with a physical lesion (as a tumor), inflammation, pregnancy, or drug or device – probably a mixture of etiologies including defects of local hemostasis, predominantly in ovulatory women, and abnormal bleeding secondary to disorders of ovulation. Because there has been so much confusion regarding this term, many suggest that it be abandoned
EA	See Endometrial ablation

EB	See Endometrial biopsy
EEC	See Endometrial echo complex
Endocervical canal	The passageway through the uterine cervix between the endometrial cavity and the vagina – the most cephalad border is termed the internal cervical os and the most caudal boundary is the exocervical os
Endometrial ablation (EA)	A surgical procedure targeted to destroy the endometrium; may be performed using a resectoscope (resectoscopic endometrial ablation; REA); or with nonresectoscopic devices (nonresectoscopic endometrial ablation; NREA)
Endometrial biopsy (EB, "EMB")	A sample taken from the endometrium, either blindly with a curette or suction catheter, or under hysteroscopic direction
Endometrial echo complex (EEC)	The sonographically-determined two layer thickness of endometrium, from the endomyometrial junction of one layer to that of the other, as measured in the sagittal plane
Endometrial polyp	A projecting mass of swollen and hypertrophied or tumorous endometrium
Endometrial sampling	The process of obtaining a sample of endometrium irrespective of technique
Endometriosis	The presence and growth of functioning endometrial-like tissue in places other than the uterus that may result in pain, infertility, and ovarian masses
Endometrium	The mucous membrane lining the uterus that comprises two main layers – the basalis and the functionalis, that sheds with normal menstruation
Endothelin-1	An endothelium-derived peptide with potent vasoconstrictor and proliferative properties
ER	See Estrogen receptor
Estradiol (17-β estradiol)	A natural estrogenic hormone that is a phenolic alcohol ($C_{18}H_{24}O_2$) secreted chiefly by the ovaries; is the most potent of the naturally occurring estrogens
Estrogen	Any of various natural steroids (as estradiol) that are formed from androgen precursors, that are secreted chiefly by the ovaries, placenta, adipose tissue, and testes, and that stimulate the development of female secondary sex characteristics and promote the growth and maintenance of the female reproductive system; *also*: any of various synthetic or semisynthetic steroids (such as ethinyl estradiol) that mimic the physiological effect of natural estrogens

Estrogen receptor (ER)	Estrogen receptor refers to a group of receptors, most commonly found in the cytoplasm, which are activated by the hormone 17-β estradiol and other molecules with estrogen activity. There are two, usually referred to as α and β and there are a number of isoforms of each. The α version is found in abundance in the endometrium
Estrone	A natural estrogenic hormone that is a ketone ($C_{18}H_{22}O_2$) found in the body chiefly as a metabolite of estradiol, is also secreted especially by the ovaries
External os (of the cervix)	The opening of the cervix into the vagina
FDA	See Food and Drug Administration
Fibroid	See Leiomyoma
Flexion (of the uterine corpus)	One of the two descriptors (along with version) of uterine position. The relationship of the long axis of the uterine corpus to the long axis of the cervix; anteflexed when the corpus is at an angle directed anterior to the axis of the cervix and retroflexed when the corpus is oriented at an angle posterior to the long axis of the cervix
Follicle stimulating hormone (FSH)	A hormone from an anterior lobe of the pituitary gland that stimulates the growth of the ovum-containing follicles in the ovary and that activates sperm-forming cells
Follicular phase	The first portion of the ovarian cycle characterized by the presence and growth of ovarian follicles and the production of estradiol
Food and Drug Administration (FDA)	An agency of the US Department of Health and Human Services responsible for the safety regulation of most types of foods, dietary supplements, drugs, vaccines, biological medical products, blood products, medical devices, radiation-emitting devices, veterinary products, and cosmetics
Fr	See French
French (Fr)	The French catheter scale is commonly used to measure the outer diameter of cylindrical medical instruments including catheters. The diameter in millimeters of the catheter can be determined by dividing the French size by three, thus an increasing French size corresponds with a larger diameter catheter
FSH	See Follicle stimulating hormone
Functionalis (of the endometrium)	The superficial layer(s) of the endometrium which undergo cyclical stimulation by gonadal steroids and which slough during the process of menstruation if pregnancy does not occur
GnRH	See Gonadotropin releasing hormone

GnRHa	See Gonadotropin releasing hormone agonist
Gonadotropin releasing hormone (GnRH)	A decapeptide hormone responsible for the release of FSH and LH from the anterior pituitary. It is synthesized and released from neurons within the hypothalamus
Gonadotropin releasing hormone agonist (GnRHa)	A synthetic peptide modeled after the hypothalamic neurohormone GnRH that interacts with the GnRH receptor to elicit its biologic response, the release of the pituitary hormones FSH and LH. For management of AUB, GnRHa is generally used to induce a temporary menopausal state
Heavy menstrual bleeding (HMB)	Menstrual bleeding that is excessive either in duration, or in volume per unit time, or both. In this book, HMB is a symptom, not a diagnosis, and does not in itself reflect any specific etiology
Her Option®	A medical device designed for the performance of hypothermic NREA by the insertion of a probe into the endometrial cavity that is attached to a controller that reduces local uterine temperature thereby freezing the endometrium. The procedure is typically performed under transabdominal ultrasound guidance
HIFU	See High-intensity focused ultrasound
High-intensity focused ultrasound (HIFU)	A medical procedure that uses high-intensity focused ultrasound energy to heat and destroy pathological tissue
HMB	See Heavy menstrual bleeding
HSG	See Hysterosalpingogram
HTA	See Hydrothermablation
Hydrothermablation (HTA)	A hyperthermic NREA technique that uses hysteroscopically-guided positioning of a specialized sheath connected to a controller unit that heats the circulating distending media thereby destroying the endometrium
Hypermenorrhea	Abnormally profuse or prolonged menstrual flow
Hypomenorrhea	Decreased menstrual flow
Hysterectomy	Surgical removal of the uterus
Hysterosalpingogram (HSG)	A radiograph made by hysterosalpingography which is performed by instilling oil or water soluble radiologic contrast material into the endometrial cavity that is visualized by fluoroscopic techniques. The technique has primary value in demonstrating patency of the Fallopian tube, but has some value in detecting congenital and acquired abnormalities in uterine structure
Hysteroscope	An endoscope used for the visual examination of the cervical canal and interior of the uterus

IMB	See Intermenstrual bleeding
Inhibin	A peptide, from the transforming growth factor β family, that, in the female, is produced in the granulosa cells and which has multiple functions in the menstrual cycle but most importantly inhibition of FSH synthesis and secretion, and, possibly, the induction of LH receptors on the granulose cells. There are two forms, Inhibin A and B that differ in their beta subunits
Intermenstrual bleeding (IMB)	Uterine bleeding between normal menses
Internal os (of the cervix)	The opening of the cervical canal into the body of the uterus
Intramural leiomyoma (myoma, fibroid)	A leiomyoma that exists within the boundaries of the myometrium; between the serosa and the endometrium
Intrauterine device (IUD)	A device inserted and left in the uterus, typically to provide effective contraception, but when impregnated with pharmaceutical agents may have additional therapeutic value, especially for heavy menstrual bleeding – called also an intrauterine contraceptive device, or IUCD. Intrauterine device is a synonym for an intrauterine system (IUS)
Intrauterine system (IUS)	Similar to an IUD, a device, implicitly comprising an inert component and a delayed releasing pharmaceutical component, that is inserted and left in the uterus to provide contraception or a therapeutic effect – see Levonorgestrel-releasing intrauterine system
Isthmus (of the cervix)	A contracted anatomical part or passage connecting two larger structures or cavities: the lower portion of the uterine corpus
IUD	See Intrauterine device
IUS	See Intrauterine system
Junctional zone	The zone that exists at the juxtaposition of the endometrium and the myometrium, which can be appreciated on imaging studies such as transvaginal ultrasound and MRI
Laparoscope	A usually rigid endoscope that is inserted through an incision in the abdominal wall and is used to examine visually the interior of the peritoneal cavity – called also a *peritoneoscope*
Laparoscopic hysterectomy (LH)	Total hysterectomy performed in part or in total under the direction of a laparoscope
Laparoscopic supracervical hysterectomy (LSH)	Subtotal hysterectomy characterized by removal of the uterine corpus with retention of the cervix performed entirely under laparoscopic direction

Leiomyoma (myoma, fibroid)	Benign tumor comprising smooth (nonstriated) muscle fibers most commonly found in the myometrium of the uterus. Approximately 70% of all women are shown to have leiomyomas by the age of 50. Leiomyomas vary greatly in volume and in sonographic echodensity
Levonorgestrel-releasing intrauterine system (LNG-IUS)	The most available device, known by the trade name "Mirena®" is an intrauterine releasing system that comprises a T-shaped inert radioopaque polydimethylsiloxane frame 32 mm long, and a capsule, encompassing the stem that allows slow release of a total of 52 mg of levonorgestrel at a rate of 11–20 µg/day over a period of 5 years. The system provides effective contraception and has been shown effective in the treatment of the symptom of HMB as well as pain associated with adenomyosis and endometriosis. It is removed by pulling on the nylon string attached to the base of the stem that is left accessible in the vagina
LH	See Lutenizing hormone or Laparoscopic hysterectomy
LNG-IUS	See Levonorgestrel-releasing intrauterine system
LSH	See Laparoscopic supracervical hysterectomy
Luteal phase	The phase of the ovarian cycle that follows ovulation and which is characterized by the production of estradiol and progesterone from the corpus luteum
Luteinizing hormone (LH)	A glycoprotein hormone that is secreted by the adenohypophysis. In the female stimulates ovulation and the development of the corpora lutea and, together with follicle-stimulating hormone, the secretion of estrogen from developing ovarian follicles. In the male LH stimulates the development of interstitial tissue in the testis and the secretion of testosterone
Matrix metalloproteinases (MMPs)	These are zinc-dependent endopeptidases capable of degrading all kinds of extracellular matrix proteins, but also can process a number of bioactive molecules. They are known to be involved in the cleavage of cell surface receptors, the release of apoptotic ligands (such as the FAS ligand), and chemokine in/activation. A number of MMPs are found in abundance starting at the end of the luteal phase, and they are thought to be important factors in initiating the process of menstruation
MEA®	See Microwave endometrial ablation
Medroxyprogesterone acetate	A synthetic steroid progestational hormone ($C_{24}H_{34}O_4$)
Menarche	The beginning of menstrual function; *especially*: the first menstrual period of an individual
Menometrorrhagia	A combination of menorrhagia and metrorrhagia

Menopause	The natural cessation of menstruation occurring usually between the ages of 45 and 55 with a mean in Western cultures of approximately 51. The World Health Organization defines menopause as the permanent cessation of menstruation resulting from the loss of ovarian follicular activity
Menorrhagia	An abnormally profuse menstrual flow in the context of predictable menses with a normal cycle length. Nominally a symptom, it is used in some constituencies as a diagnosis as well. A term that, like "dysfunctional uterine bleeding" should be abandoned
Menstruation	A discharging of blood, secretions, and tissue debris from the uterus that recurs in nonpregnant human and other primate females of breeding age at approximately monthly intervals; is initiated by the involution of the corpus luteum and the resultant dramatic decrease of circulating estradiol and progesterone.
Metrorrhagia	Spontaneous uterine bleeding between menstrual periods another term that should likely be abandoned.
Microwave endometrial ablation (MEA®)	Hyperthermic NREA system that uses a microwave transmitter on an intrauterine probe attached to a controller. The surgeon moves the probe over the endometrial surface at a rate that maintains a predetermined therapeutic temperature
Mirena®	See Levonorgestrel-releasing intrauterine system
MMP	See Matrix metalloproteinases
Molimina	The periodic symptoms (as tension or discomfort) associated with the physiological stress preceding or accompanying menstruation
Monophasic oral contraceptive	A combined oral contraceptive (COC) that comprises pills of identical composition in both formulation and dose; e.g., 35 µg of ethinyl estradiol and 1 mg norethindrone in each active pill
Morcellation	Division and removal in small pieces (as of a tumor on the uterus to facilitate hysterectomy)
MRgFUS (MR-guided focused ultrasound)	High intensity focused ultrasound (HIFU) targeted and monitored using magnetic resonance imaging (MRI) techniques
Myolysis	See Myoma ablation
Myoma	See Leiomyoma
Myoma ablation	A surgical procedure designed to destroy leiomyomas using hyperthermic (laser, radiofrequency electricity), or hypothermic (cryosurgical) techniques. Myoma ablation

237

	is still under clinical evaluation to determine efficacy and the appropriate patient selection process
Myomectomy	Surgical excision of a leiomyoma (myoma or fibroid)
Myometrium	The muscular layer of the wall of the uterus
Nonresectoscopic endometrial ablation (NREA)	see Endometrial ablation performed with a device other than a resectoscope
Nonsteroidal anti-inflammatory drug (NSAID)	A family of anti-inflammatory agents, generally administered orally, that act by inhibition of cyclooxygenase, and which have particular roles in the treatment of primary dysmenorrhea and heavy menstrual bleeding that is often associated with abnormal local prostaglandin production (HMB-E) – see COX-inhibitors
Norethindrone	A synthetic progestational hormone ($C_{20}H_{26}O_2$) used in birth control pills, often used in the form of norethindrone acetate ($C_{22}H_{28}O_3$)
Norgestrel	A synthetic progestagen $C_{21}H_{28}O_2$ having two optically active forms of which the biologically active levorotatory form is used in birth control pills
NovaSure®	A hyperthermic NREA system that uses a uterine probe with an integrated and semiconforming bipolar radio-frequency electrode, which, when activated by the controller unit, results in endometrial desiccation and vaporization
NREA	Nonresectoscopic endometrial ablation – see Endometrial ablation
NSAID	See Nonsteroidal anti-inflammatory drug
NuvaRing®	The trade name for a combined hormonal contraceptive vaginal ring comprising a flexible plastic (ethylene-vinyl acetate copolymer) ring that releases a low dose of a progestin and an estrogen over three weeks
OD	See Outside diameter
Oligomenorrhea	Abnormally infrequent or scanty menstrual flow usually infers a cycle interval of more than 35 days.
Oligo-ovulatory	Infrequent ovulation
Os-Finder®	A cervical dilator with a narrow tip made of extremely smooth and malleable teflon-like material
Outside diameter (OD)	The diameter of a cylindrical device as measured from the external surfaces. The inside diameter (ID) of the channel is smaller by twice the thickness of the cylinder wall
Ovarian artery	Either of two arteries in the female that correspond to the testicular arteries in the male, arise from the aorta below the renal arteries with one on each side, and are

distributed to the ovaries with branches supplying the ureters, the fallopian tubes, the labia majora, and the groin

Ovulation	The discharge of a mature ovum from the ovary
PA	See Plasminogen activator
PAI	See Plasminogen activator inhibitor
PBAC (or PBLAC)	See Pictorial blood loss assessment chart
Perimenopause	The period around the onset of menopause that is often marked by various physical signs (as hot flashes and menstrual irregularity) – also called the climacteric
Phasic oral contraceptive	Oral contraceptives comprising pills that vary in the dose of either the estrogenic component, the progestin component or both
Pictorial blood loss assessment chart (PBAC)	A measurement of menstrual blood loss whereby the patient compares the amount of blood "staining" on her menstrual tampons and/or pads and compares and records each one to a chart with pictures (pictogram) that allow for the calculation of a score for the period that corresponds with blood loss. Abnormal scores are typically those more than 150 and many trials require that patients achieve scores of 75–100 to determine success. It is thought that scores less than 75 are consistent with normal menstrual blood loss
Pipelle®	A disposable device consisting of a plastic core and a drinking-straw-like sheath, used to obtain endometrial biopsies through gentle suction
Plasminogen activator (PA)	Any of a group of substances (as urokinase) that convert plasminogen to plasmin
Plasminogen activator inhibitor (PAI)	Is the principal inhibitor of tissue plasminogen activator (tPA) and urokinase (uPA), the activators of plasminogen and hence fibrinolysis (the physiological breakdown of blood clots)
Polymenorrhea	Menstruation at abnormally frequent intervals generally considered to be less than 22 days.
Polyp	A projecting mass of swollen and hypertrophied or tumorous membrane
Portio vaginalis (of the cervix)	The part of the uterine cervix that protrudes into the vagina
Postmenopausal bleeding	Spontaneous vaginal bleeding following menopause
PR	See Progesterone receptor
Progesterone	A female steroid sex hormone ($C_{21}H_{30}O_2$) that is secreted by the corpus luteum to prepare the endometrium for implantation and later by the placenta during pregnancy

Progesterone receptor (PR)	An intracellular steroid receptor that specifically binds progesterone. It has two main forms, A and B; the PR-A isoform is necessary to oppose estrogen-induced proliferation as well as PR-B-dependent proliferation
Progestin	A natural or synthetic analog progestational substance that mimics some or all of the actions of progesterone. Progestins are used in a variety of situations including hormonal contraception (either alone or with an estrogen); to prevent endometrial hyperplasia from unopposed estrogen in hormone replacement therapy; to treat secondary amenorrhea; abnormal uterine bleeding; endometriosis, breast, endometrial, prostate, and renal cell carcinoma; as well as anorexia, cachexia and AIDS-related wasting
Proliferative endometrium	The endometrium that results from unopposed estradiol secreted from the ovary in the follicular phase
Prostacyclin (Prostaglandin I_2)	A prostaglandin that is a metabolite of arachidonic acid, inhibits aggregation of platelets, and dilates blood vessels. It is increased in the presence of heavy menstrual bleeding
Prostaglandin	The name "prostaglandin" derives from the prostate gland from which the compounds were originally thought to originate. A prostaglandin refers to any member of a group of 20-carbon lipid compounds that are derived enzymatically from arachadonic acid and are technically hormones, although they are rarely classified as such. Arachadonic acid is released from plasma membrane phospholipids or dietary fats and reduced to the intermediary prostaglandin H_2 by COX enzymes. PGH_2 then becomes the substrate for terminal prostinoid synthase enzymes specific for a given prostaglandin (e.g., $PGF_{2\alpha}$, PGE_2, thromboxane, PGI_2, etc.)
Prostaglandin E_1	Available as the pharmacologic agent "misoprostol" that has value in the preparation of the cervix for dilation
Prostaglandin E_2	A prostaglandin with a spectrum of activity including endometrial vasodilation and variable effects on smooth muscle elsewhere; also seems critical to ovulation and may be associated with dysmenorrhea. It may contribute to the genesis of heavy menstrual bleeding in ovulatory women
Prostaglandin $F_{2\alpha}$	A prostaglandin that causes bronchoconstriction in addition to being a potent vasoconstrictor of the myometrium (contributing both to primary dysmenorrheal and labor) and of the endometrial blood vessels; it thought to be an important initiator of the endometrial ischemia that precedes menstruation, and equally important in the process of endometrial hemostasis at the time of menstruation

Prostaglandin I_2	See Prostacyclin
Provera[®]	See Medroxyprogesterone acetate
Randomized clinical/controlled trial (RCT)	A clinical trial in which the subjects are randomly distributed into groups which are either subjected to the experimental procedure (as use of a drug) or which serve as controls
RCT	See Randomized clinical/controlled trial
REA	Resectoscopic endometrial ablation (See Endometrial ablation).
Resectoscope	An instrument consisting of a tubular fenestrated sheath with a sliding electrode within it that is used for surgery within cavities (as of the endometrial cavity through the cervix)
Retroversion	A condition of being retroverted, when used to describe the uterus means the long axis of the cervix is posterior to the long axis of the vagina
Round ligament	Either of a pair of rounded fibromuscular cords arising from each side of the uterus and traceable through the inguinal canal to the tissue of the labia majora into which they merge
Saline infusion sonography (SIS)	An office-based technique for performing uterine ultrasound (usually transvaginally) using saline (or other sterile fluid) injected into the endometrial cavity, via the cervical canal, for the purpose of identifying and characterizing intracavitary pathology such as polyps and submucosal leiomyomas
Secretory endometrium	The endometrium that results from both estradiol and progesterone secreted from the ovary in the phase of the ovarian cycle following ovulation
Secretory phase	See Luteal phase
SIS	See Saline infusion sonography
Sonohysterography	See Saline infusion sonography
Sound n	An elongated instrument for exploring or examining body cavities
Sound v	To explore or examine a body cavity (e.g., the uterus) with a sound, usually to determine length
Spotting	To experience abnormal and sporadic bleeding in small amounts from the uterus
Submucosal leiomyoma (myoma, fibroid)	A leiomyoma that extends from the myometrium to be in direct contact with the endometrium. Such leiomyomas may be attached by a narrow stalk (pedunculated submucosal myoma) or have a variable proportion of their volume extending into the myometrium. A classification system is based on the proportion of the

myoma that is in the endometrial cavity – type 0 if the myoma is pedunculated, type 1 if less than 50% of the diameter is intramural, type 2 if more than or equal to 50% of the diameter is intramural

Subserosal leiomyoma (myoma, fibroid)

A leiomyoma that extends from the myometrium to be in direct contact with the uterine serosa. Such leiomyomas may be attached to the uterus by a narrow stalk (pedunculated subserosal myoma) or have a variable proportion of their volume extending into the myometrium

Subtotal hysterectomy

See Supracervical hysterectomy

Supracervical abdominal hysterectomy

Supracervical hysterectomy performed via laparotomy

Supracervical hysterectomy

Surgical removal of the uterine corpus with retention of the uterine cervix. Usually accomplished via laparotomy or under laparoscopic direction, it is possible to perform the procedure vaginally

TAH

See Total abdominal hysterectomy

Tenaculum

A forceps-like instrument with two opposing sharp-pointed hooks attached to handles used mainly in surgery for seizing and holding the uterine cervix

Thelarche

The first stage of secondary (postnatal) breast development, usually occurring at the beginning of puberty in girls characterized by a firm, tender lump directly under the center of the nipple (papilla and areola). Thelarche is also referred to as a "breast bud," or as as Tanner stage 2 breast development (Tanner stage 1 being the entirely undeveloped prepubertal state)

Thermachoice®

Hyperthermic nonresectoscopic endometrial ablation (NREA) system comprising a balloon tipped catheter attached to a controller, which, when placed in the endometrial cavity, is distended with fluid that is subsequently heated and results in thermal destruction of the endometrium

Thromboxane (TXA_2)

Any of several prostinoid substances that are produced especially by platelets, are formed from endoperoxides, cause constriction of vascular and bronchial smooth muscle, and promote blood clotting

TNF

See Tumor necrosis factor

Total abdominal hysterectomy

Surgical removal of the entire uterus (corpus and cervix) through a laparotomy incision

Total hysterectomy

Surgical removal of the entire uterus (corpus and cervix) either vaginally, via a laparotomy incision, or under laparoscopic direction

Transmural	Passing or administered through an anatomical wall, e.g., "*transmural* leiomyoma"
Transvaginal sonography (TVS)	An ultrasound examination of the pelvis performed with an elongated, narrow, vaginal transducer
Tumor necrosis factor (TNF)	A protein that is produced chiefly by monocytes and macrophages in response especially to endotoxins, that mediates inflammation, and that induces the destruction of some tumor cells and the activation of white blood cells
TVS	See Transvaginal sonography
Uterine artery	An artery that arises from the internal iliac artery and after following a course between the layers of the broad ligament reaches the uterus at the cervix and supplies the uterus and adjacent parts
Uterine corpus	The body of the uterus cephalad to the uterine cervix that contains the endometrial cavity
Uterine sound ("Sound")	See Sound (*n*)
Uterosacral ligament	A fibrous fascial band on each side of the uterus that passes along the lateral wall of the pelvis from the uterine cervix to the sacrum and that serves to support the uterus and hold it in place – called also *sacrouterine ligament*
Uterus	An organ in female mammals for containing and usually for nourishing the young during development prior to birth that consists of a greatly modified and enlarged section of an oviduct (as in rodents and marsupials) or of the two oviducts united (as in the higher primates including humans), that has thick walls consisting of an outer serous layer, a very thick middle layer of smooth muscle, and an inner mucous layer containing numerous glands, and that during pregnancy undergoes great increase in size and change in the condition of its walls
Vaginal hysterectomy (VH)	Removal of the entire uterus through a vaginal incision
Vasculoendothelial growth factor (VEGF)	An angiogenic factor that is a major specific stimulator of endothelial cell proliferation and vascular permeability in the endometrium
VEGF	See Vasculoendothelial growth factor
Version (of the uterus)	One of the two descriptors (along with flexion) of uterine position. The orientation of the axis of the uterine cervix that deviates either anteriorly or posteriorly from the vaginal axis; see Anteversion and Retroversion
VH	See Vaginal hysterectomy

Index